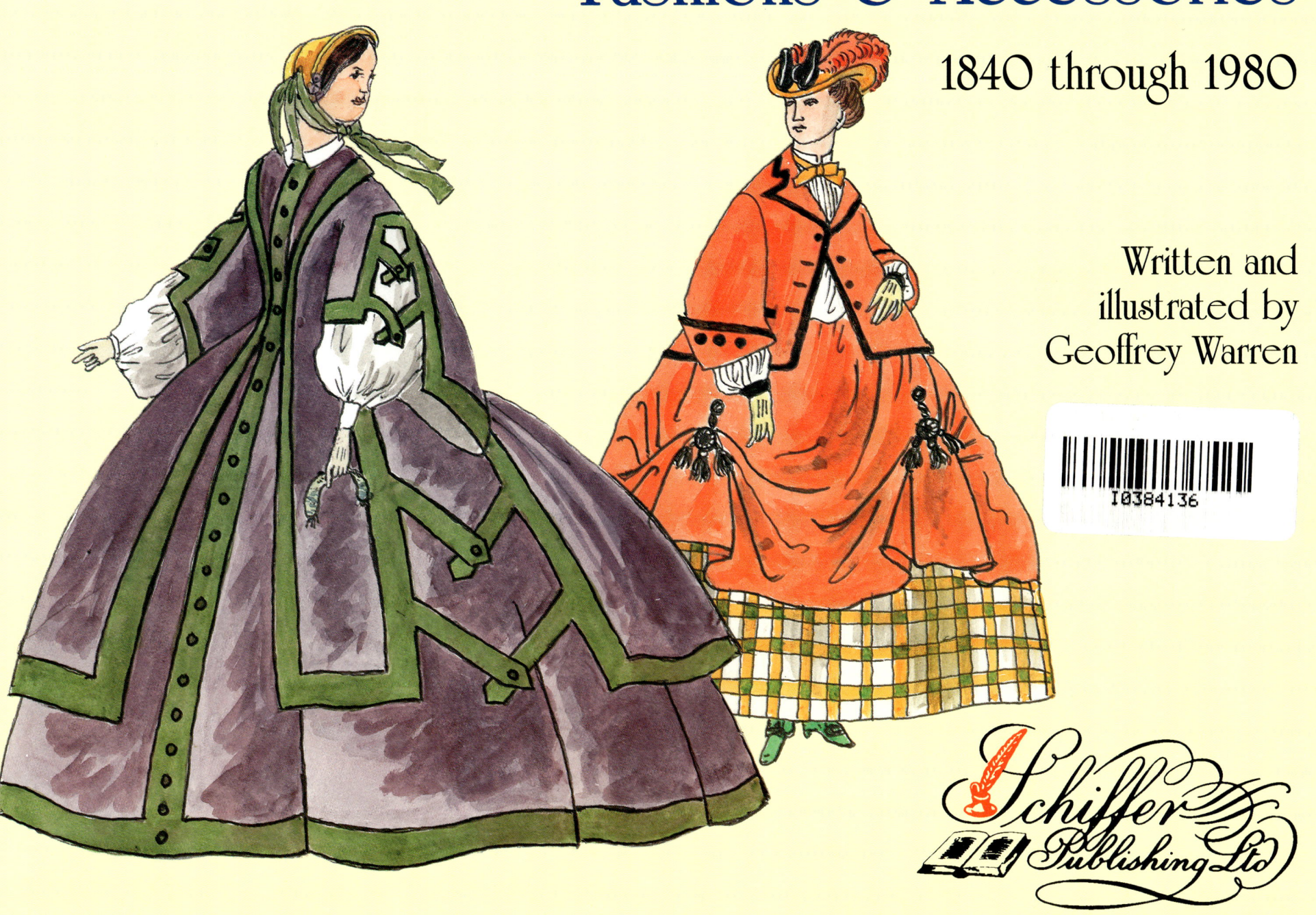

Fashions & Accessories
1840 through 1980

Written and illustrated by Geoffrey Warren

Schiffer Publishing Ltd

4880 Lower Valley Road, Atglen, PA 19310 USA

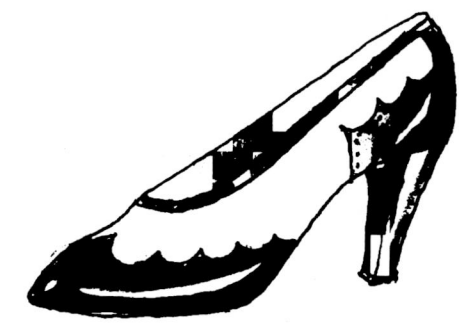

Dedication

For my great-nephew James Warren Dempster

Acknowledgments

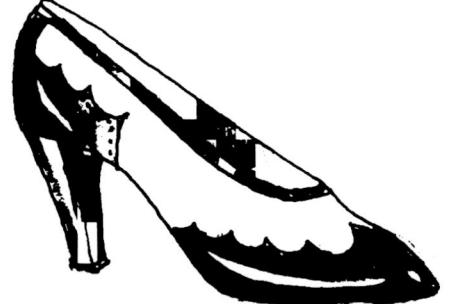

Library of Congress Cataloging--in-Publication Data

Warren, Geoffrey.
    Fashions & accessories, 1840 through 1980/written and illustrated by Geoffrey Warren.
       p.   cm.
    Includes bibliographial references.
    ISBN 0-7643-0309-0 (paper)
    1. Costume--United States--History--19th century.
2. Costume--United States--History--20th century. 3. Dress accessories--United States--History--19th century. 4. Dress accessories--United States--History--20th century. I. Title.
GT610.W37 1997
391'.00973--dc21   97-20311
                              CIP

Copyright © 1997 by Geoffrey Warren

All rights reserved. No part of this work may be reproduced or used in any form or by any means—graphic, electronic, or mechanical, including photocopying or information storage and retrieval systems—without written permission from the copyright holder.

Designed by "Sue"

ISBN: 0-7643-0309-0
Printed in Hong Kong

    The author wishes to thank Nancy and Peter Schiffer for their support; Ray Lavender for his encouragement; William Lawford for his helpful comments regarding the illustrations; Jane Deverson, James Harding, and Vincent McQueen for lending items; and the London Library for supplying much useful information.

Back cover, author photo by Robert Field

Published by Schiffer Publishing Ltd.
4880 Lower Valley Road
Atglen, PA 19310
Phone: (610) 593-1777; Fax: (610) 593-2002
E-mail: Schifferbk@aol.com
Please write for a free catalog.
This book may be purchased from the publisher.
Please include $3.95 for shipping.
Try your bookstore first.

We are interested in hearing from authors
with book ideas on related subjects.

Contents

Introduction 4
WOMEN
1840-1850 Day Wear 6
1850-1855 Day Wear 10
1840-1855 Evening Wear 13
1855-1864 Day Wear 17
1855-1864 Evening Wear 20
1864-1868 Day Wear 22
1864-1868 Evening Wear 25
1868-1870 Day Wear 27
1868-1870 Evening Wear 29
1870-1875 Day Wear 31
1870-1875 Evening Wear 34
1875-1880 Day Wear 36
1875-1880 Evening Wear 40
1880-1883 Day Wear 42
1880-1883 Evening Wear 44
1883-1888 Day Wear 46
1883-1888 Evening Wear 50
1888-1892 Day Wear 52
1888-1892 Evening Wear 54
1892-1897 Day wear 56
1892-1897 Evening Wear 59
1897-1902 Day Wear 61
1897-1902 Evening Wear 63
1902-1908 Day Wear 66
1902-1908 Evening Wear 70
1908-1911 Day Wear 72
1908-1911 Evening Wear 75
1911-1915 Day Wear 77
1911-1915 Evening Wear 81
1915-1919 Day wear 84
1915-1919 Evening Wear 88
1919-1923 Day Wear 91
1919-1923 Evening Wear 93
1923-1929 Day Wear 95
1923-1929 Evening Wear 99
1929-1937 Day Wear 101
1929-1939 Evening Wear 105
1937-1939 Day Wear 107
1940-1945 Day Wear 110
1945-1947 Day Wear 113
1947-1948 Day Wear 115
1947-1950 Day Wear 117
1945-1950 Evening Wear 119
1950-1955 Day Wear 121
1950-1955 Evening Wear 125
1955-1960 Day Wear 127
1955-1960 Evening Wear 129
1960-1970 Day Wear 131
1960-1970 Evening Wear 135
1970-1980 Day Wear .... 137 & 139
1970-1980 Evening Wear 141

MEN
1840-1850 Day Wear 144
1840-1850 Day & Evening Wear 145
1850-1860 Day Wear 146
1870-1880 Day Wear 148
1890-1900 Day Wear 154
1900-1910 Day Wear 156
1910-1920 Day Wear 158
1920-1930 Day Wear 160
1930-1940 Day Wear 162
1940-1950 Day Wear 164
1950-1960 Day Wear 166
1960-1970 Day Wear 168
1970-1980 Day Wear 171
Select Bibliography 174
Price Guide 175

Introduction

There is an old English saying: "Manners maketh man." One can also claim that "Accessories maketh clothes." Or, as British *Vogue* stated in 1965: "We've always stressed the power of accessories to change the whole look." These are the factors this book sets out to demonstrate.

Fashion has always reflected the social, sexual, and economic spirit of its age. Clothing and accessories also express the status, aspirations, and wealth of the wearer. New fashions develop from these reasons and from a natural need for change. Change such as this—particularly in this century—is fostered by the fashion industry, for the sake of being different or for financial and competitive reasons, and introduces new styles as frequently as possible, encouraging many women and men to become "slaves of fashion."

Most books on fashion tend to divide clothing and accessories into decades. Fashion cannot always be so clearly demarcated. For instance, the first crinoline appeared in 1855 and the trend lasted until 1864. The 1890s can be divided into three sections, and several other 10-year periods can be divided into two. Many view the entire decade of the 1920s as the era of short skirts, short hair, and the cloche hat; however, this look did not hit the mainstream until the mid-1920s and ceased abruptly in 1929. The style of men's two-toned brogue shoes began in the late 1920s and continued into the late 1930s. Some styles lasted for only a few years, others for a great many, and so on.

All accessories—be they necessary, such as shoes, or decorative, such as jewelry—ideally must be seen in the context of the clothing with which they are worn or carried. For this reason, and to give a brief history of fashion covered herein, I have included full-length figures with explanatory text.

I have also concentrated on the upper sections of society. In earlier ages, there was a very distinct sartorial difference between the fashions of the upper and lower section of society, but after about 1840, people lower down the social scale simply donned cheaper, less extravagant versions of upper-society fashions. Fashion usually percolates downward. In particular, the period covered by this book saw greater changes in the economic climate than any other time in history. The Industrial Revolution created a new, affluent middle class; by 1840, this group was anxious to display its wealth, status, and power. One of the best ways to do so was through fashion, especially for women. Throughout the rest of the century and up to 1914 and beyond, quality clothing and accessories became readily available to those who had "new" money.

After the upheaval of the First World War (among other changes), fully-emancipated women emerged in greater numbers to create a new fashion market. This market was amply fed through the explosion of mass production. In the 1920s and 1930s, the women's "emancipation" movement, which also applied to men, proliferated. This revolution extended well into the 1940s, when wealth in general also increased.

By the 1960s, the scales of fashion had tipped. Many of the styles of the time originated in the bottom strata of society and spread upward. This was quite the opposite of earlier trends, which mostly were generated in high-society wear and then filtered downward. The fashions of the 1970s saw even greater evidence of this trend.

Throughout the ages, there were fewer men's fashions accessories to speak of, and those there were usually accompanied men's casual wear. Therefore, I have not included full-length drawings of men in formal clothes, such as frock coats, morning coats, and trousers or formal evening wear, because the accompanying accessories (i.e., top hats, gloves, shoes) did not change a great deal.

For those readers who are designing costumes for the stage, movies, or television, this book is intended to couple the proper accessory with the proper costume or fashion. For example, this book illustrates that an 1840s bonnet was not worn after 1855; a "My Fair Lady" hat was rarely seen before 1908 and not after 1911; a bowler (derby) was not worn before approximately 1860 but a long time afterward, and so on.

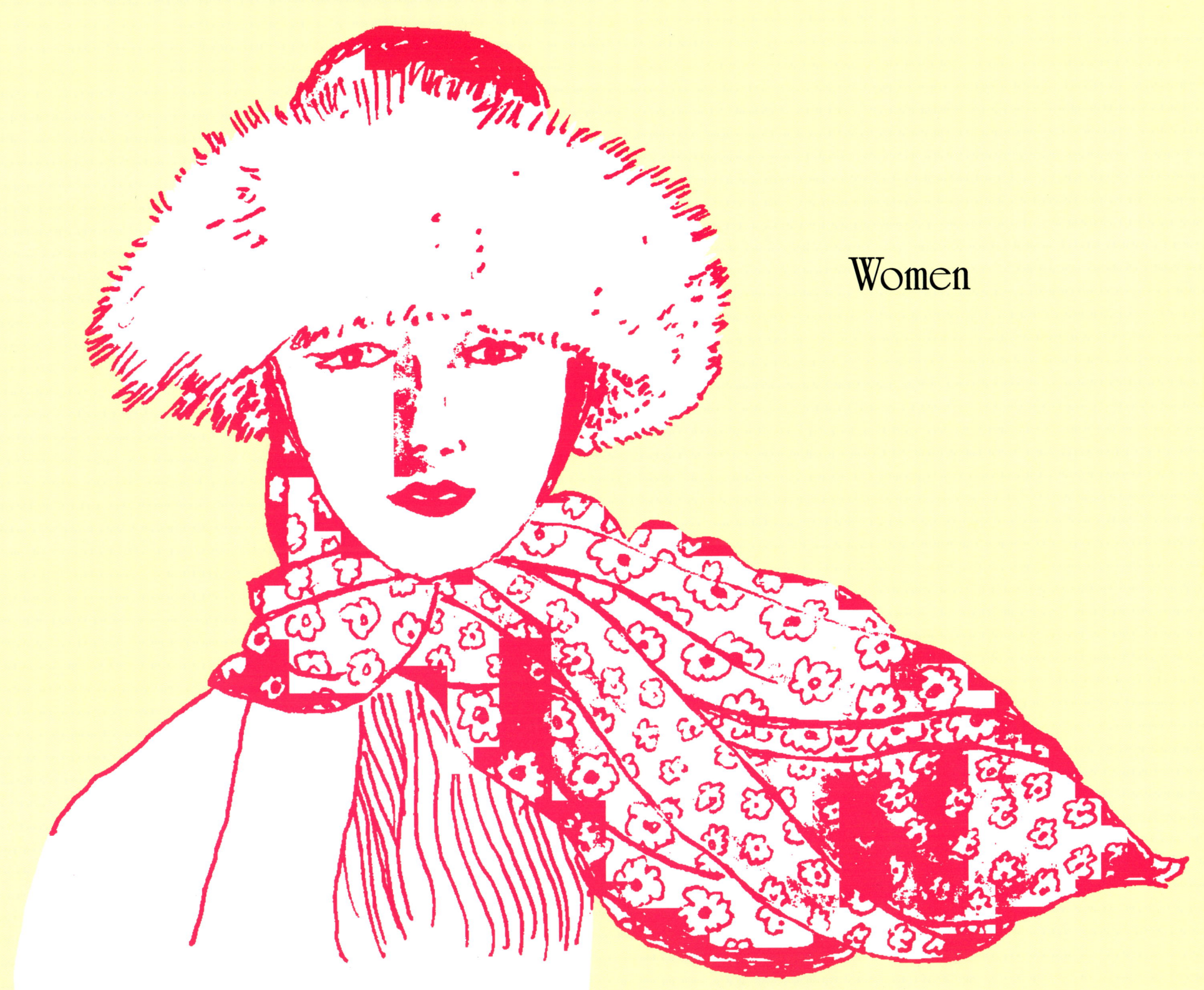

Women

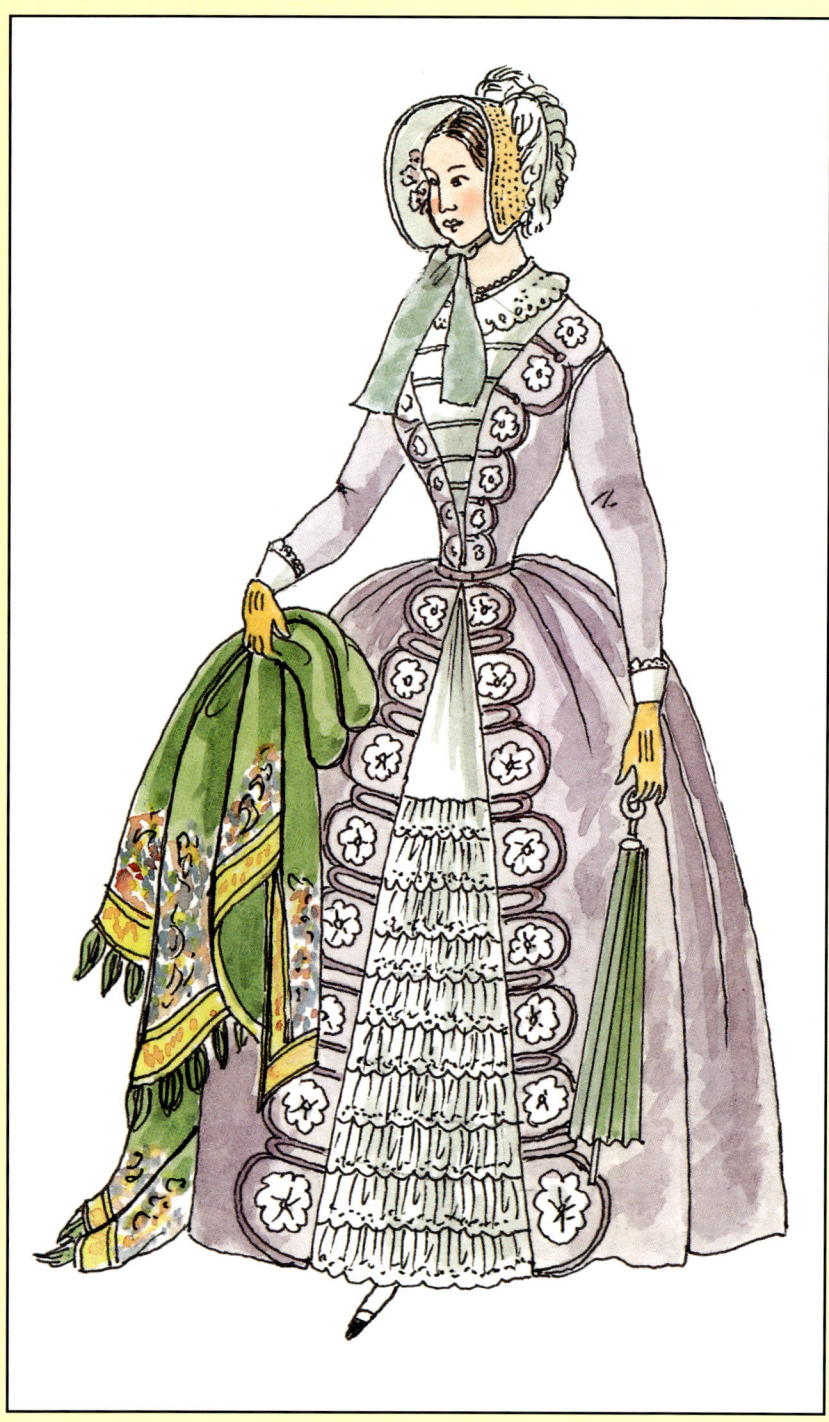

1840-1850 Day Wear

    Never in the history of fashion have clothing and accessories been designed to make women appear so helpless, modest, and subservient to men.
    In clothing everything was done to promote this image. The bodice, worn over very tight corsets, was long and narrow with a pinched-in waist, the corsage was usually high, the sleeves were tight and restricting. Full skirts, supported by many petticoats, were equally restricting. Everything drooped. Dresses were either closed or, as in the illustration, open to reveal a filled-in bodice and petticoat. Trimming consisted of lace and ribbons; colors were mostly muted, and materials were soft. Short kid gloves were worn even indoors—a sign that high-society women did no work. Bonnets hid the face, and large shawls, embroidered in silk for summer and woollen cashmere for winter, were either worn or carried.

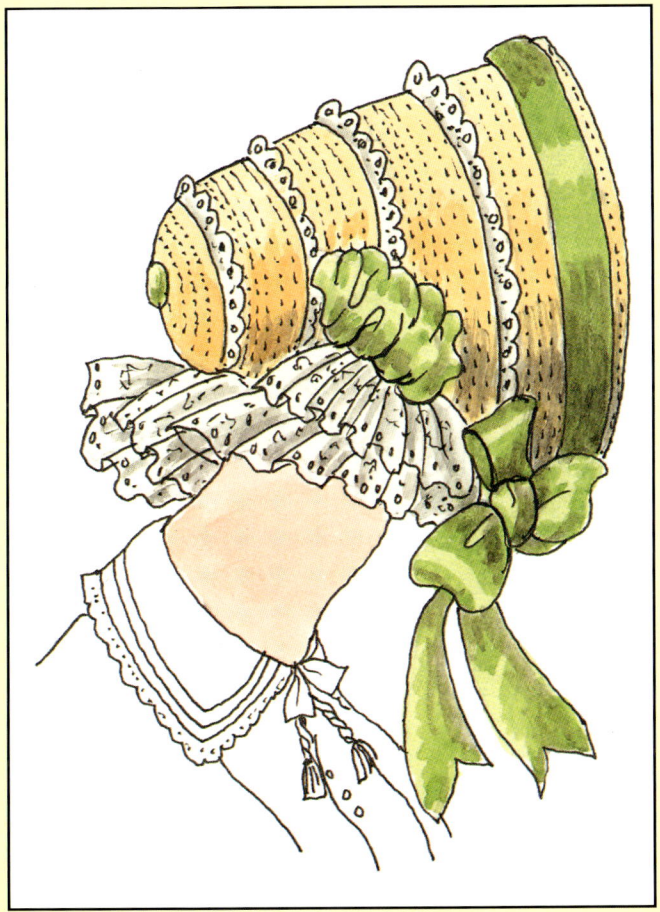

For all bonnets during this period, the crown and brim merged into a horizonal line, forming a "coal scuttle" shape. The brim usually sat so low over the ears and projected so far forward, to prevent women from looking sideways or being seen, except from the front. Most bonnets, such as this straw example, had frills at the nape of the neck called bavolets.

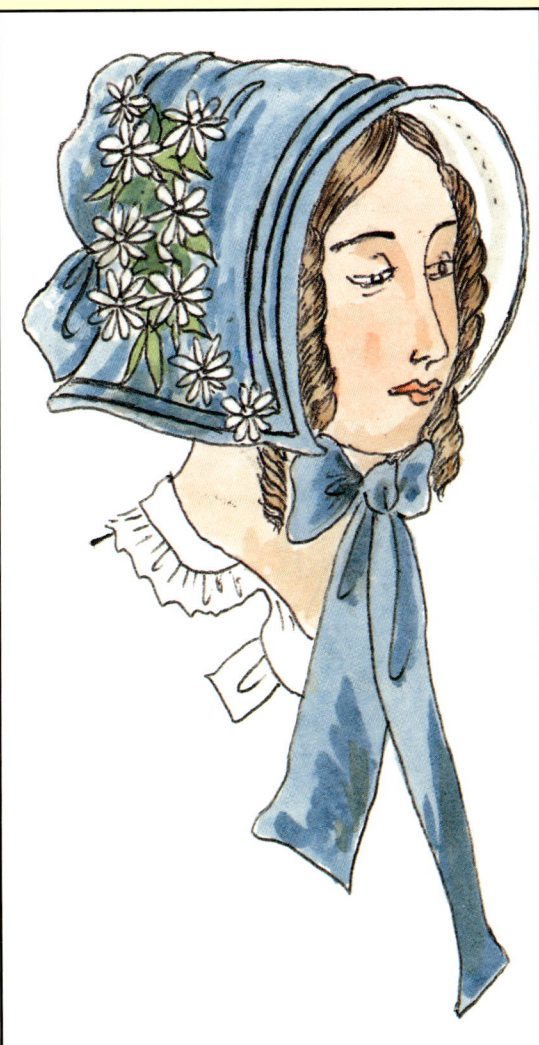

Silk-trimmed bonnet with artificial flowers and leaves.

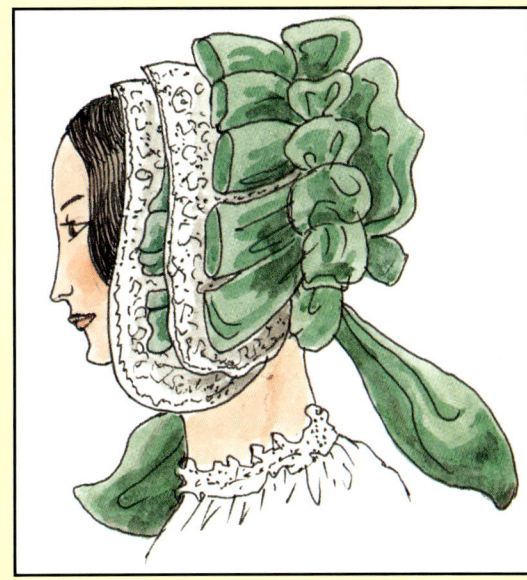

A more face-revealing bonnet made of stiffened lace.

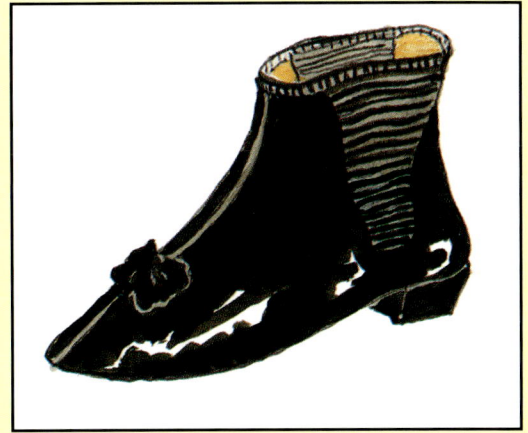

An outdoor satin boot with elastic gussets.

Although skirts were given pockets, some women carried reticules, such as this silk example, which hooked on to the waist.

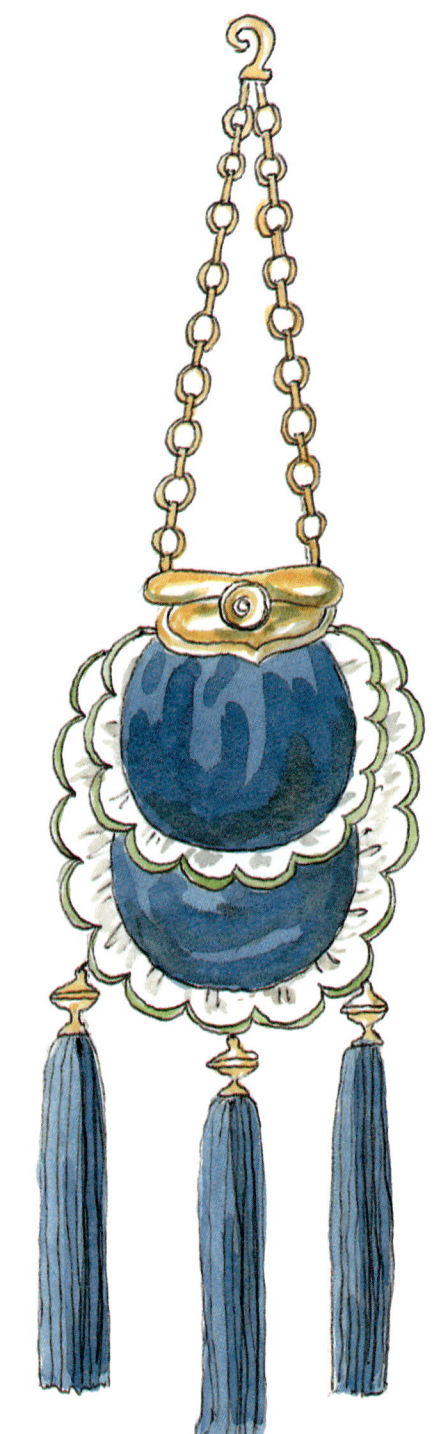

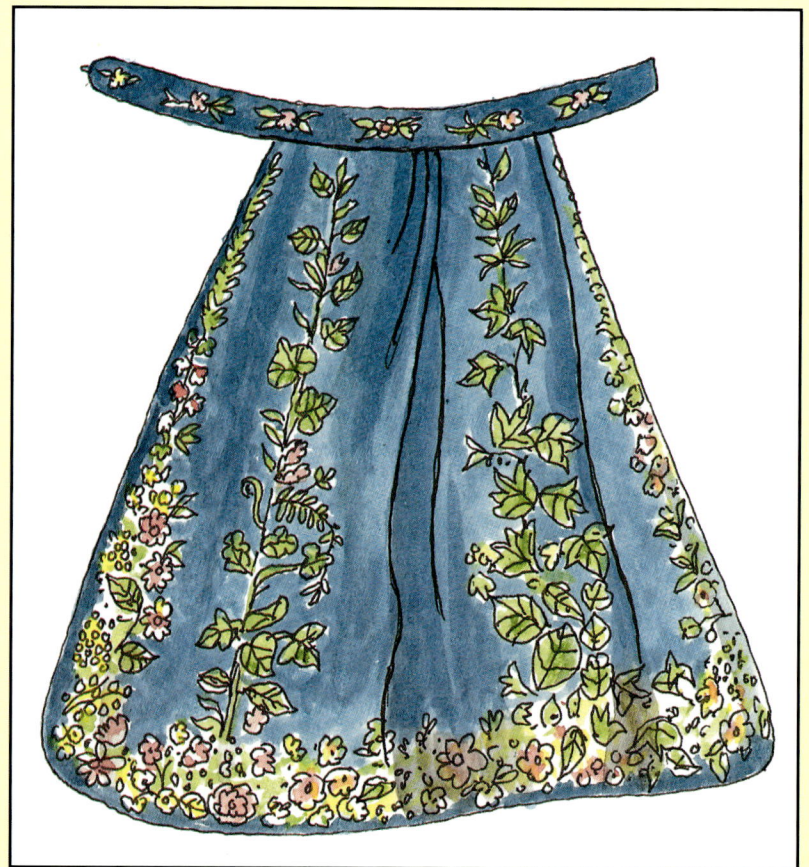

A silk apron embroidered with ribbon work. Such aprons were purely decorative, because the only "work" that genteel ladies ever did was needlework or watercolors.

Ancient or new cameos, carved out of lava or shells, very popular throughout the century and now, were mounted to form necklaces, bracelets, and brooches. Most pieces were set in plain gold mounts, but this one has an elaborate vine leaf and grape mount set with pearls.

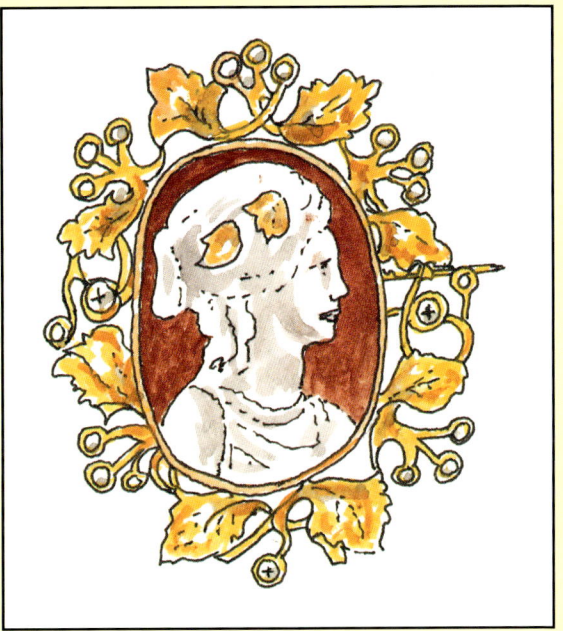

Since the late eighteenth century, human hair has been used for jewelry: plaited on its own (even for men's watch chains) or set into miniatures, lockets, and brooches. The hair was often that of a lost loved one, making the object an *momento mori*, which was very popular during the Romantic period up to the 1870s. After this time, it was considered bad taste by high society to make a public show of grief, and hair was hidden in separate compartments in jewelry. The plaited hair in this brooch is set in gold and diamonds.

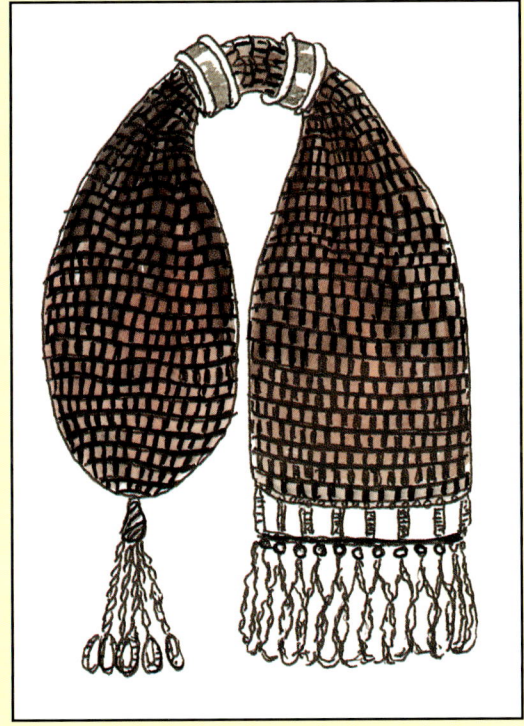

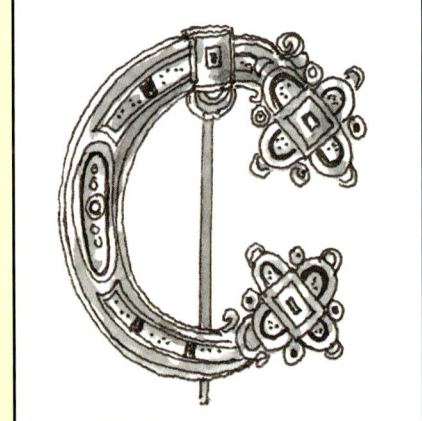

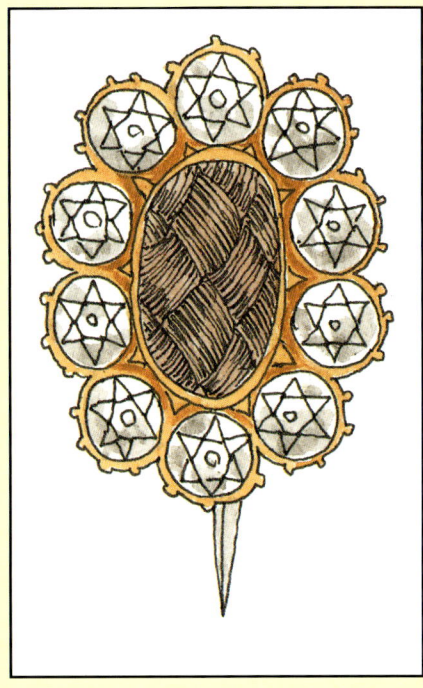

The "stocking," "long," "sausage," or "miser" purse first appeared in approximately 1800 and was in use until 1880, only to lapse in fashion until the 1920s, when it was used for bridge. Made of kid, silk, plush, knitting, or crochet, the purse had a central opening which could be closed by metal rings. Most had rounded ends, but in this crochet example one shaped end was for gold coins, the other for silver. The tassel and fringe are made of steel beads.

Archeological finds in Ireland in the 1940s set the fashion for Celtic-style jewelry in gold, silver, silver-gilt or parcel-gilt, often set with turquoises. This example is in silver.

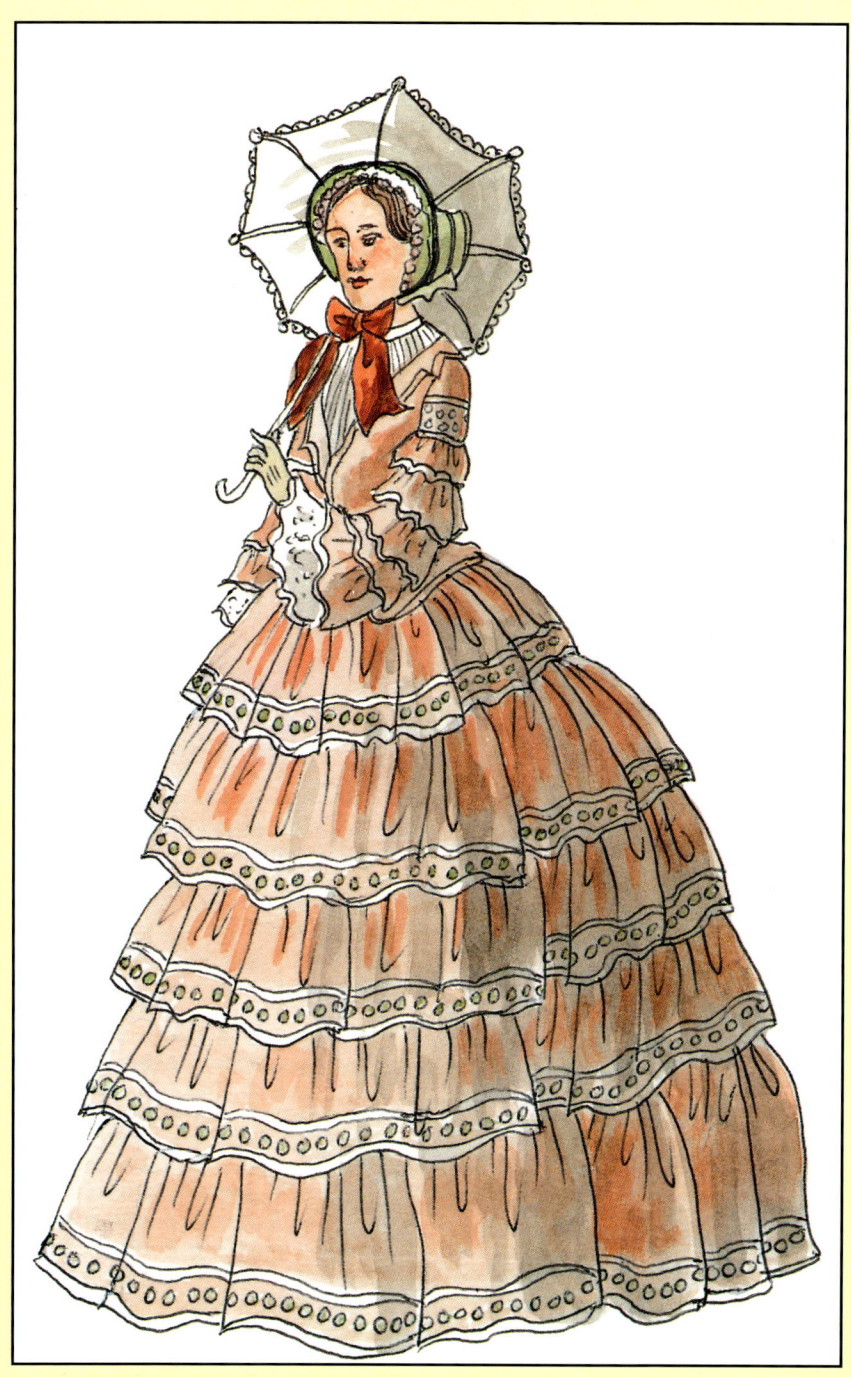

1850-1855 Day Wear

Although just as full, skirts of this period were more frilled with matching sleeves in "pagoda" shapes, revealing deep lace undersleeves. In an attempt to relieve the weight of the skirts, some petticoats were stiffened with hoops of horsehair, metal, and even rubber tubes but to little avail.

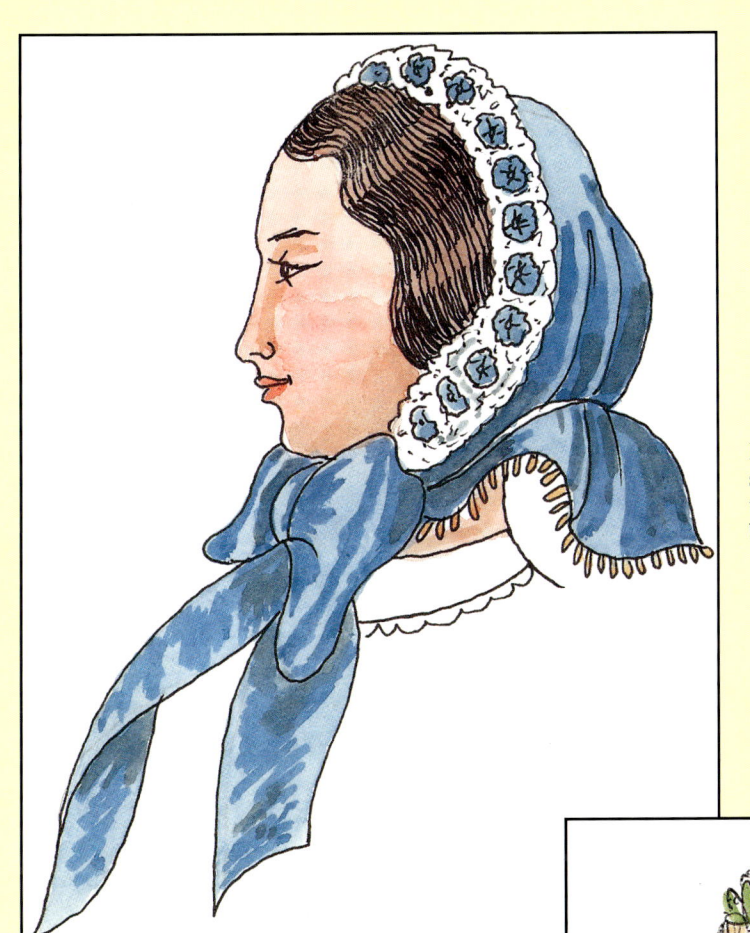

By the late 1840s, the bonnet was set much further back on the head; this bavolet is stiffened with buckram.

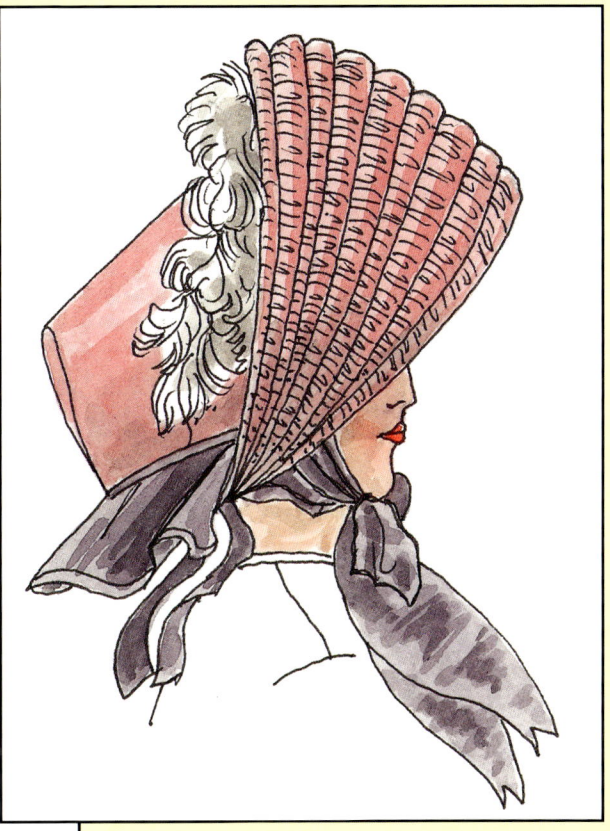

A bonnet called an "ugly;" its large brim is made of padded and ruched silk; this bonnet was worn mostly by young girls and older women.

Silk decorated with artificial flowers and leaves in and outside the brim, with a soft muslin and lace bavolet.

During the day indoors, women wore muslin and lace caps with long lappets and much decoration.

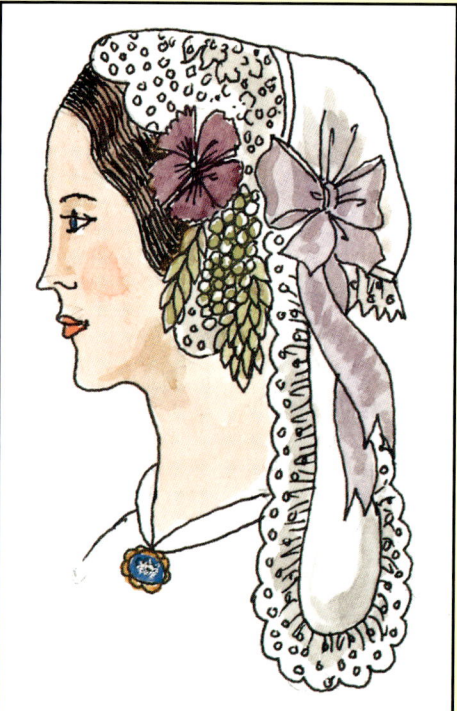

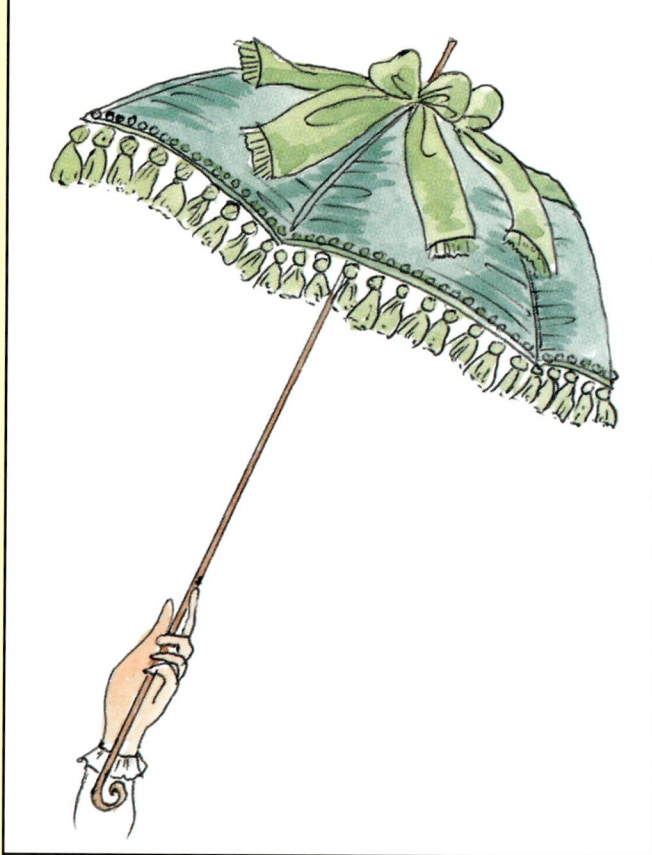

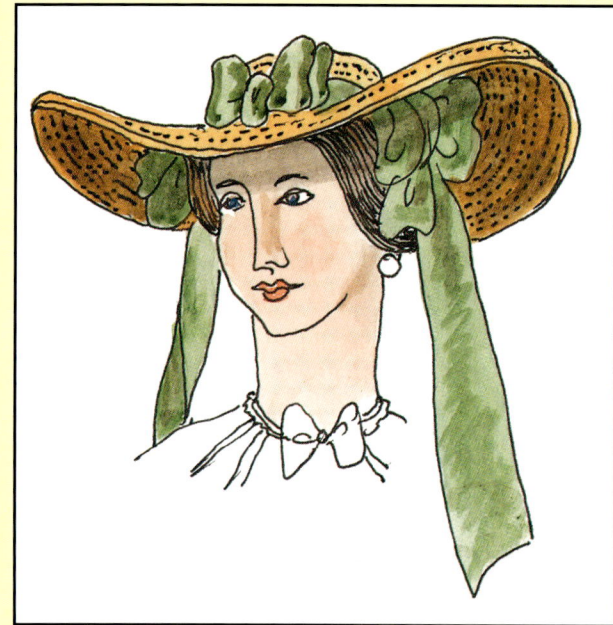

The beautiful leader of fashion, the French Empress Eugénie, wife of Napoleon III, made it acceptable to wear hats, such as this straw example, but only in the garden or in the country.

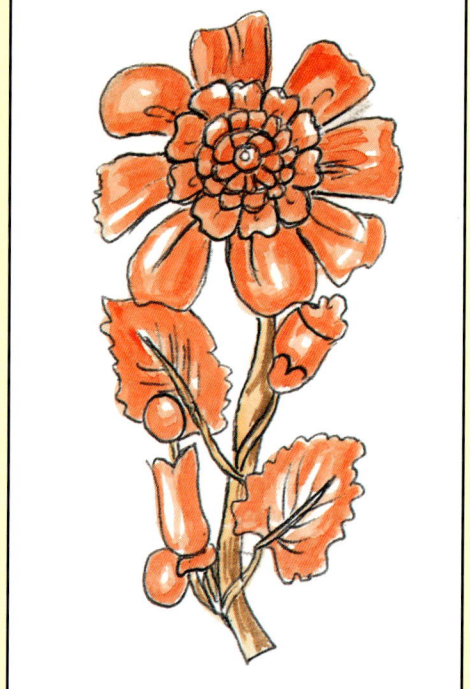

Silk parasols were either very small, as in the full-length figure, or of a more "sensible" size.

Coral jewelry was very popular during the 1850s. At a time when naturalism was in favor, this flower, bud, and leaf brooch with a gold stem is typical of the style.

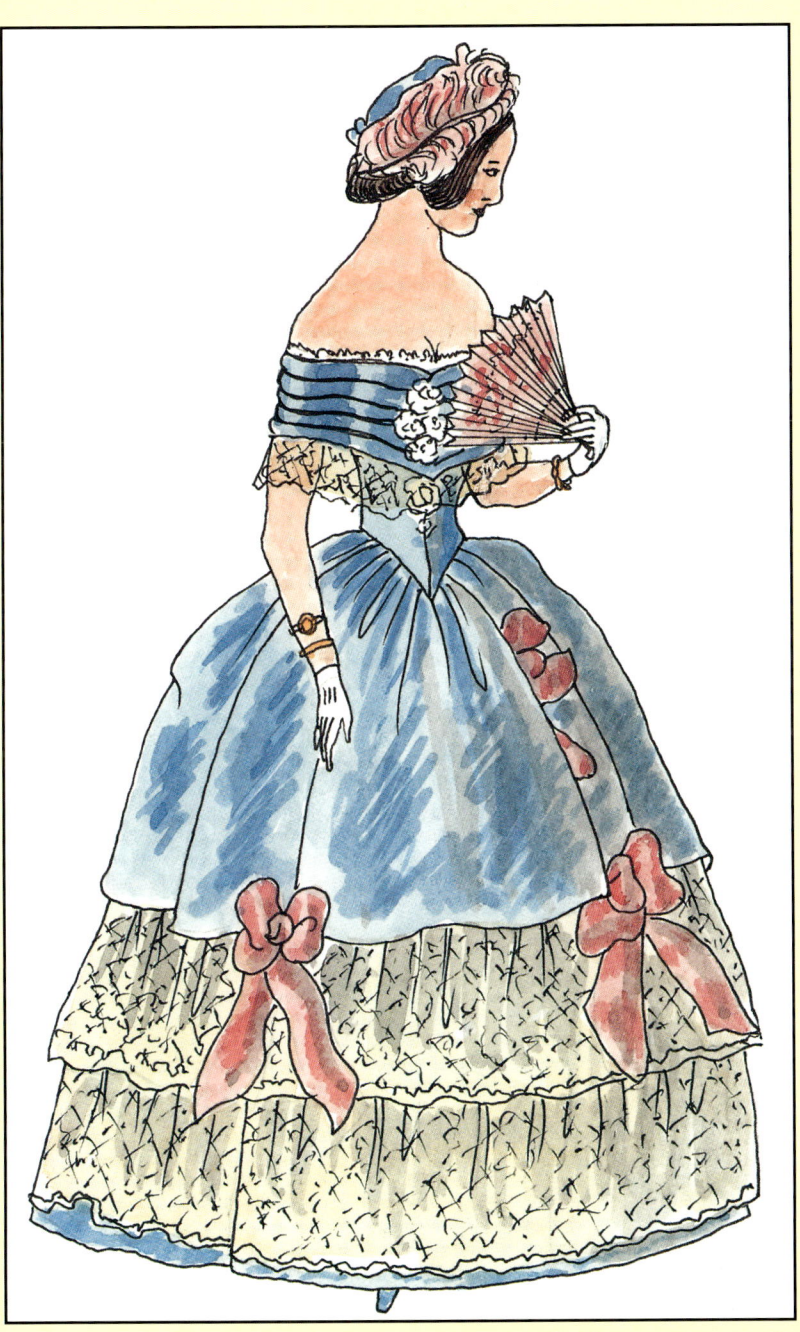

1840-1855 Evening Wear

If women were too covered by day, they were very much uncovered for the evening, in fashions showing bare shoulders and low necklines from shoulder to shoulder. The bodice was as tight as those were by day, extravagantly trimmed and with short sleeves. Arms were bare, apart from short gloves and many bracelets. Skirts were flounced in layers, trimmed with ribbons, lace, and artificial flowers.

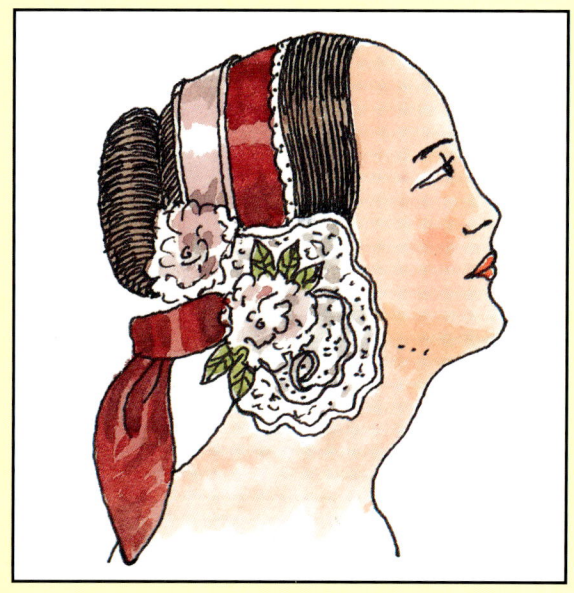

Because evening dresses between 1840 and 1855 changed very little, accessories also remained much the same. Head coverings were mere scraps of lace, ribbons, and flowers.

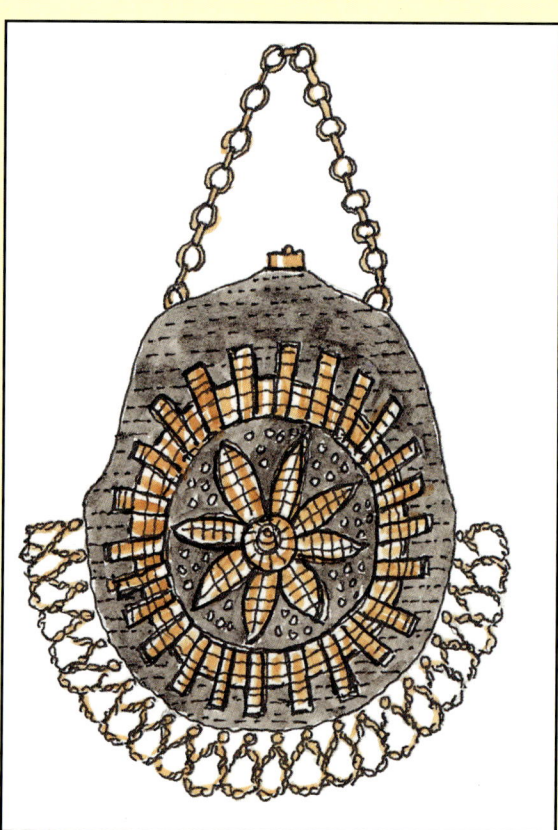

A crochet reticule, thickly sewn with beads, given a bead fringe.

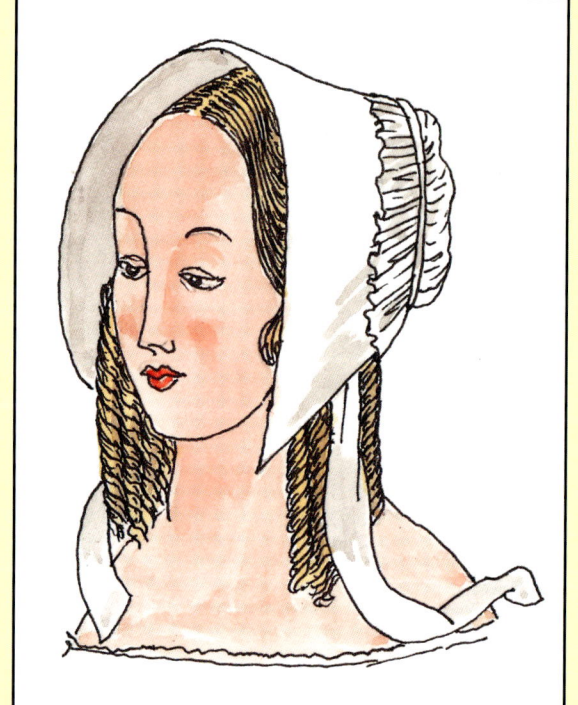

An unusual "milkmaid" stiffened silk bonnet.

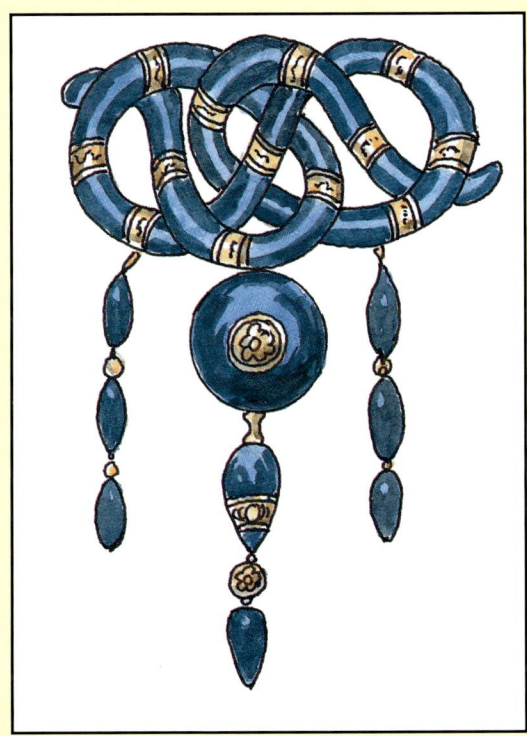

Despite women's traditional aversion to the reptile, snakes have inspired jewelry of all kinds since ancient Greek and Roman times. This enameled silver brooch is set with gold and diamonds.

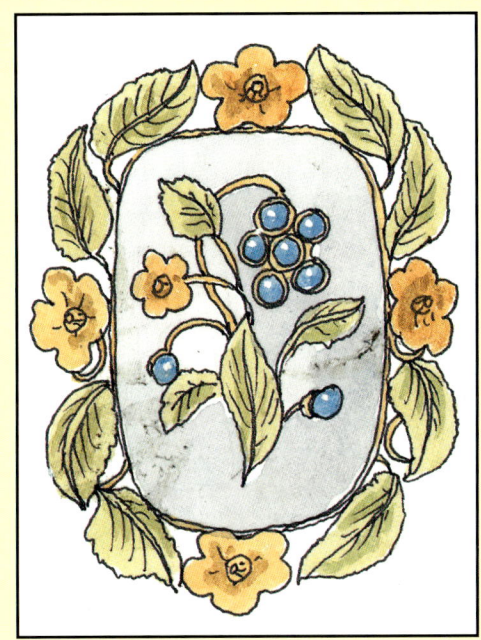

A brooch made of chalcedony decorated with two shades of gold.

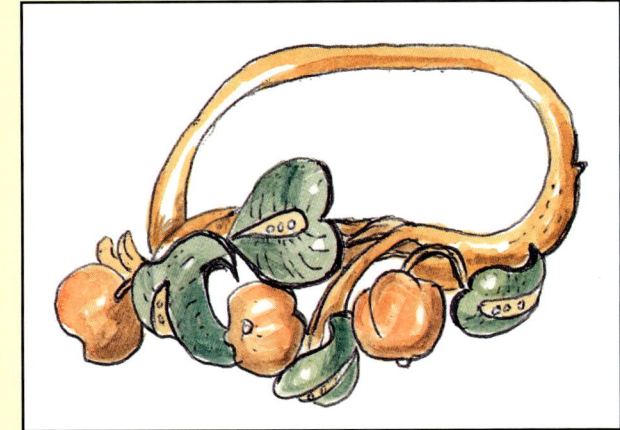

Another example of the fashion for naturalism: a bracelet consisting of a gold twig and enameled fruit and leaves set with tiny diamonds.

A flexible gold bracelet; its center decoration an oval of Italian mosaic or inlay work: carved semiprecious stones, coral, and ivory, embedded in black marble.

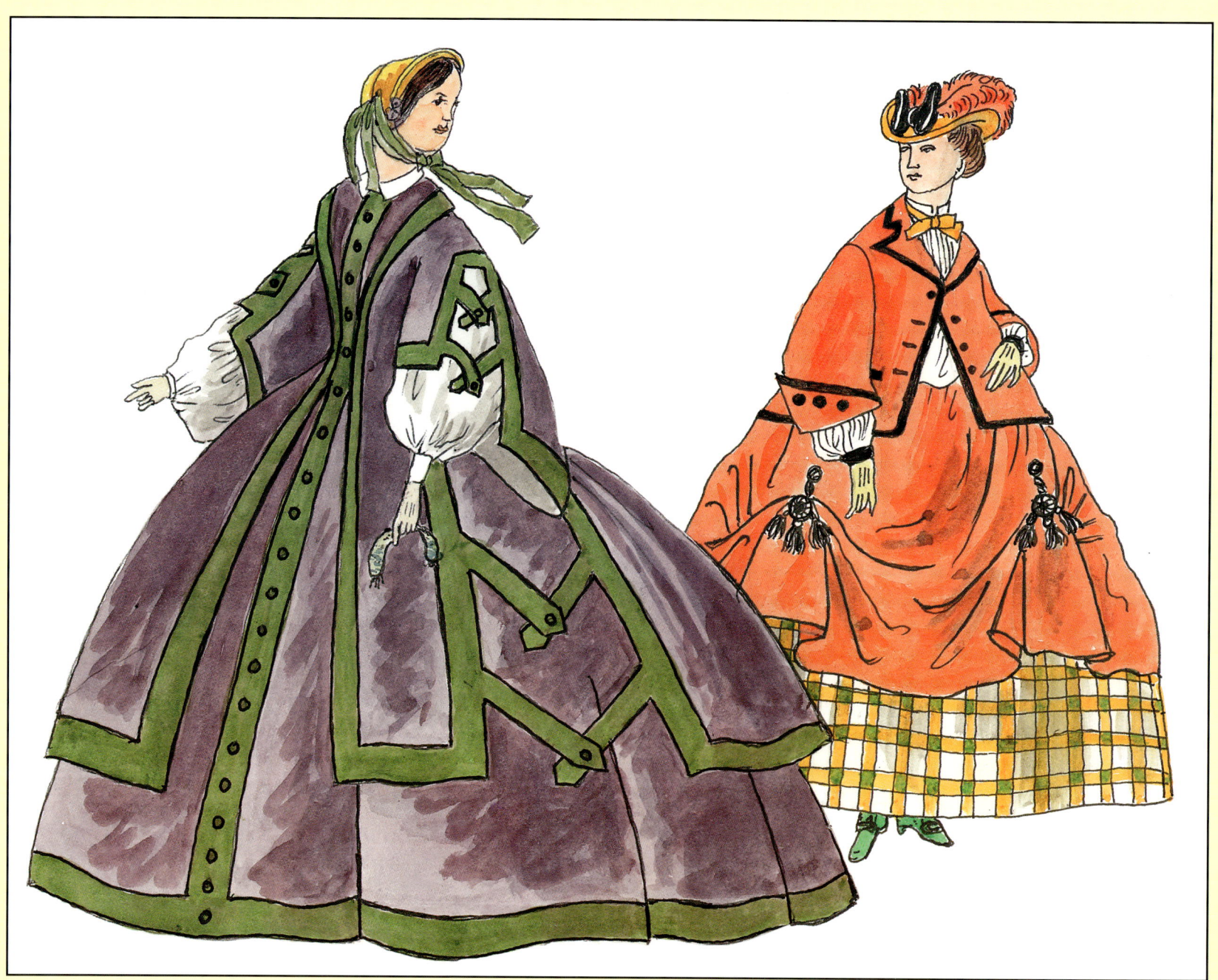

1855-1864 Day Wear

In approximately 1855, for women weighed down by heavy skirts and too many petticoats, help was at hand. The crinoline was invented. This accessory was either a dome-shaped petticoat strengthened with a series of metal, horsehair (*crin* is the French word for horsehair), or whalebone hoops or a light steel or whalebone frame which, by the late 1850s is said to have measured up to 15 feet in circumference (called a cage in France). The upper layer of the skirt could be separate from the bodice or (left) connected with it. For daring women who wore shorter skirts (right) the upper layer was hitched up over the lower.

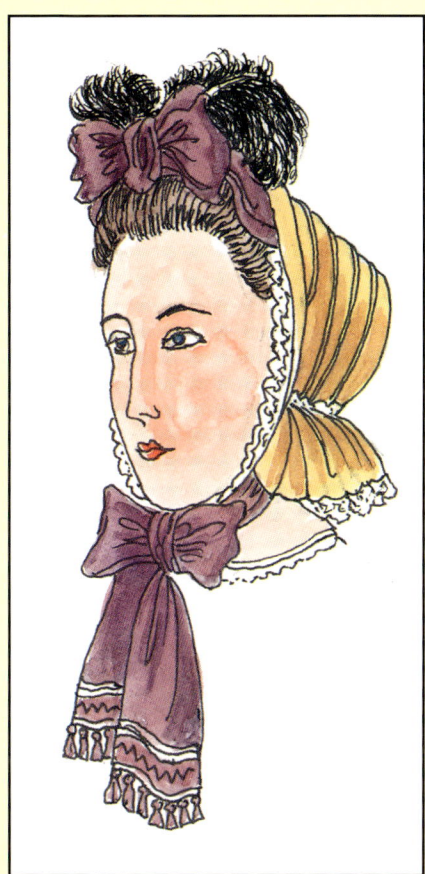

Bonnets were even smaller, set further back on the head and tied with very long ribbons.

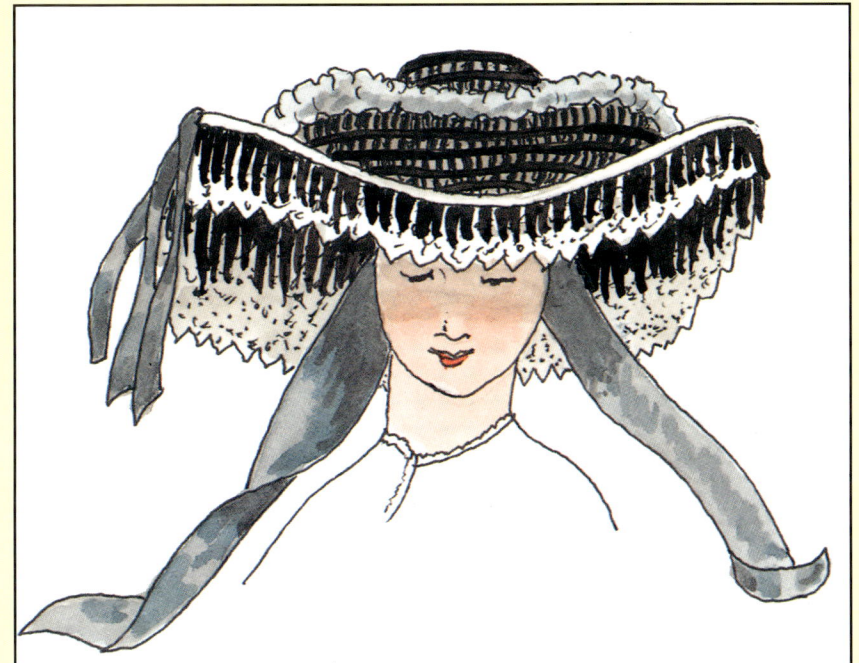

A brown straw *Mosquetaire* hat, deeply fringed with lace and feathers, its tie-ribbons left unfastened...again for the garden or country only.

This ruched silk round hat echoes the domed shape of the crinoline.

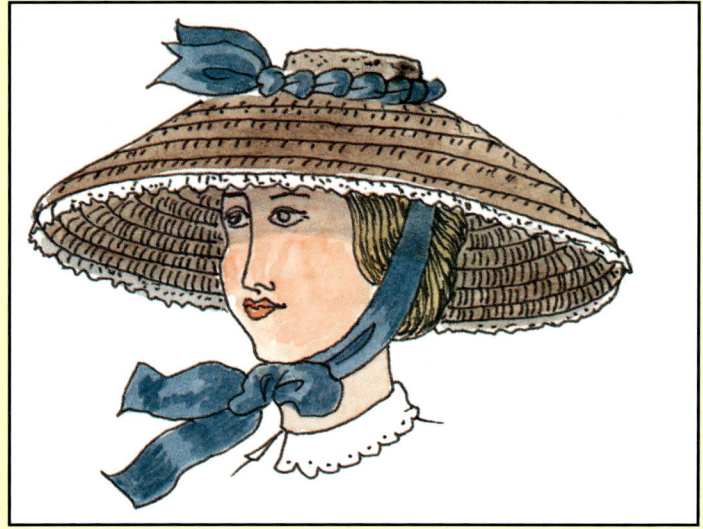

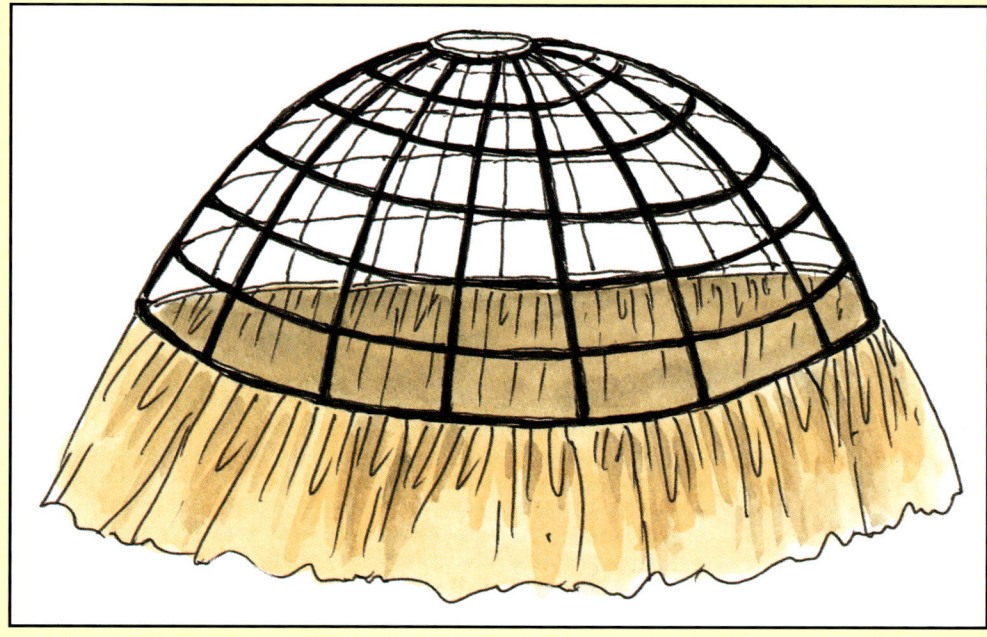

The lightest of crinolines: the French cage made of steel; here given a cotton flounce.

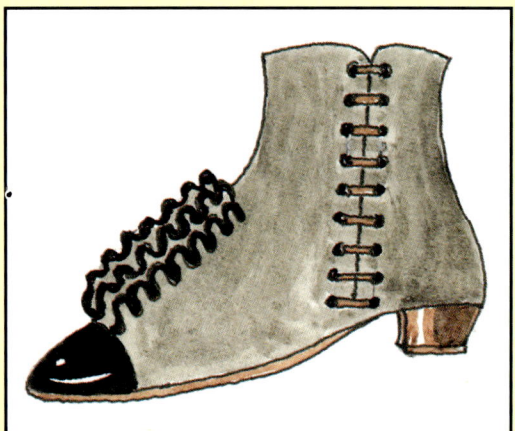

A suede boot with a patent leather toe cap which laces up the side.

A "dressy" silk boot generously trimmed with gold galloon braid and a gilt buckle; to be seen on women who wore the shorter skirts.

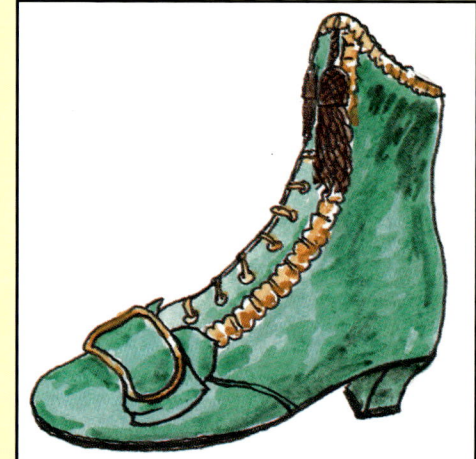

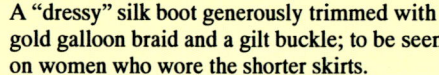

One of the simplest of crinolines: a calico petticoat threaded with whalebone, horsehair or steel hoops.

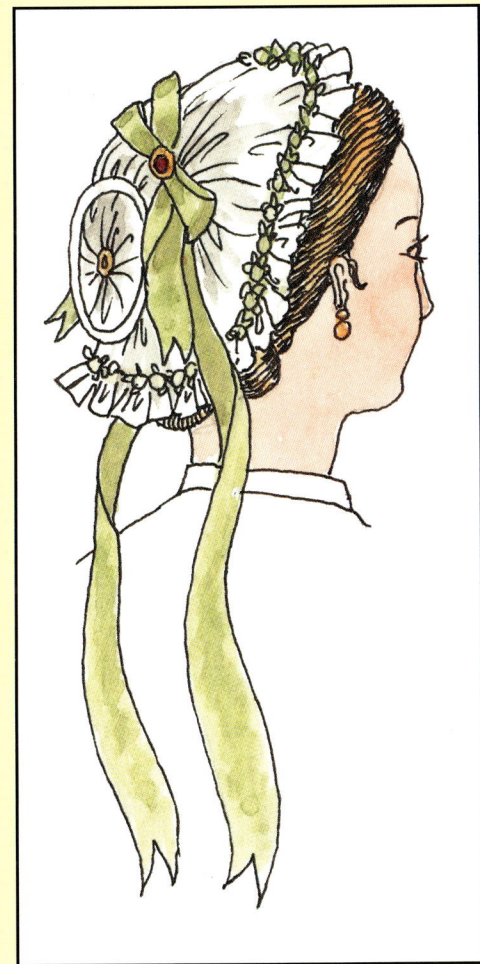

At home during the day, or as an alternative to a hat in the garden, women wore little, trimmed, muslin caps.

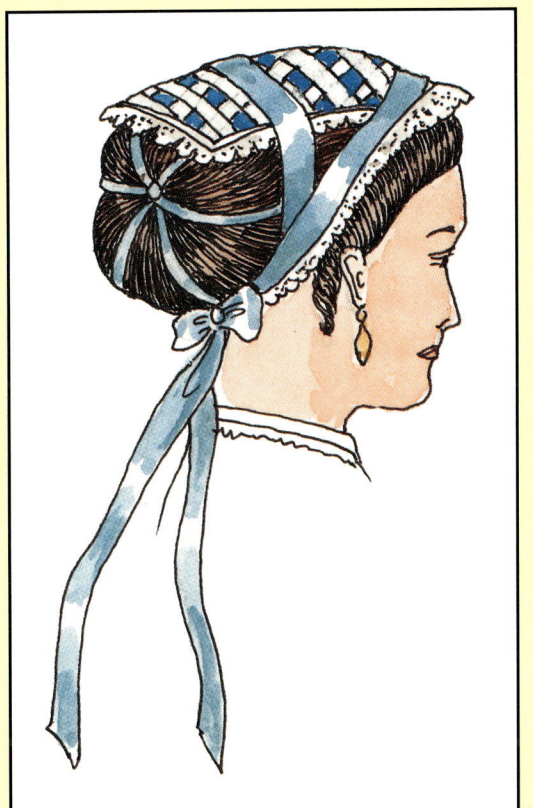

Plaited silk and lace, securely held in place with yet more ribbons; note ribbons also in the chignon.

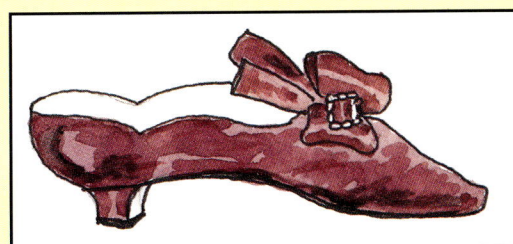

Silk shoe with a paste buckle.

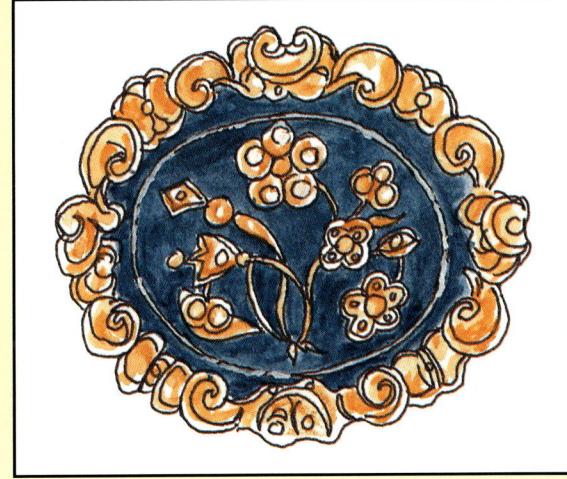

So many dresses had little turned-down collars that a brooch was an attractive accessory, such as this one in enamel, gold, and pearls.

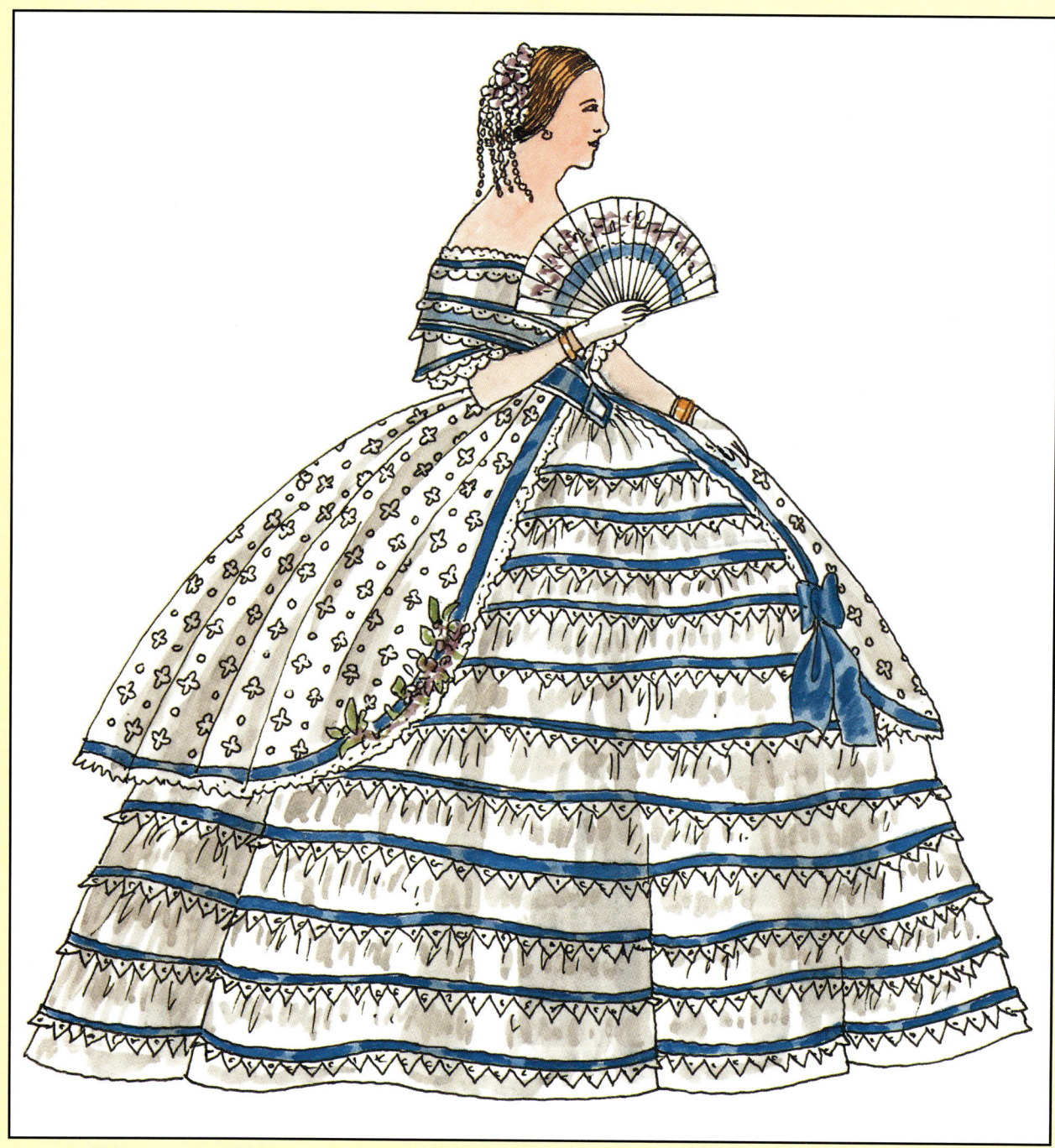

1855–1864 Evening Wear

The low bodice remained much the same with short sleeves, but the wide expanse of the crinoline allowed for many decorative materials, such as a multitude of frills or ribbons arranged in zig-zag patterns, and artificial flowers.

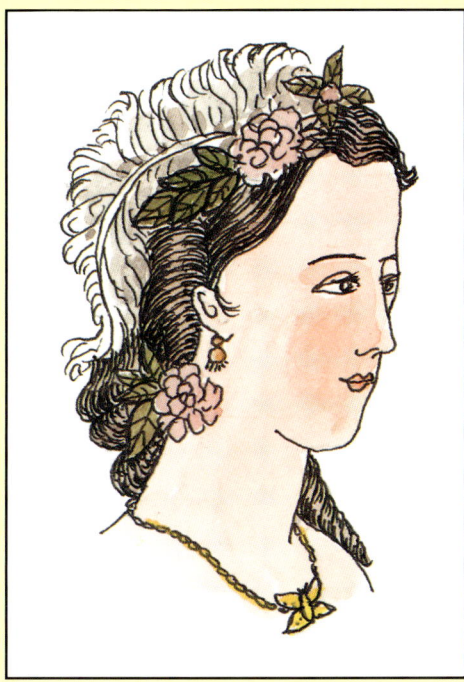

Decoration for the head consisted of concoctions of feathers, flowers, and beads.

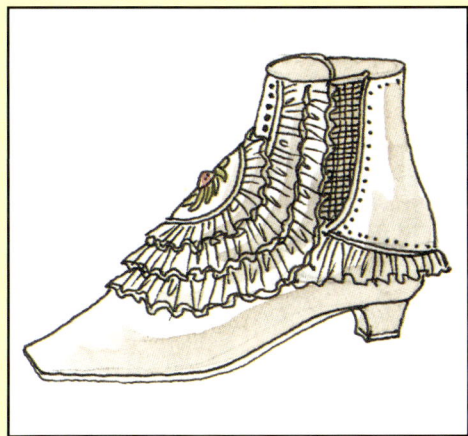

Silk evening shoes were often highly decorated, with side gussets.

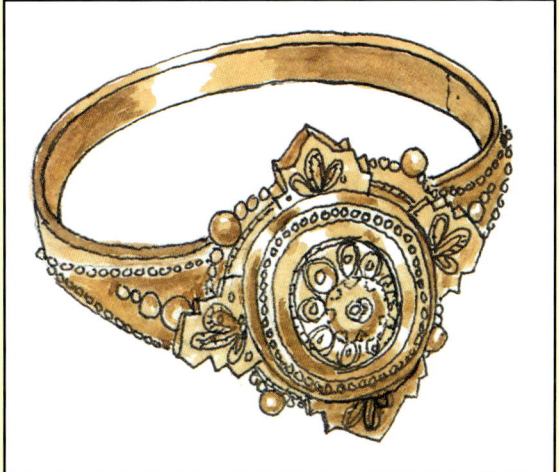

Evening jewelry was heavy and "barbaric," much of it in gold or gilt. Nineteenth-century designers were nothing if not eclectic, borrowing ideas from many past periods and countries. This gold bracelet is in "Etruscan" style.

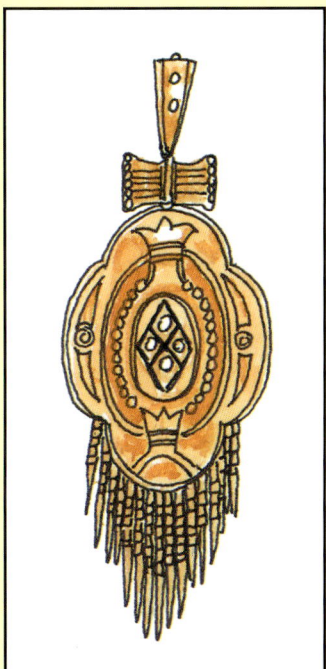

A gold ancient Greek-inspired pendant.

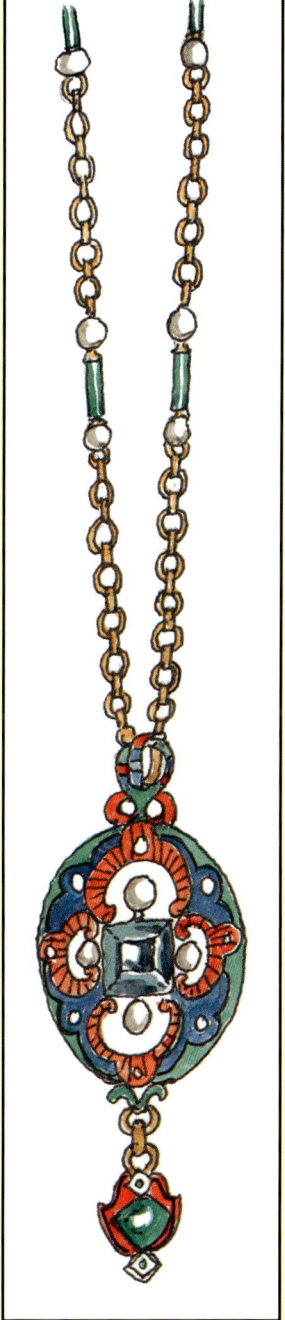

An enameled gold, emerald, diamond, and pearl "Holdbein" pendant hung from a gold, enamel, and pearl chain.

21

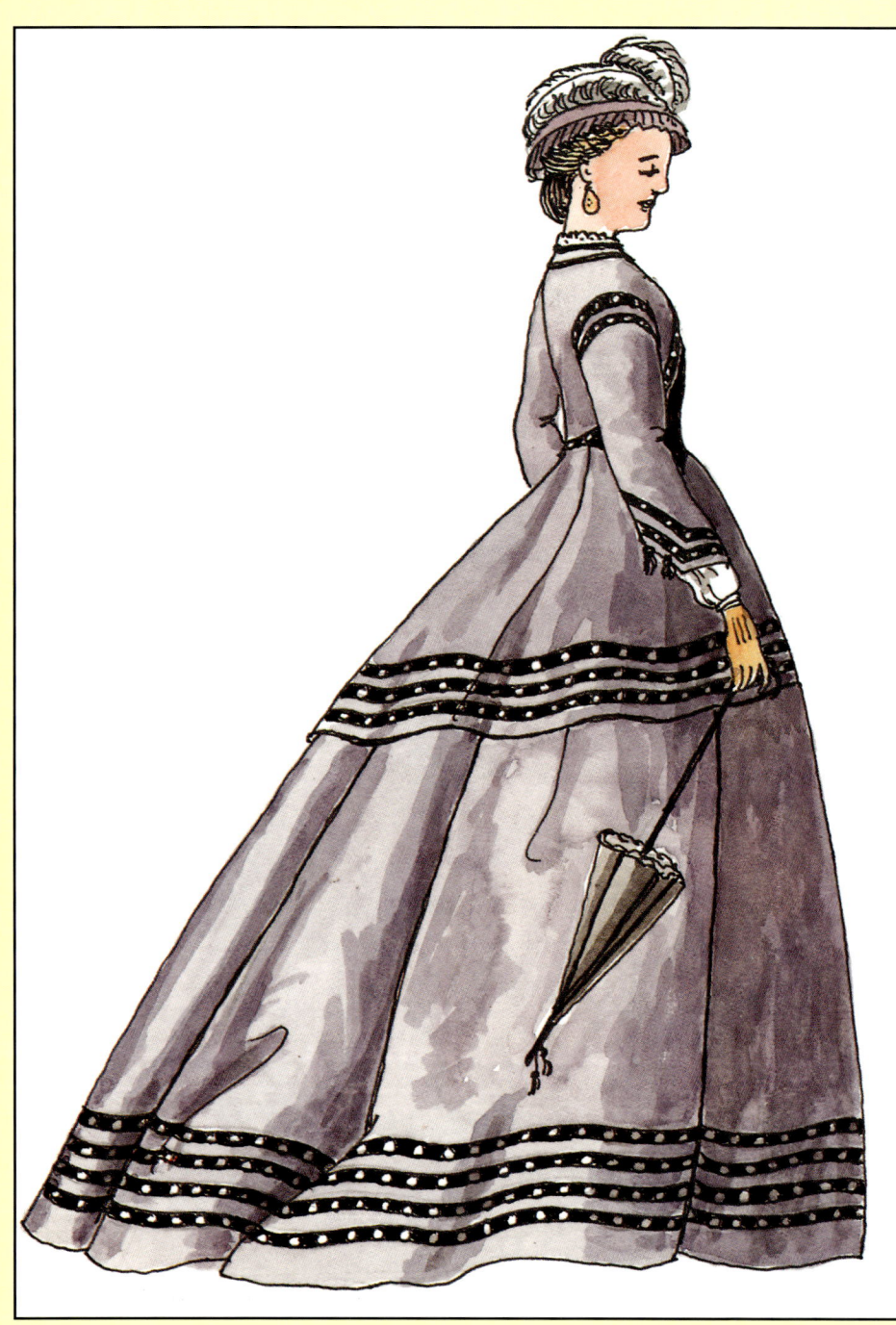

1864-1868 Day Wear

In 1864, the crinoline was flattened in the front, leaving it full at the back, with the appearance of a train. The bodice was closed at the neck, but the dress was often divided into a long jacket and skirt, both simply trimmed. Sleeves were narrower, with only a little of the chemise sleeve showing.

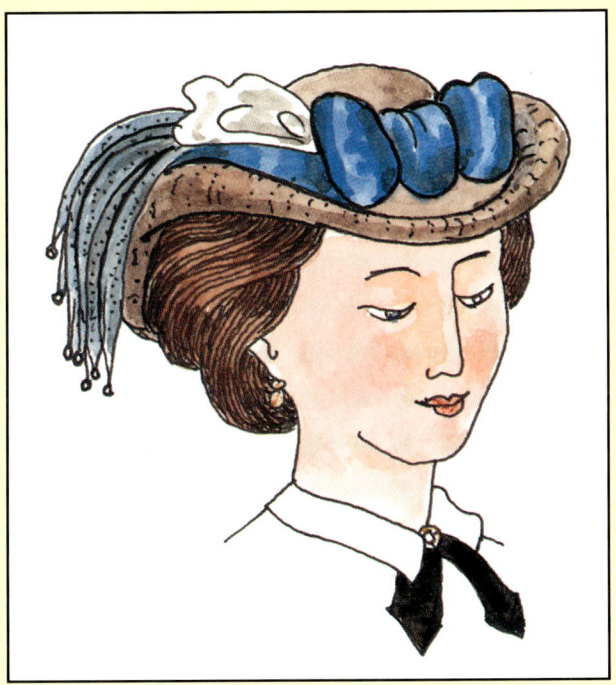

Small and jaunty hats were rapidly replacing bonnets, although it was still improper to wear them in church. This felt example was called an *imperatrice* after the Empress Eugénie.

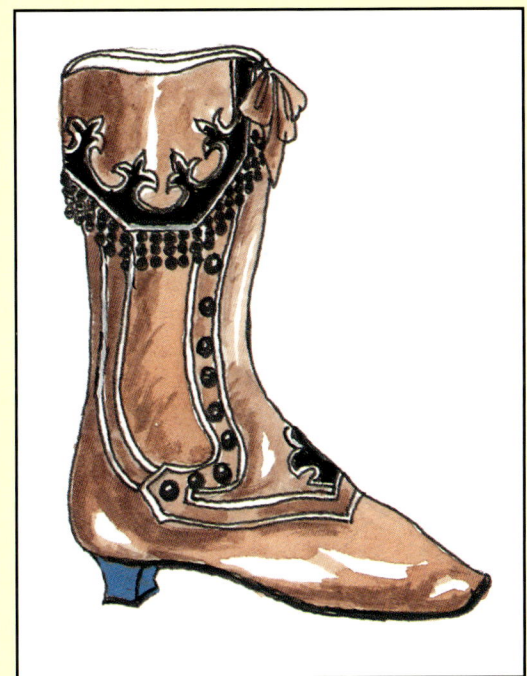

This dashing Russian leather boot is adorned with Cossack embroidery as well as tassels and buttons. Colored heels were very fashionable, certain to be admired under a lifted long crinoline or with a shorter skirt.

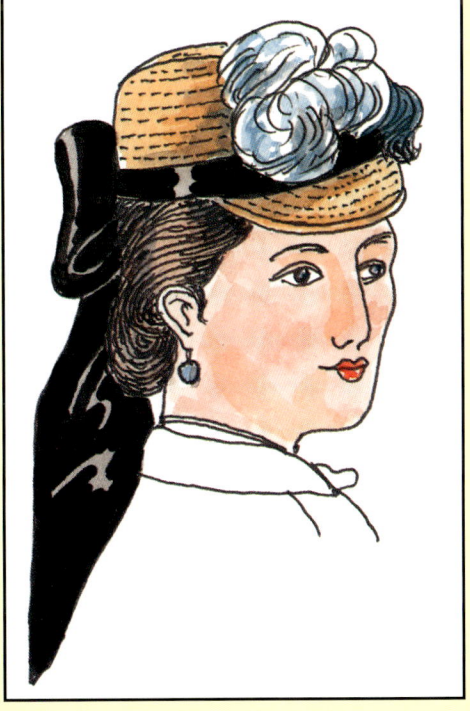

A little straw called a *Casquette*.

Patent leather and cloth outlined with cord make up this short boot.

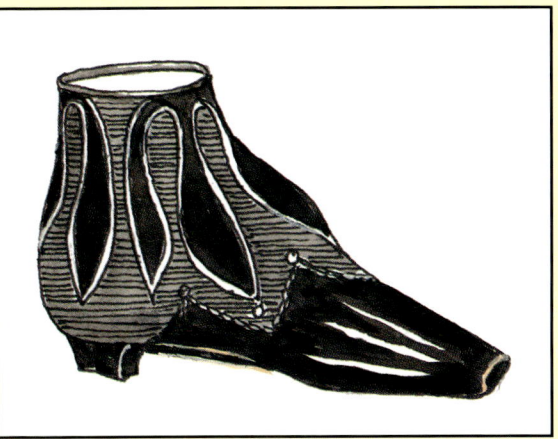

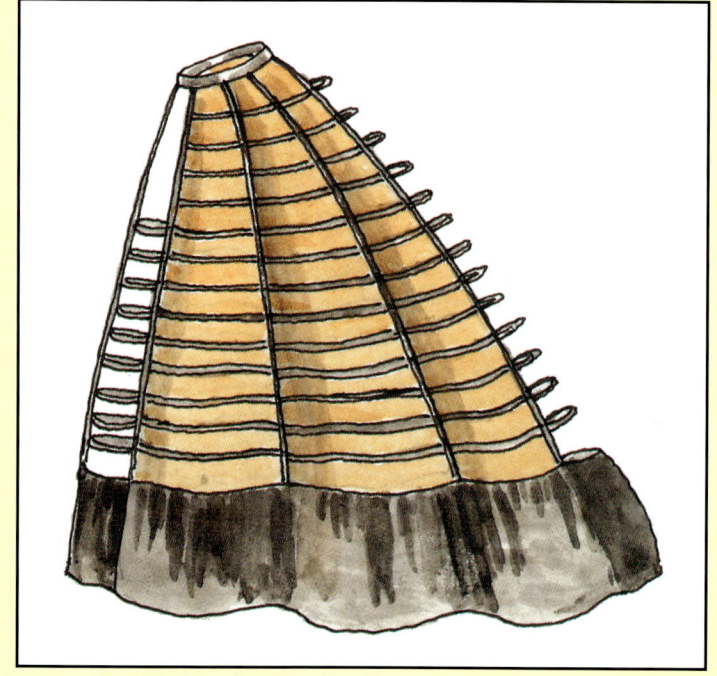

One of the many types of flat-fronted crinolines, made from calico, steel, and with a cotton flounce.

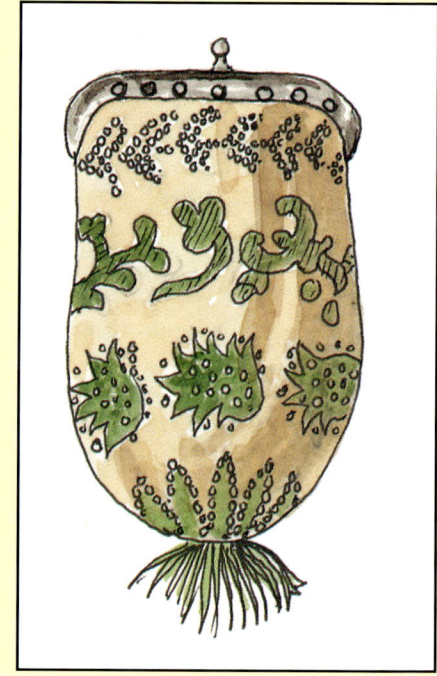

A probably homemade velvet purse, rich with beads. The frames and materials for such purses were obtainable form haberdashery stores.

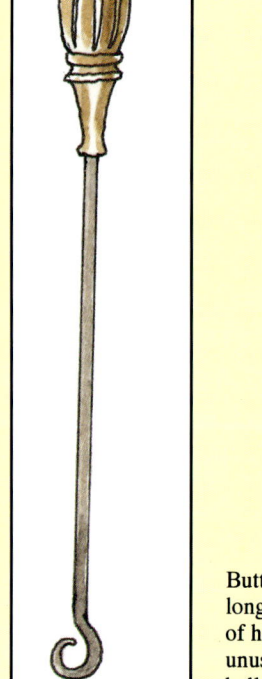

Button hooks were essential during the long life of the boot and given all kinds of handles. This example shows an unusual brass hand holding an agate ball.

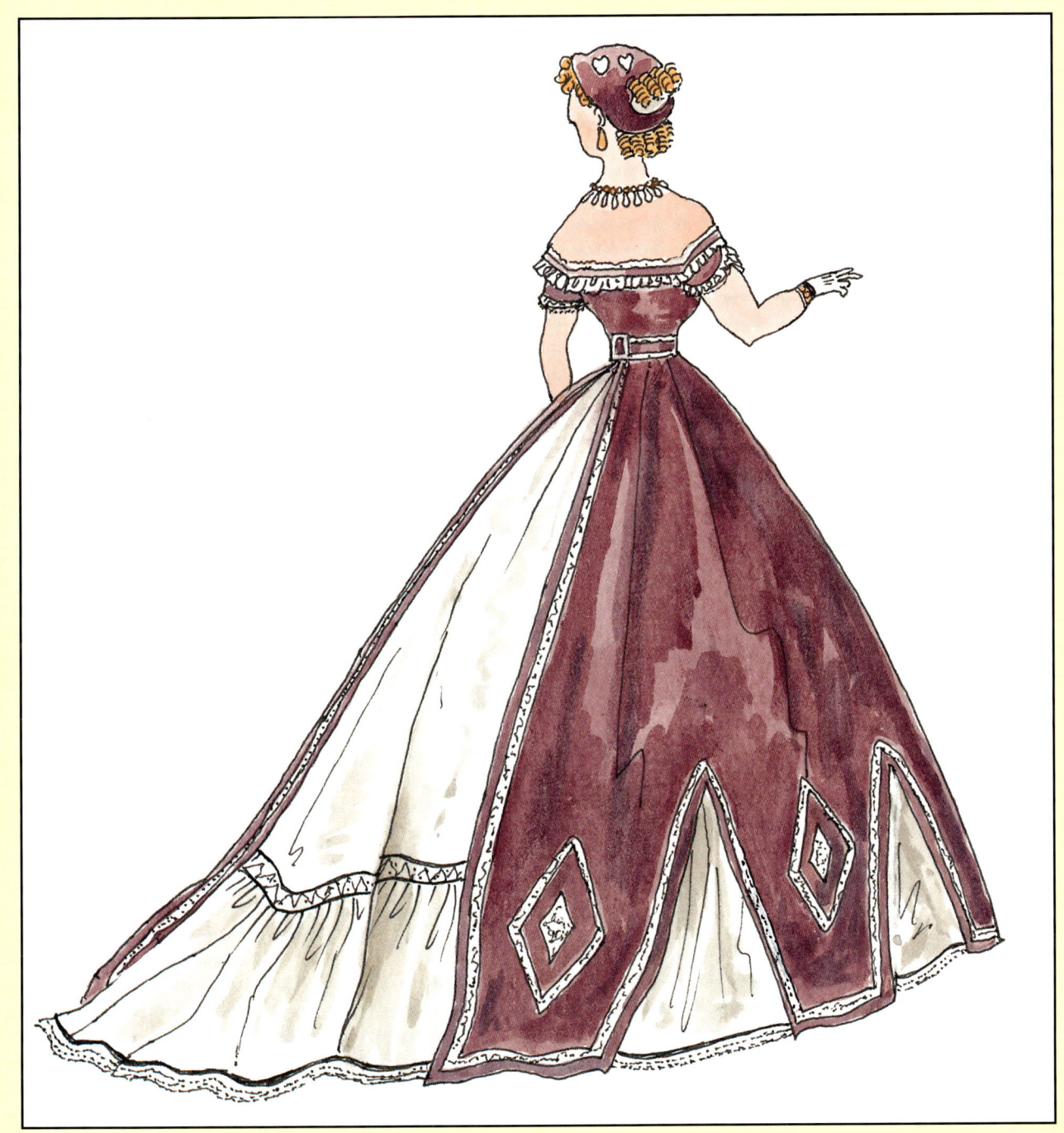

1864–1868 Evening Wear

The low neckline now exposed the upper back. Evening skirts were longer-trained than those worn by day and were mainly in two layers, often geometrically trimmed. Sleeves and gloves remained short.

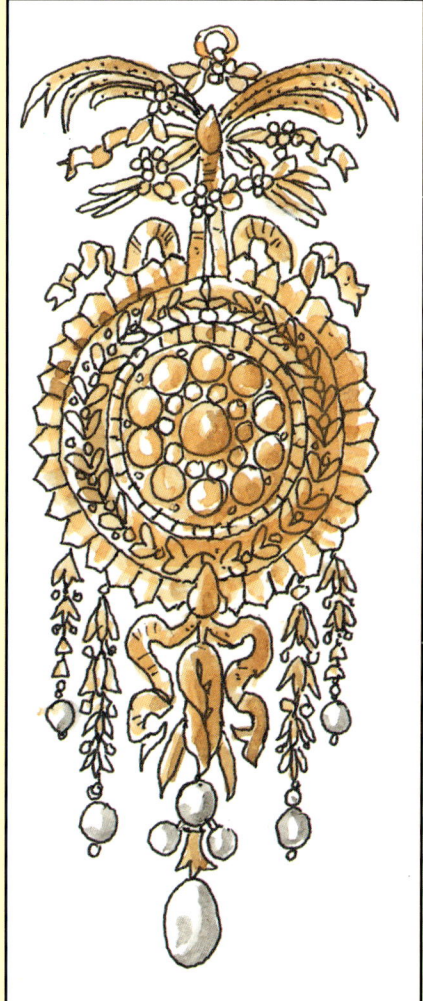

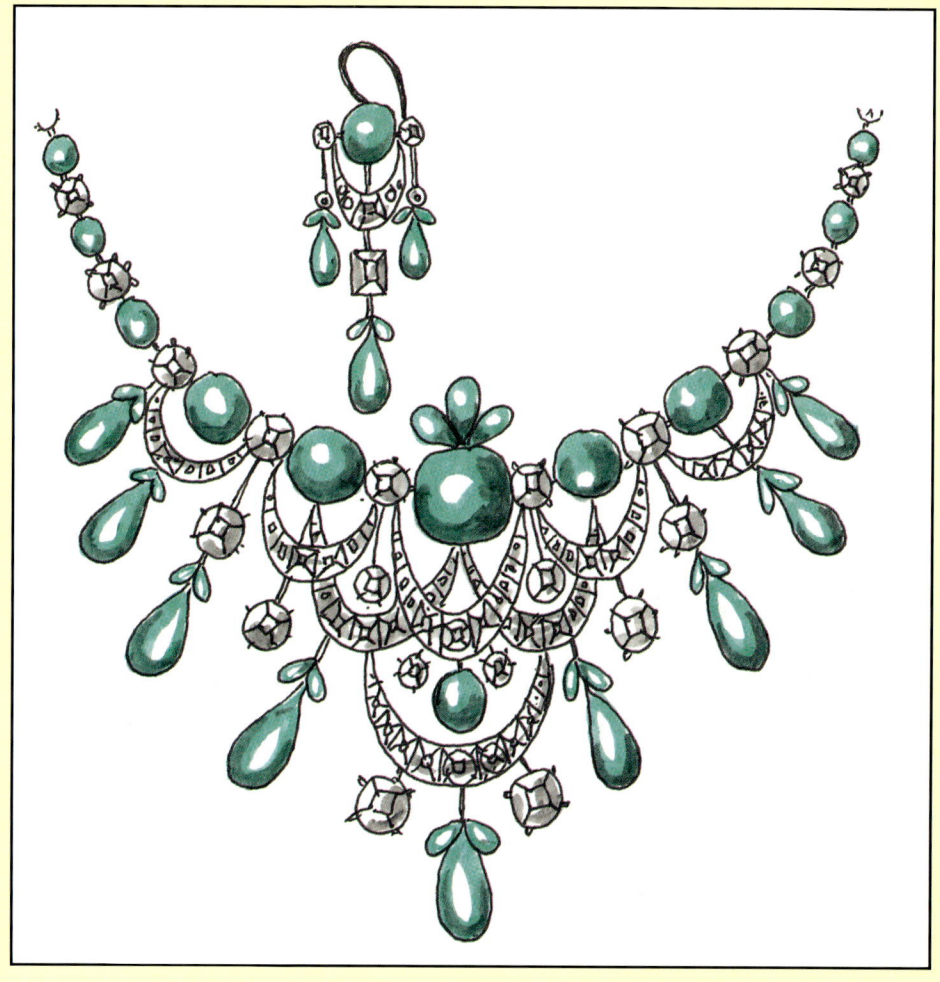

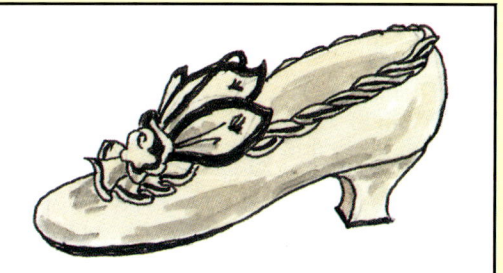

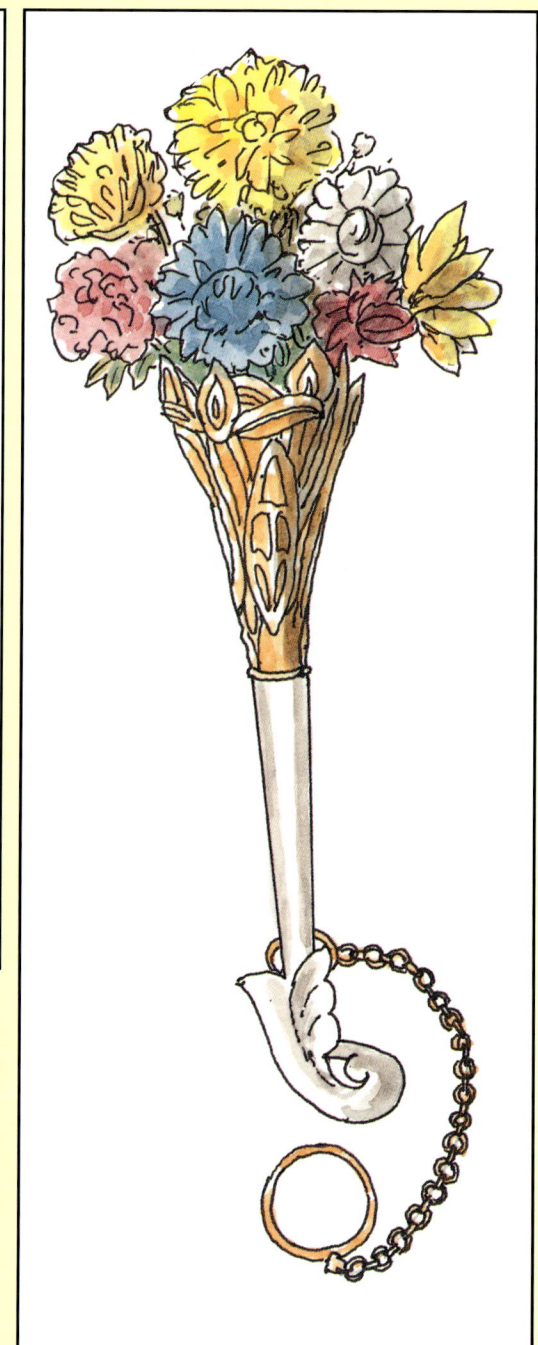

Top left: A Renaissance-style gold and pearl pendant or corsage ornament.

Bottom left: Silk shoe, decorated with metal braid-edged ribbons.

Above: A magnificent diamond and emerald necklace and earring; part of a parure or set which included a matching bracelet, brooch, and ring.

Right: At balls, from the late eighteenth century, many women and especially girls carried posies of flowers in charming flute-shaped holders, made of gold, silver, gilt, or ivory, in every style from "Egyptian" to "Gothic." This example has silver-gilt leaves and a mother-of-pearl handle carved in the shape of a lotus flower. The fashion died out in the 1880s.

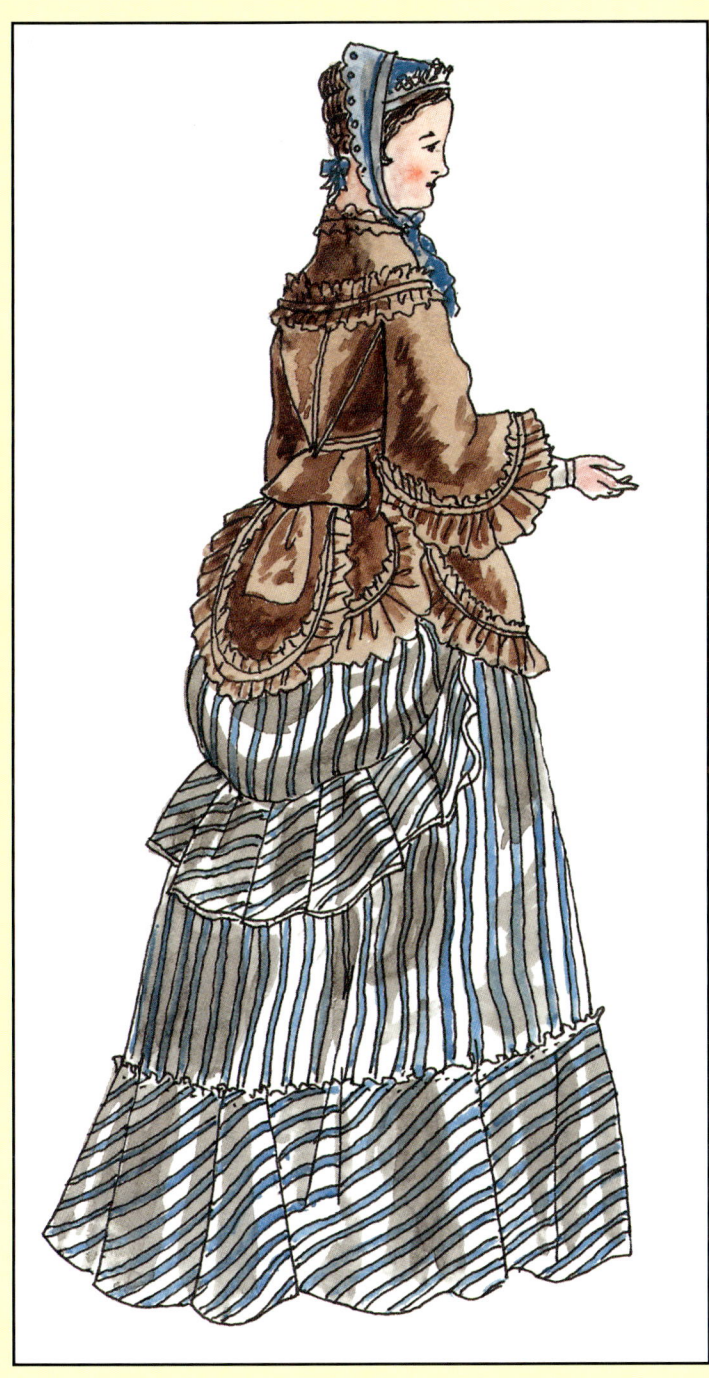

1868-1870 Day Wear

The crinoline suddenly disappeared to be replaced by dresses which were quite full or bunched up at the back—a hint of the first bustle to come. Some skirts were ankle-length. As shown here, short, elaborate hip-length capes were fashionable for winter.

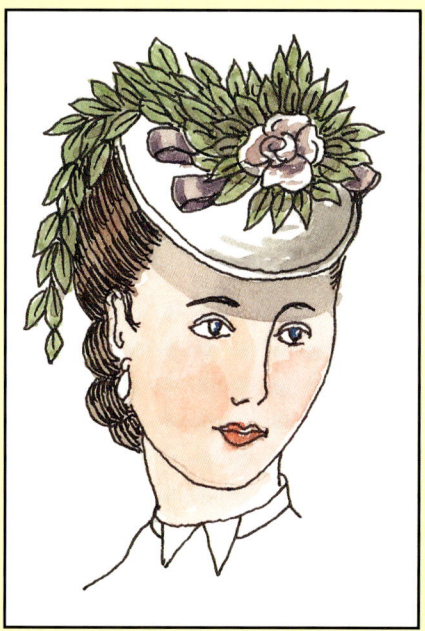

A jaunty silk hat liberally trimmed with artificial flowers and leaves.

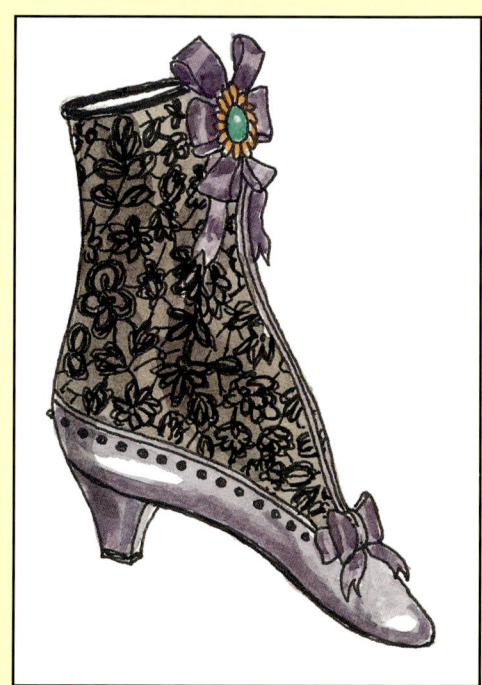

With ankle-length dresses, such an over-decorated leather, lace, and ribboned boot would have been much in evidence.

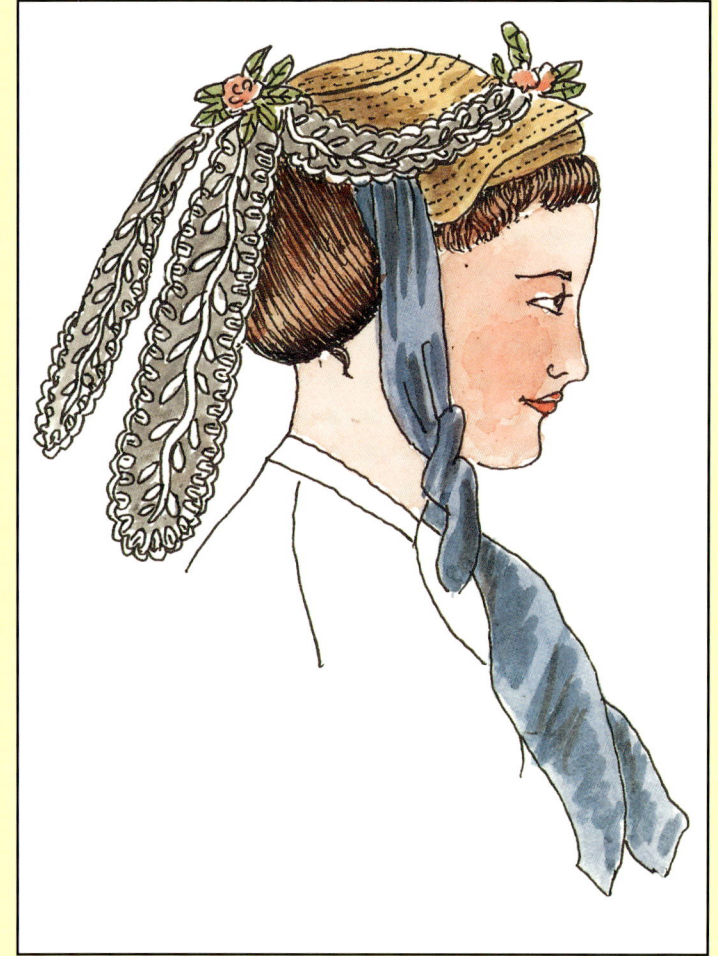

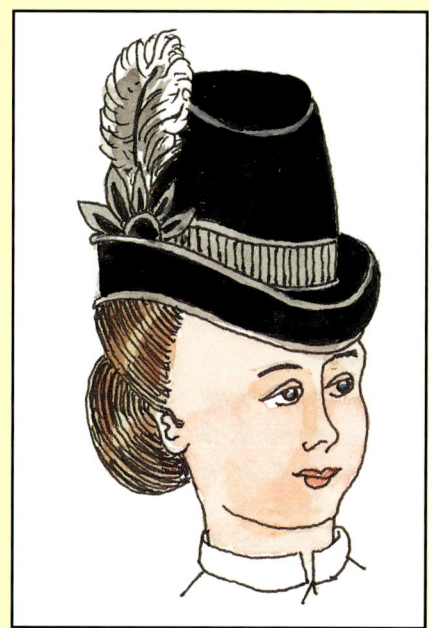

This man's-style hat is made feminine with feathers.

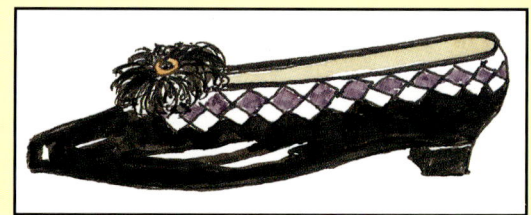

A patent-leather slipper, decorated with cloth in a fashionable checked pattern.

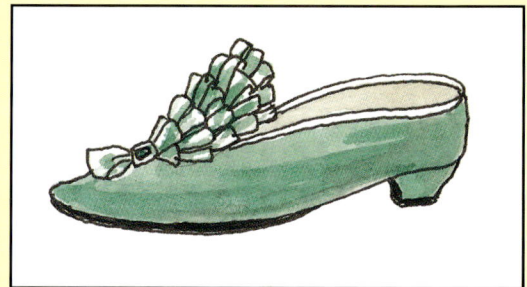

Many ribbons adorn this satin shoe.

A tiny straw hat with embroidered muslin lappets and huge bow.

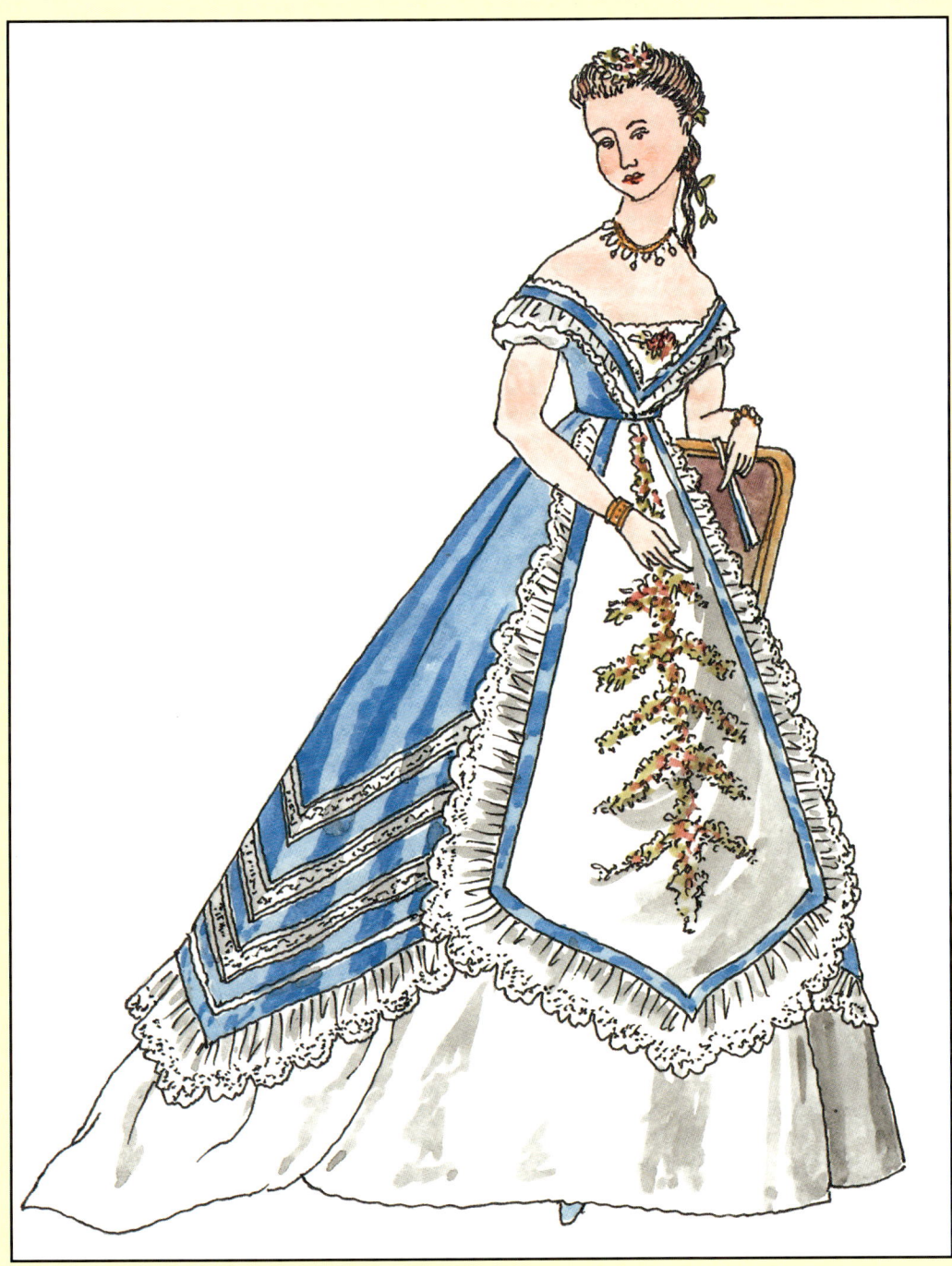

1868-1870 Evening Wear

Naturally-waisted bodices with low necklines were still the norm but skirts, still often in two layers, had shorter trains. Purely decorative aprons were frequently worn.

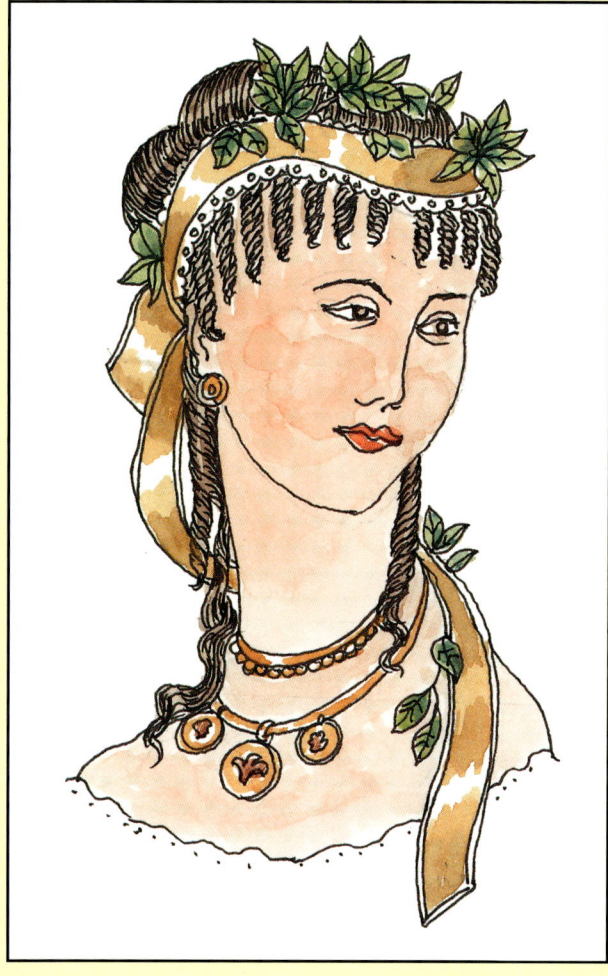

This elaborate ribbon and leaf headdress is in "Greek" French Empire or British Regency style, as are the gold necklaces and earrings.

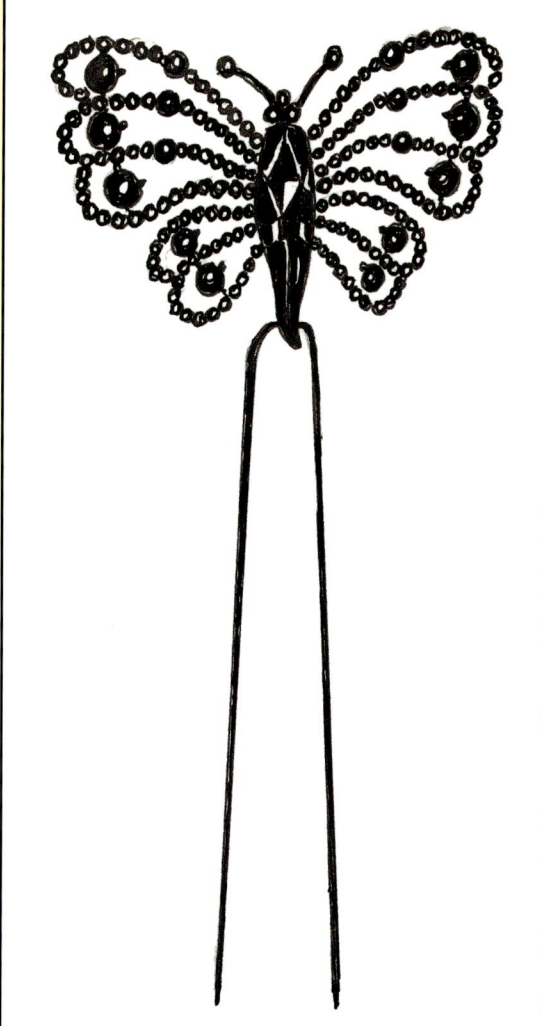

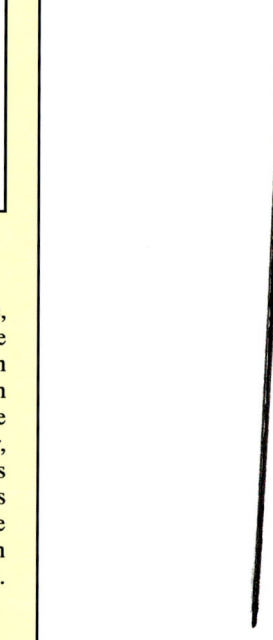

An elastically-expanded jet bracelet.

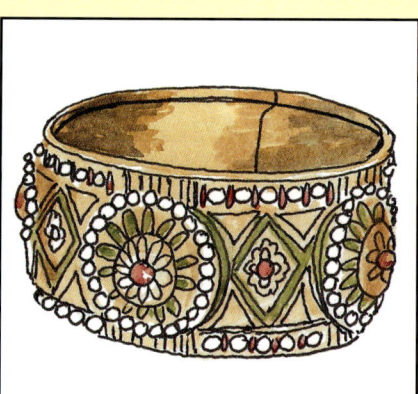

This articulated "barbaric" gold bracelet is set with enamel, rubies, and pearls.

Jet jewelry, from Whitby in Yorkshire, England, had been popular for some years, but after the death of Queen Victoria's husband, Prince Albert, in 1861, pieces became even more popular as mourning jewelry. However, jet was not confined to this use. This delicate butterfly hair ornament is mounted on a spring to make it tremble whenever the wearer moved. Imitation jet was made of French glass.

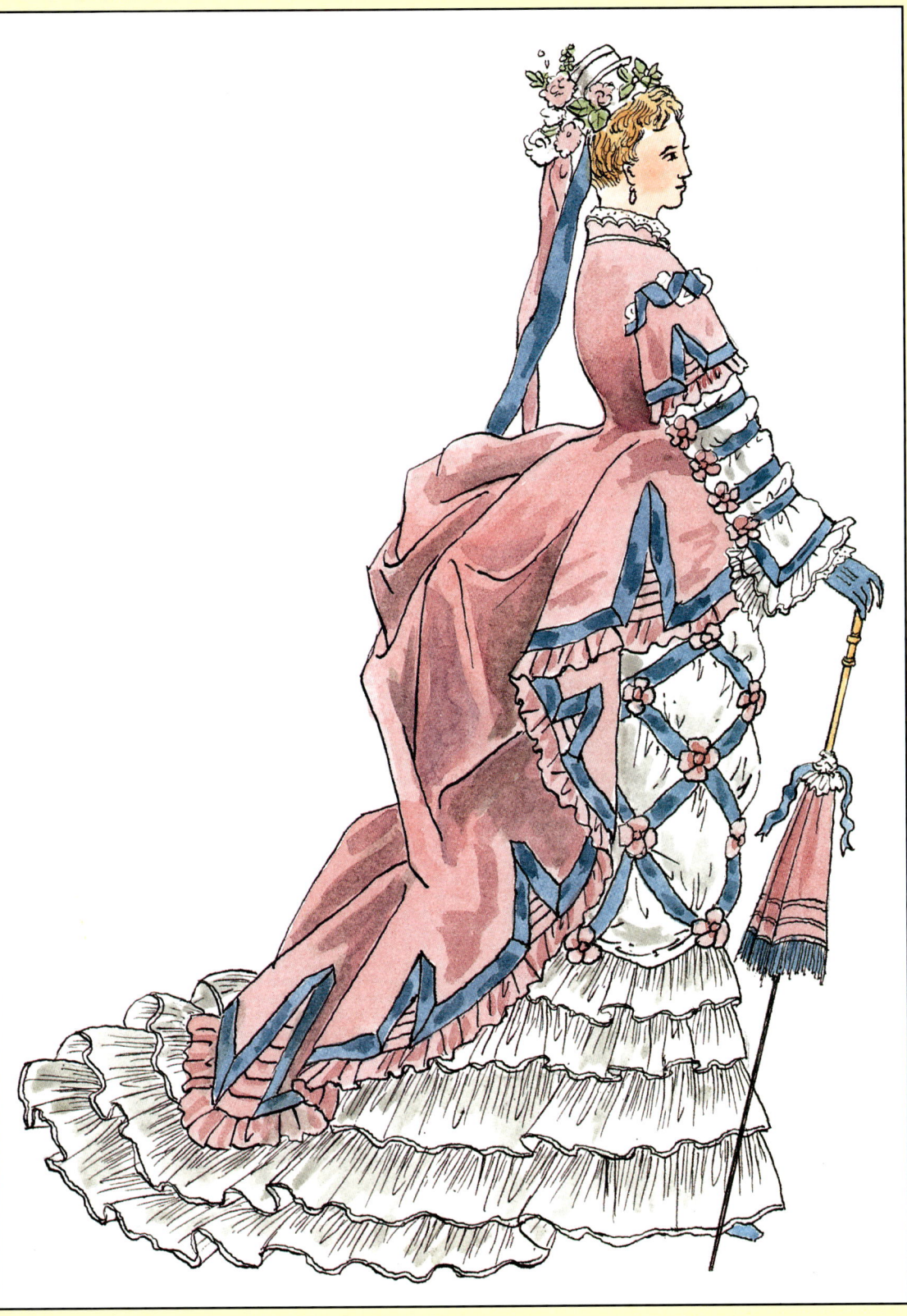

1870-1875 Day Wear

The first bustle is shown here. Rarely has there been a time when women's clothes were so bulky, so overelaborate, and so overtrimmed. The overskirt was bunched up behind in great, uneven folds, and the underskirt also had a very long train, with undersleeves of the bodice trimmed to match. (Note that, to us, the woman holds her parasol upside-down.)

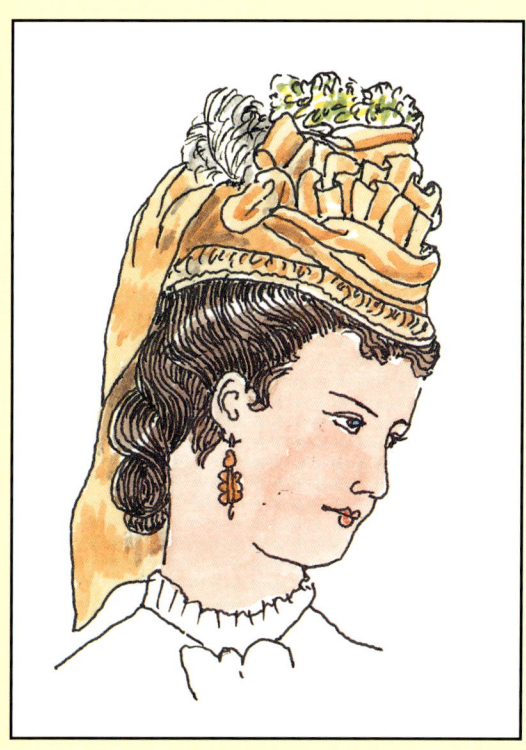

With the introduction of the first nineteenth-century bustle, hats echoed the backward raising of the skirt, here, in a swirl of satin and feathers.

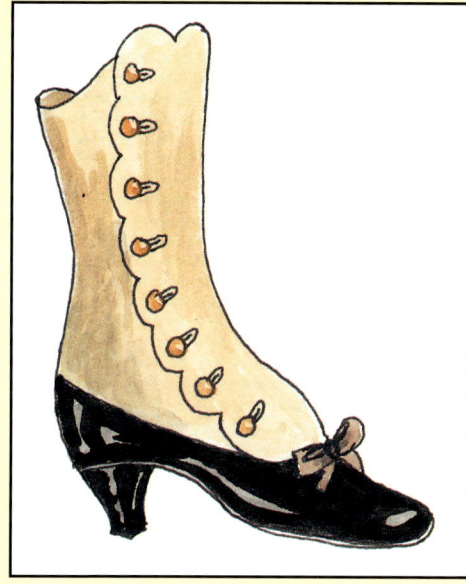

A black leather boot with buttoned suede upper; a fashion which continued well into the twentieth century.

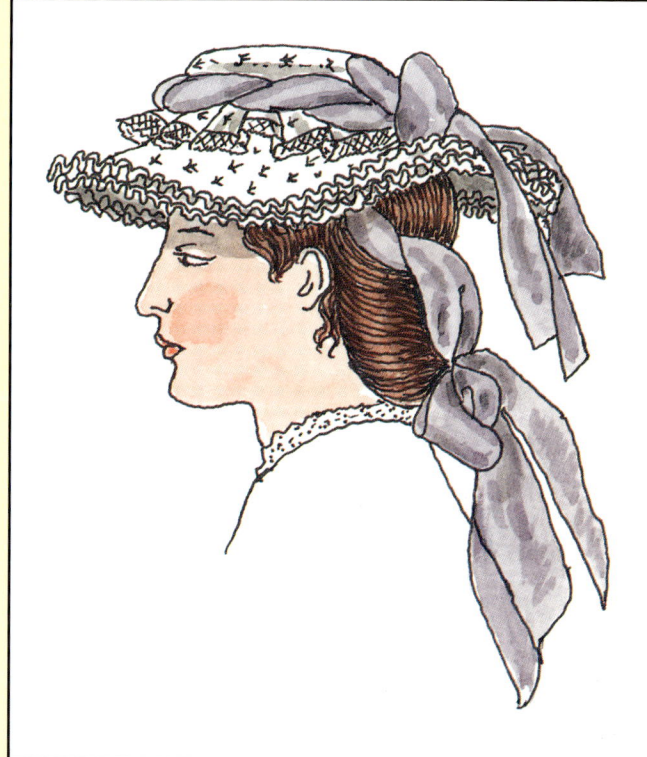

A stiffened muslin garden hat; note the matching ribbons entwined in the bunched-up hairstyle.

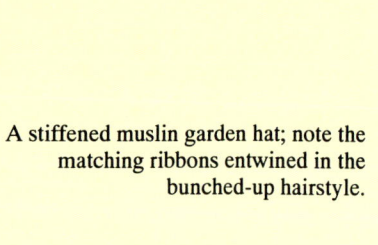

A straw "Dolly Varden" hat, named after the heroine in Charles Dickens" novel *Barnaby Rudge*. It is a revival of the French mid-Nineteenth Century *bergère* or shepherdess's hat, which was disapproved of by the "best" people.

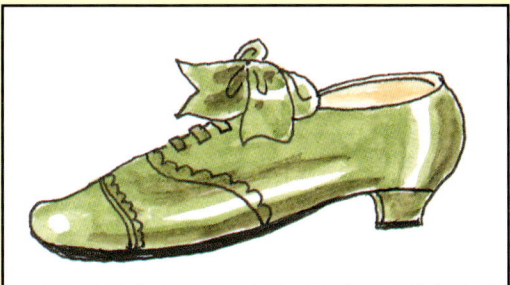

A calf walking shoe laced with a wide ribbon.

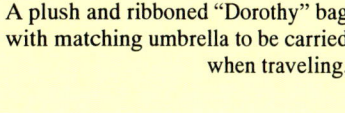

A plush and ribboned "Dorothy" bag with matching umbrella to be carried when traveling.

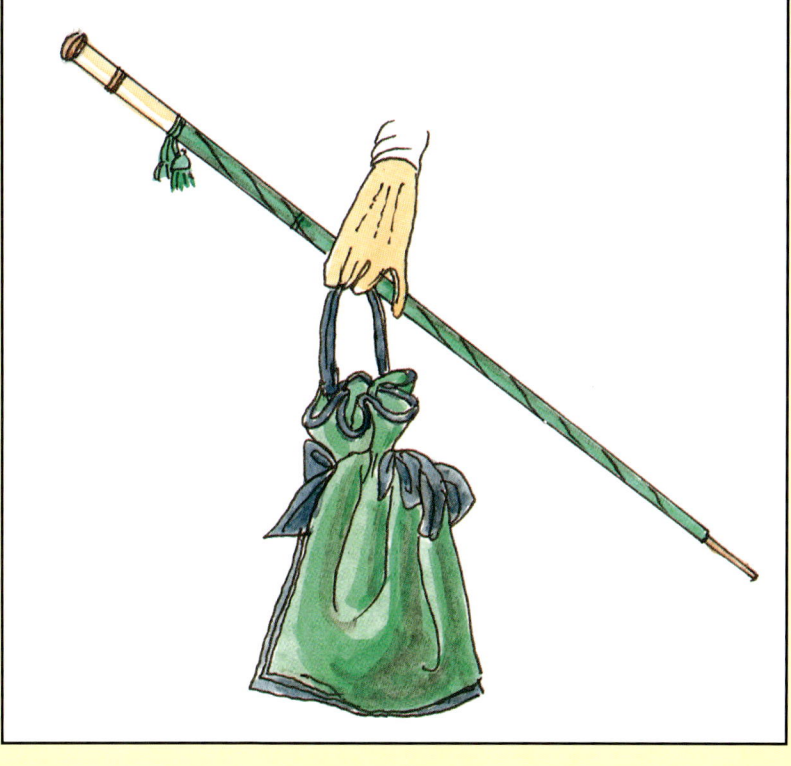

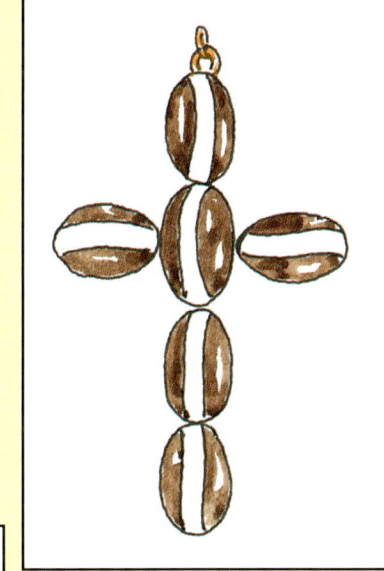

Not a great deal of jewelry was worn by day, except for such a simple piece as this onyx pendant cross.

A "crinolette" or bustle, made of horsehair, mounted on a thick calico foundation, and stiffened with whalebone.

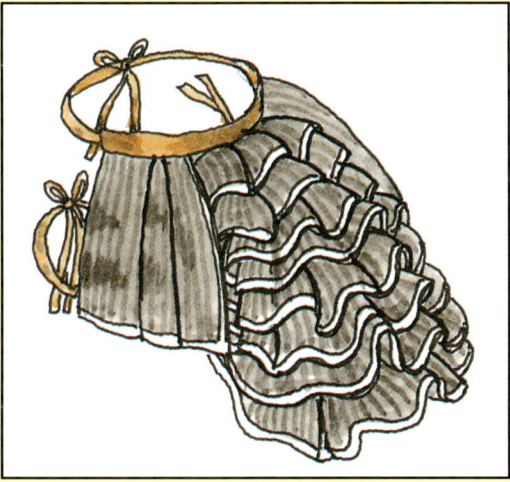

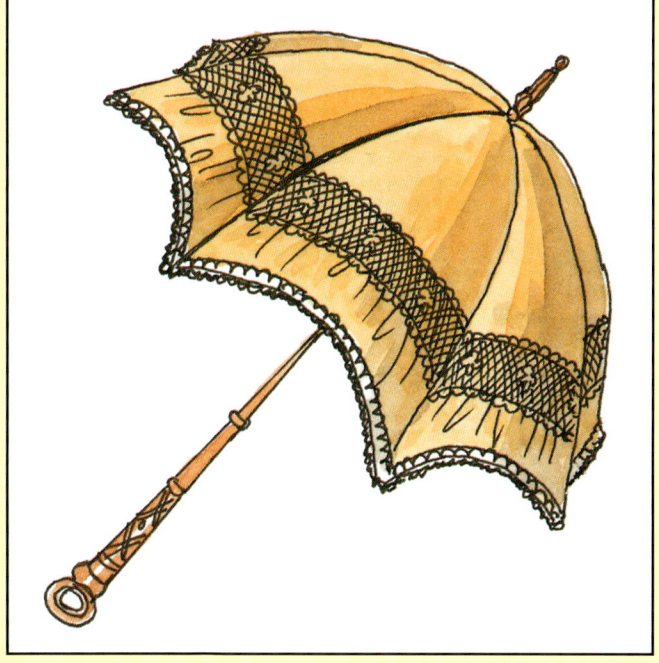

This silk parasol is trimmed with black lace and has a carved wooden handle.

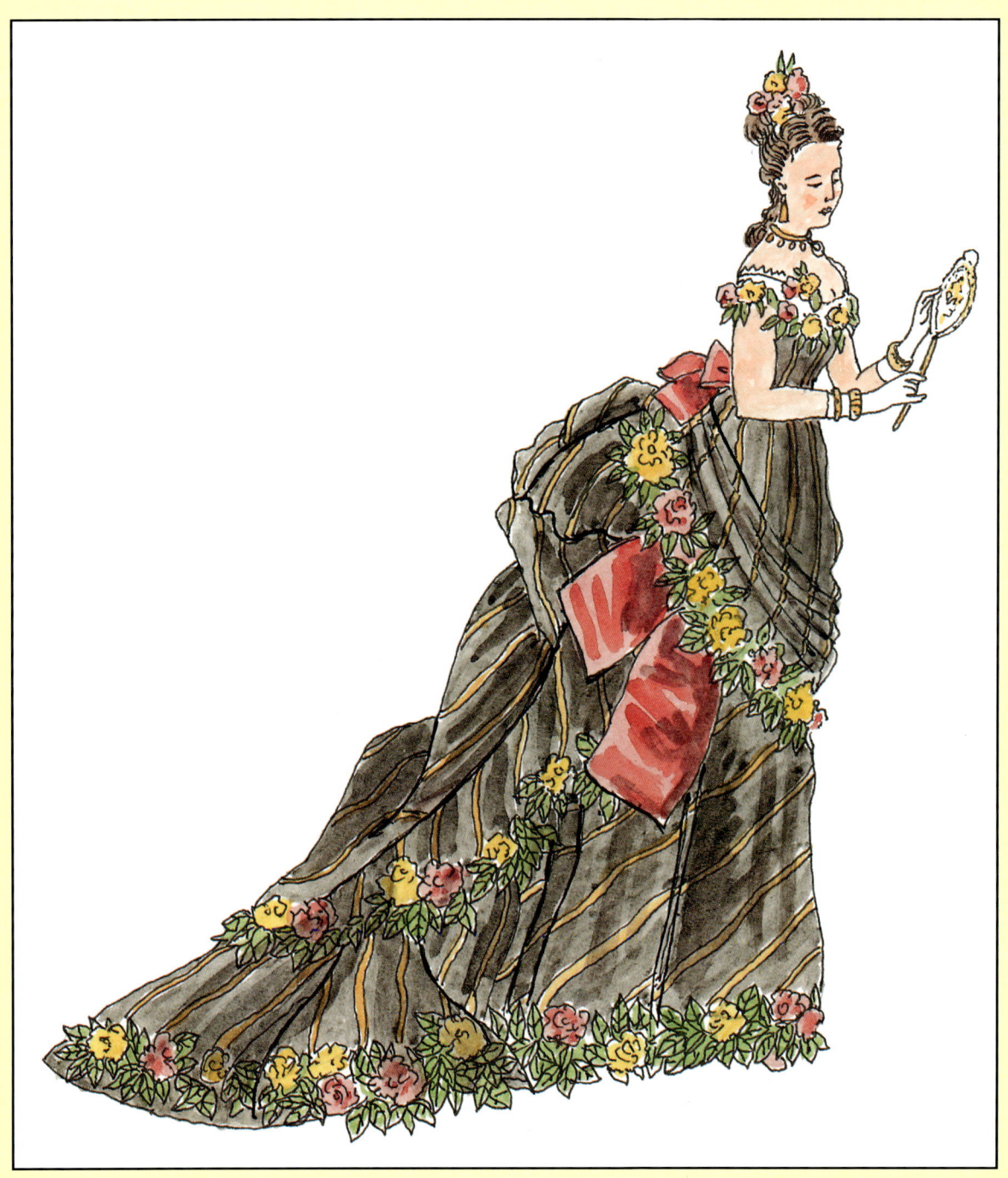

1870-1875 Evening Wear

Very long-trained evening dresses were even bulkier than dresses for day wear (making women look like badly tied up parcels), festooned with lace, ribbons, artificial flowers, buttons, and bows.

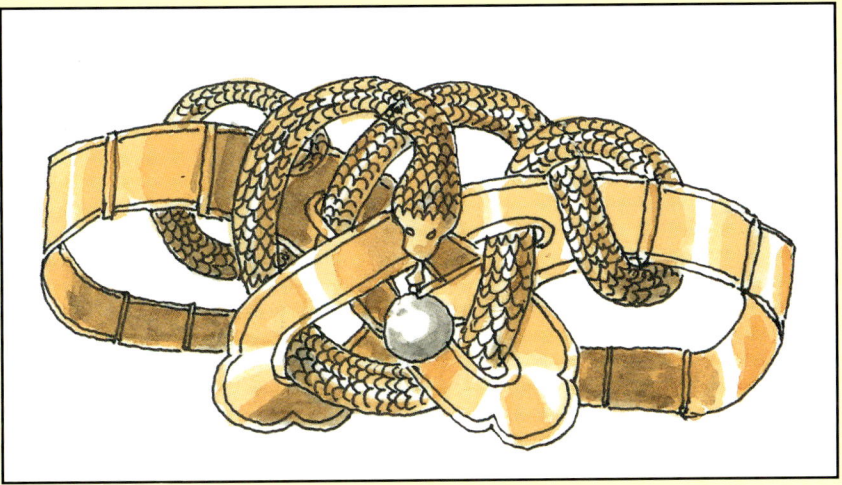

One of the most elaborate of all gold, articulated, snake bracelets; note the pearl in the serpent's mouth.

A carved coral and filigree gold earring.

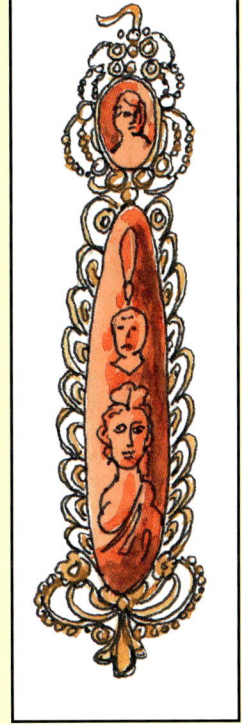

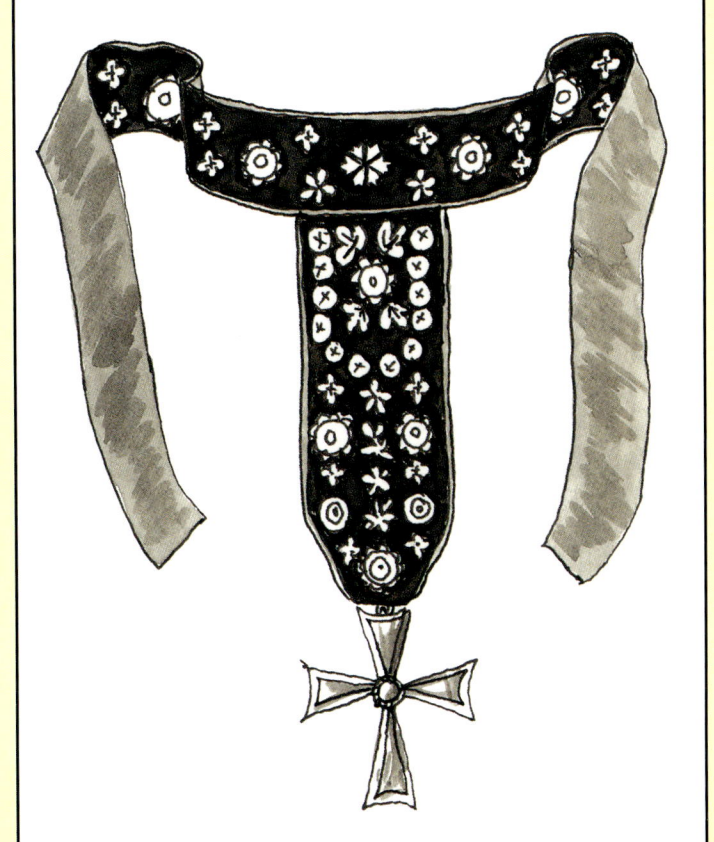

A silk-lined, velvet "dog-collar" studded with brilliants and finished with a silver cross.

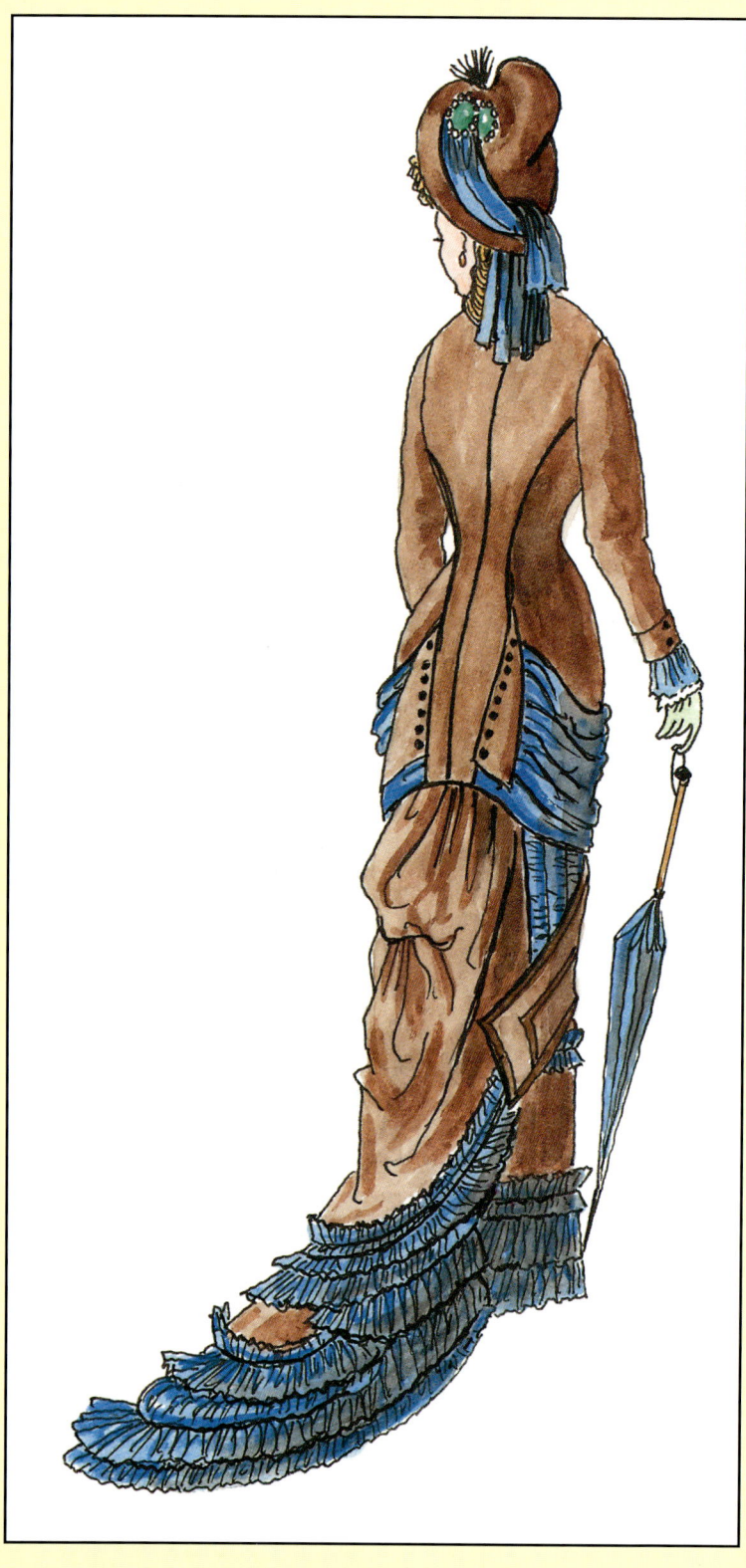

1875-1880 Day Wear

A complete change of silhouette. In the 23 October 1876, issue, American *Harper's Bazaar* announced: "The ideal figure at present is the greatest possible flatness and straightness: a woman is a pencil covered in raiment." Aided by a long, very tight corset which "molded the body to perfection" to her hips, this was the new "Princess" (named after Princess Alexandra, later Queen to King Edward VII) or cuirass line. Dresses were often made in two parts, or the effect was achieved using swathes of material. Trimming began below the hips and extended to a long, mermaid-like, fishtail train. The comparatively new sewing machine lessened the burden of hand-sewing but also encouraged yet more fanciful and complex trimming, such as frills, flounces, box-pleated panels, quilting, fluting, tasseled cords, lace, and fur. The use of only two colors and several materials was very fashionable, as the British magazine *The Queen* explained in 1887: "There is no such thing as a dress made of a single material." The dress was usually made of a dark shade and its trimmings of a lighter shade.

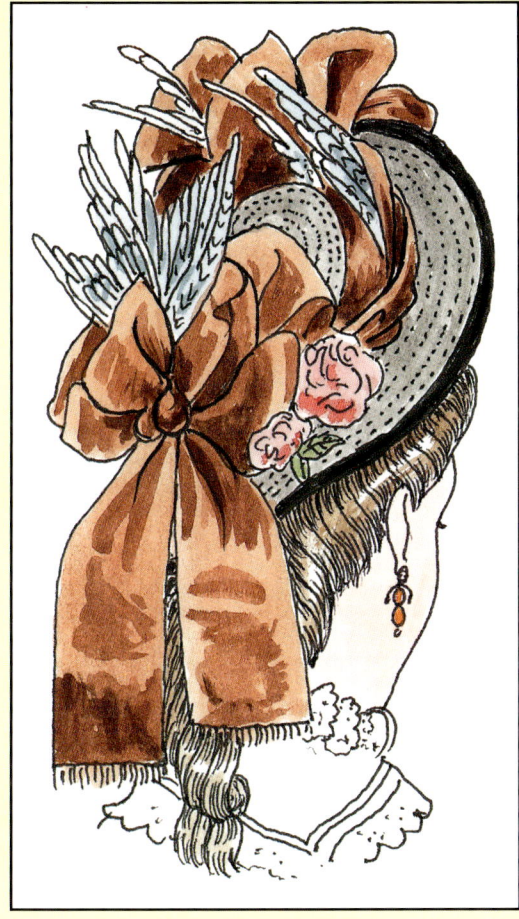

Bonnets were making a comeback; the difference was that a bonnet was tied under the chin, a hat was not. Otherwise, they looked much the same, as with this hat (echoing the "fish-tail" skirt) made of stitched felt bound with velvet ribbon and trimmed with a welter of ribbons, a rose, and real bird wings.

A surrah [a soft, twilled silk] bonnet, extravagantly trimmed; the silk tying ribbons are edged with lace.

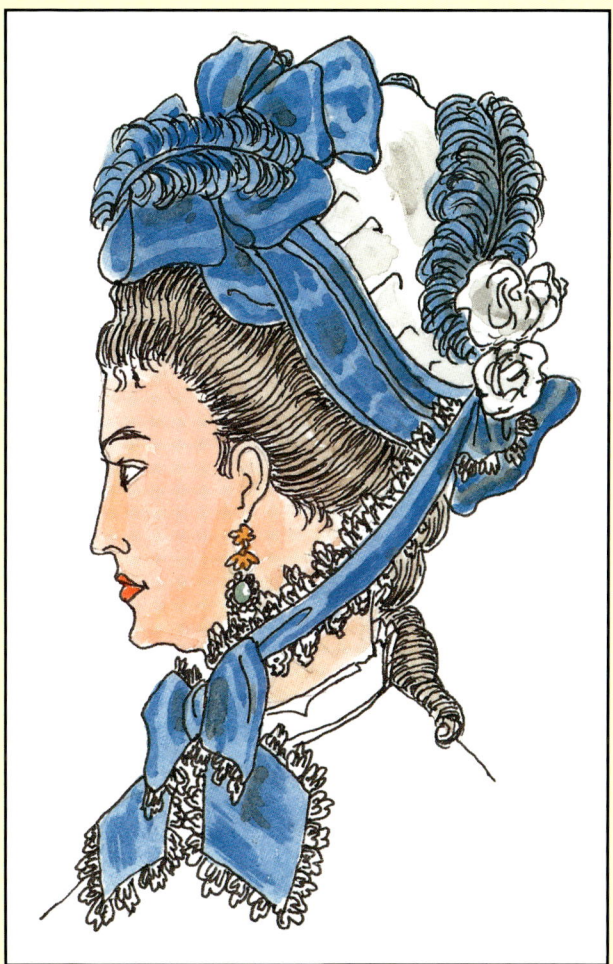

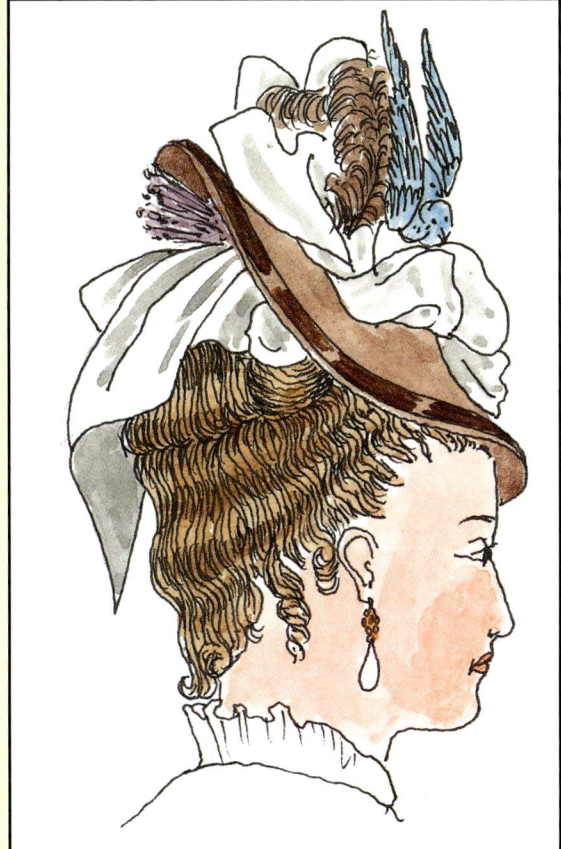

Hats could also be tilted forward; this highly trimmed example has a backward silk flounce.

37

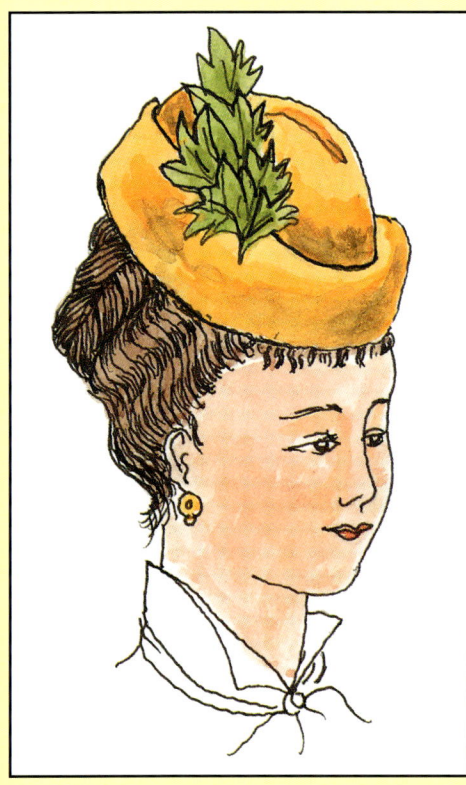

Not all women wore elaborate hats or bonnets; some preferring this little felt, man's style, "pork-pie" hat adorned with artificial leaves.

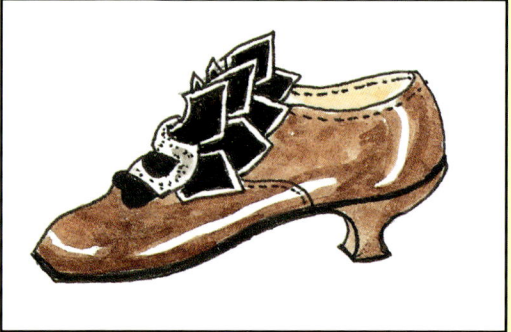

This calf walking shoe is embellished with stiffened silk ribbons and a metal buckle.

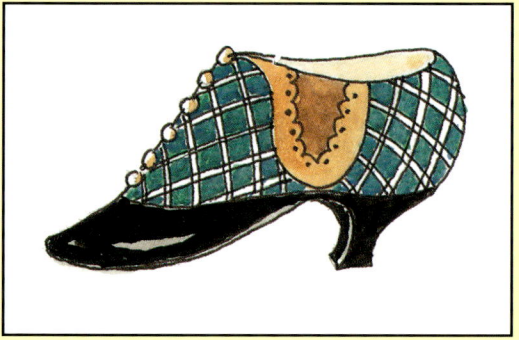

A dainty, patent-leather walking or at-home shoe, its upper covered with woollen plaid and a curve of tooled leather.

Dressy three-quarter length kid gloves. *Left:* embroidered with chain stitch, its pleated serge cuff bound with braid. *Right:* also embroidered, with a braid-bound ruffled crêpe cuff.

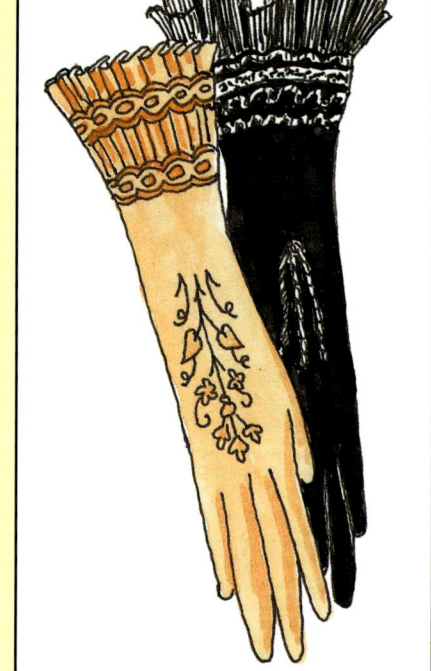

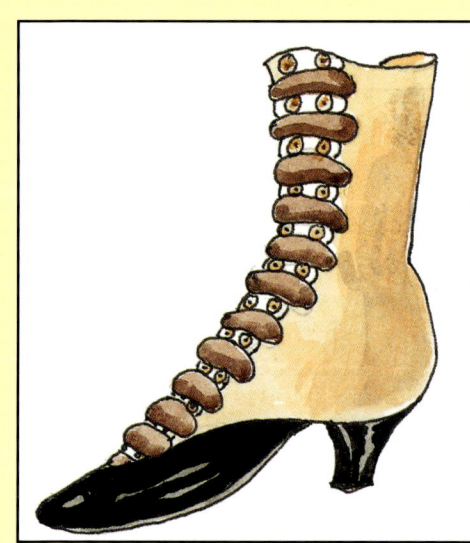

A patent leather and cloth boot heavily decorated with padded ribbons and buttons.

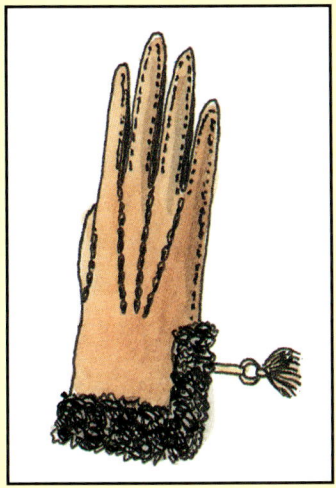

Even this everyday glove is decorated with an astrakhan cuff and a gold tassel.

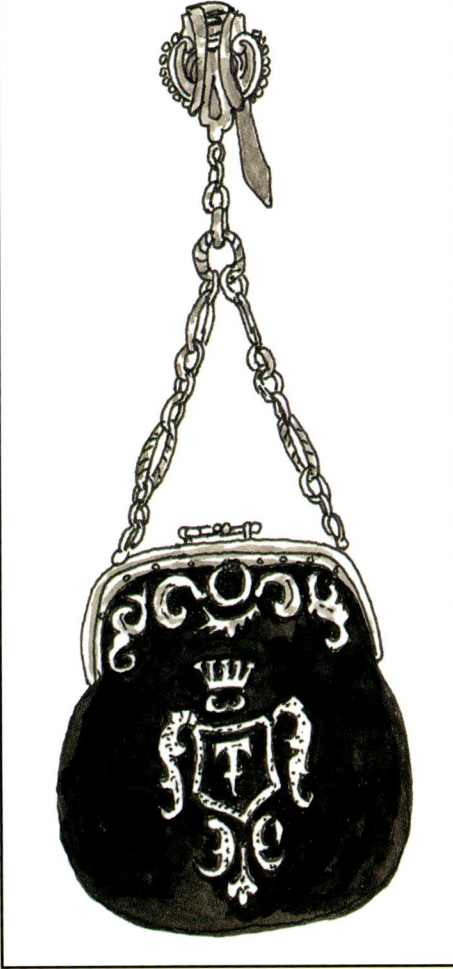

Called a "chatelaine pocket," this velvet purse is ornamented with a crest and a monogram worked in silver thread embroidery. The frame, handle, and belt hook are of chased silver.

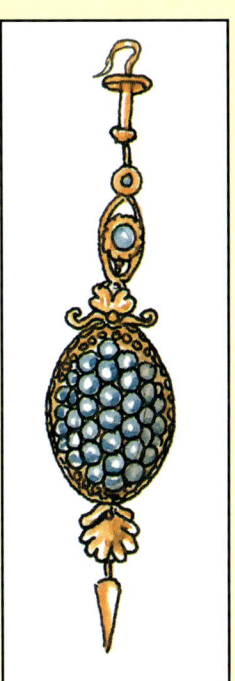

A gold and turquoise earring.

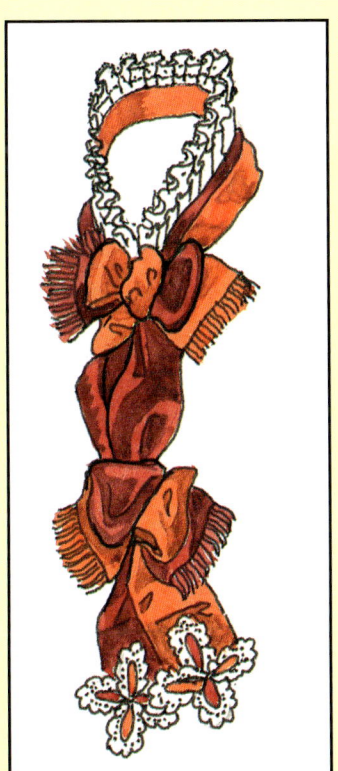

Separate jabots were worn to vary an ensemble. With a box-pleated collar, this elaborate construction is made of fringed and lace-edged wide ribbons.

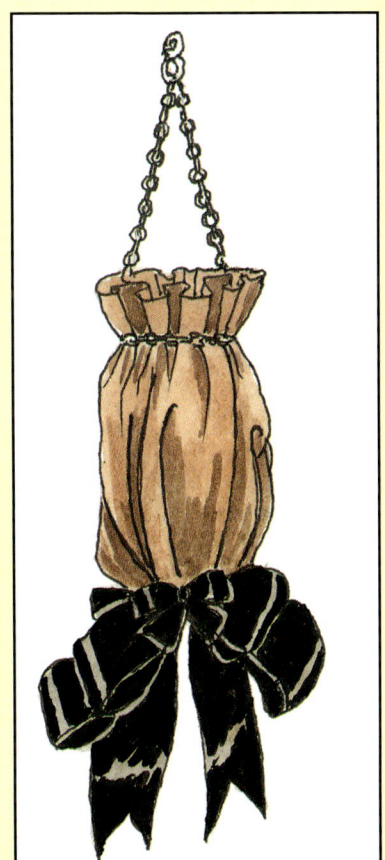

A simple plush at-home bag, made extravagant with a huge bow and given a chain to attach to a waistband or belt.

39

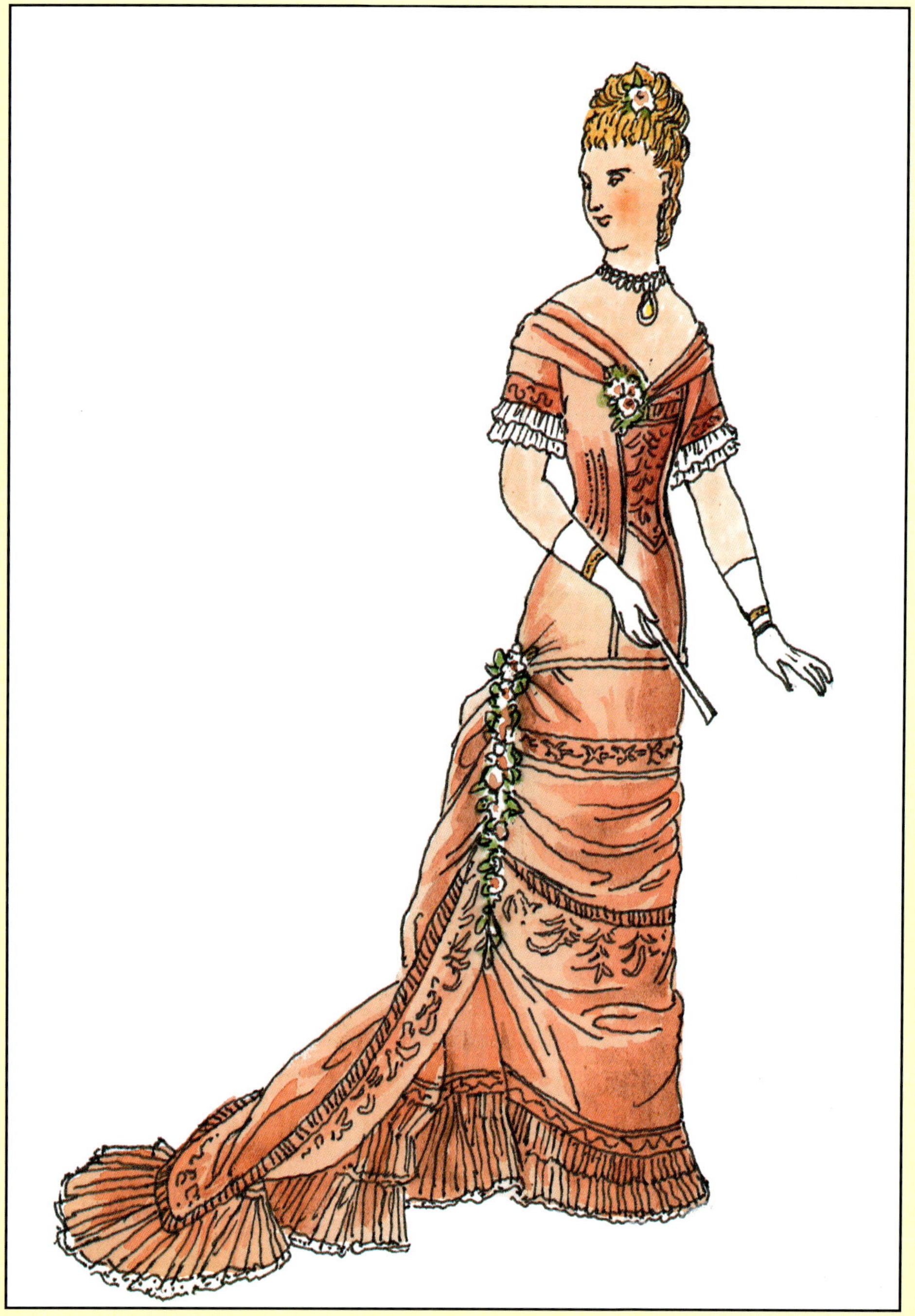

1875-1880 Evening Wear

Evening dresses followed the same line as for day with low "V" or square necklines, which were often high at the back, with slightly longer sleeves ending in ruffles. Trimming below the hips was as elaborate and excessive as on day dresses. "Mermaid" trains must have greatly restricted dancing.

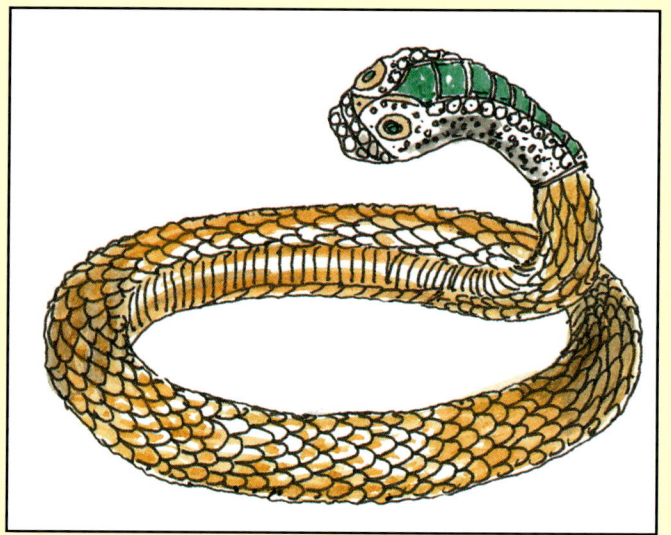

A superbly naturalistic gold, diamond, and emerald snake bracelet which could be turned into a necklace.

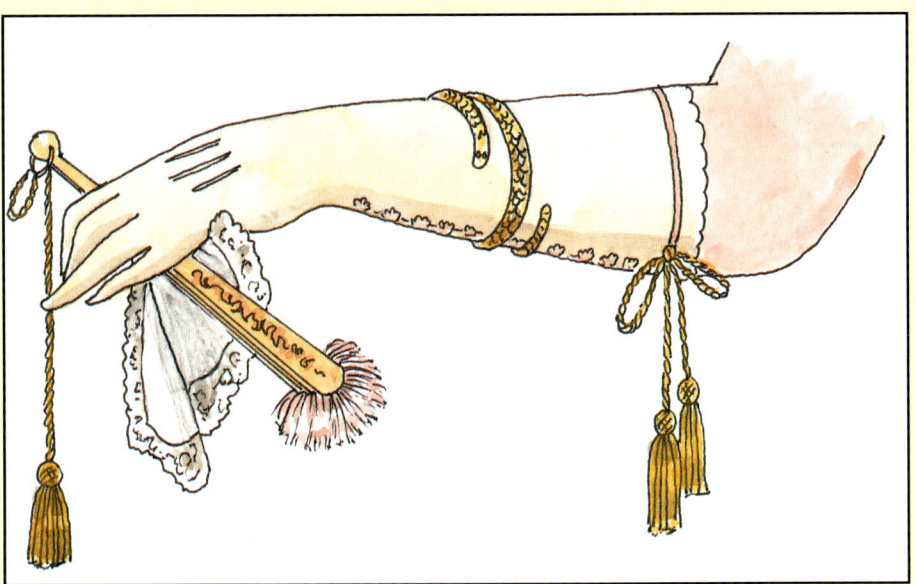

Soft kid evening gloves were increasing in length. Here, the ornamentation takes the form of a gold, tasseled cord and decorative buttons. Other evening gloves were embroidered or given beaded or ruched-silk cuffs. This woman wears not only a snake bracelet but also carries such evening necessities as a feathered fan and a lace-edged lawn handkerchief.

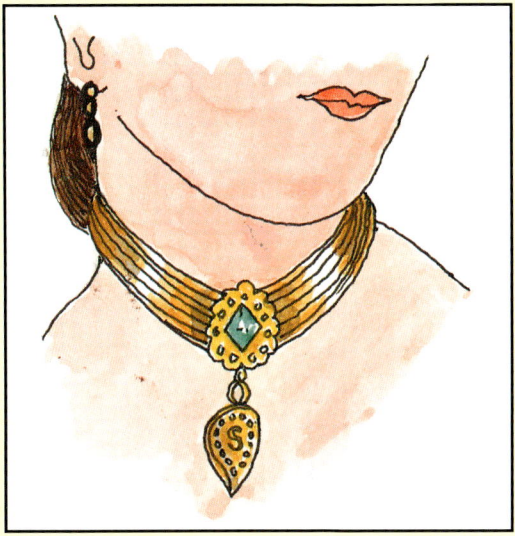

Flexible bands of gold, a medallion encrusted in gold, emerald, and pearl, and a gold locket make up this unusual necklace.

A wired bead pendant hangs from this jewel-sewn velvet "dog-collar."

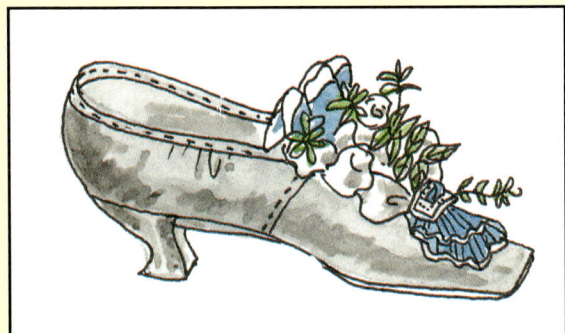

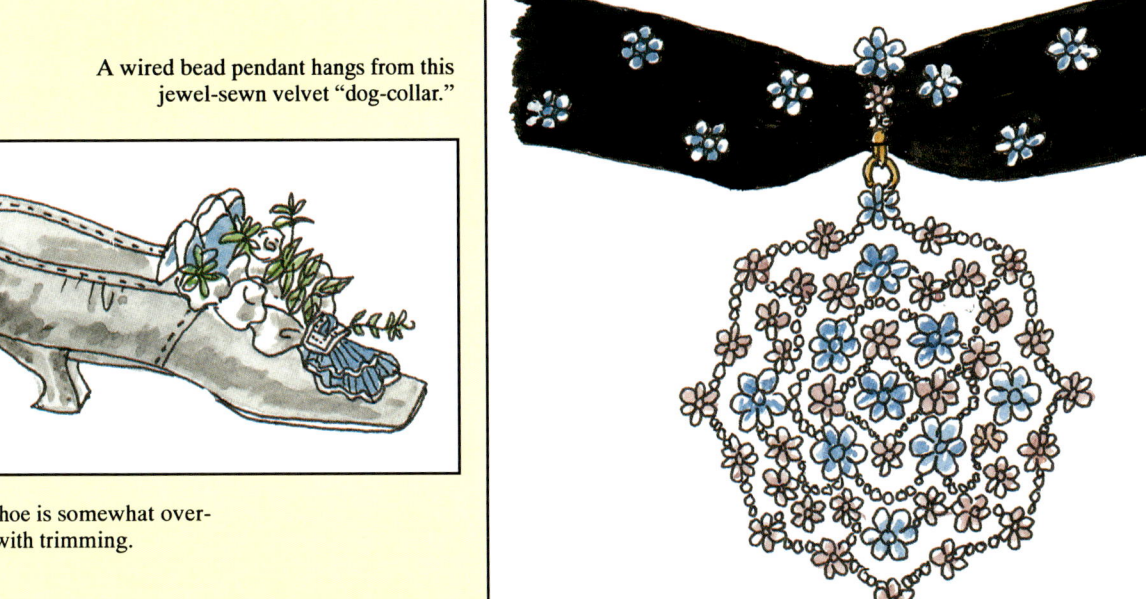

This silk shoe is somewhat overwhelmed with trimming.

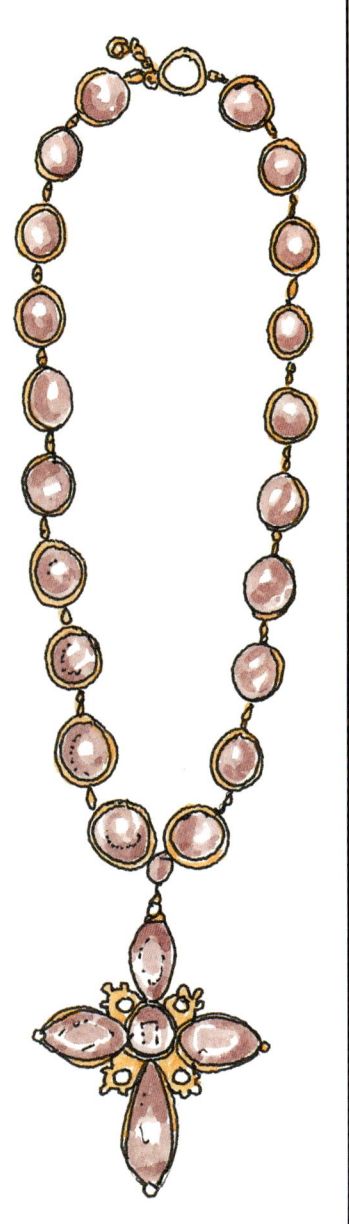

A conventional gold and amethyst necklace with an elaborate pendant to match.

41

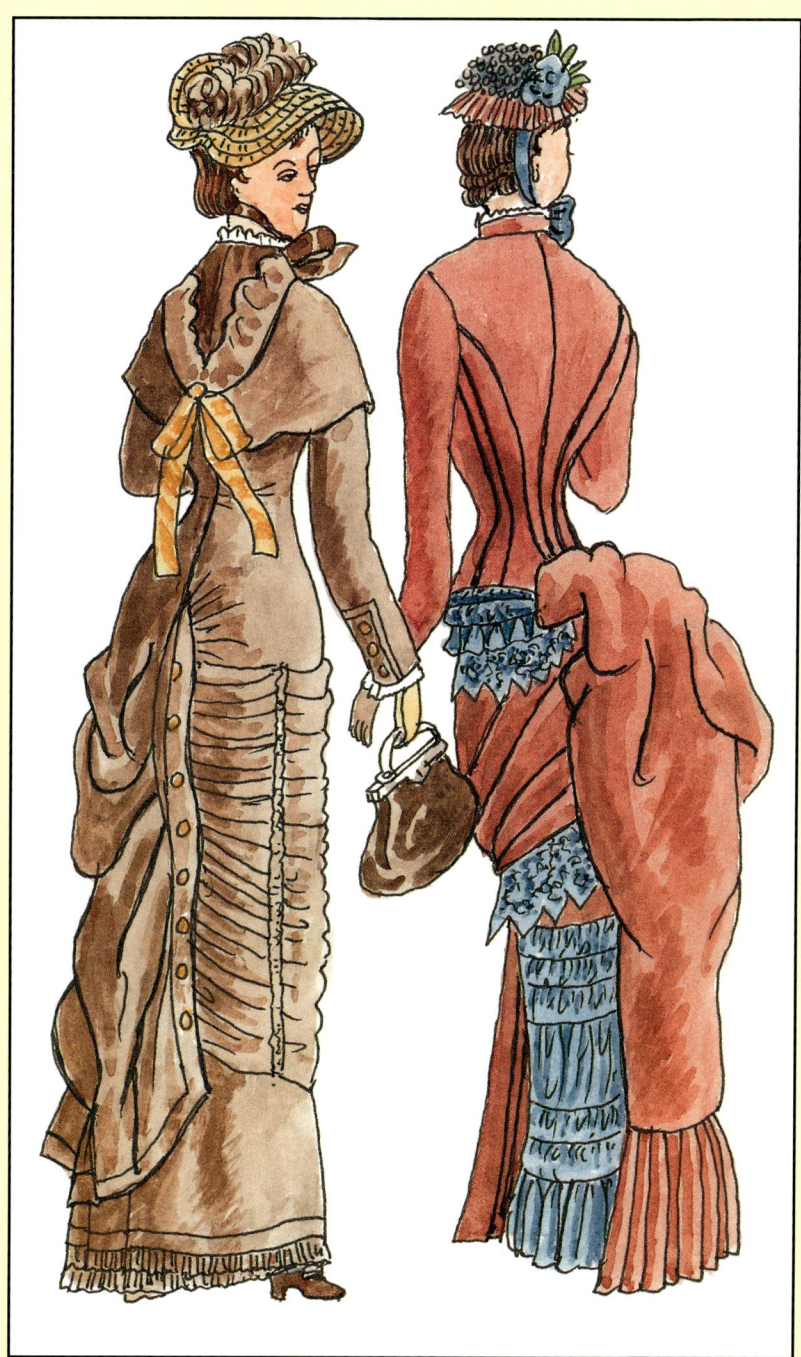

1880-1883 Day Wear

Although some women still wore long trains, two new styles appeared during this short period: still fitting to the hips, but with less trimming and untrained (at left) and the beginnings of the second bustle (at right), achieved by a "dress improver" called the "crinolette," which led many women to fear the return of the crinoline. Such dresses were narrow to the hips but, tightly bound and much trimmed below.

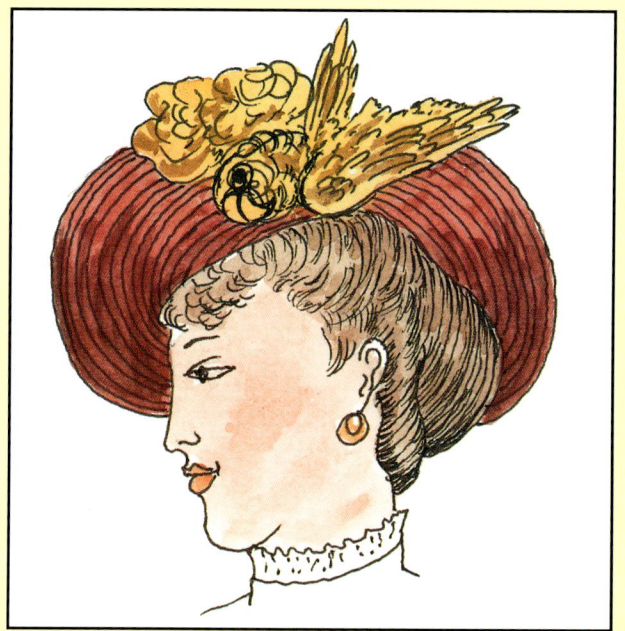

With the abandoning of the long, trained skirt, hair was cut shorter and hats, in general, were simpler and smaller. In America, hats were regarded as a symbol of emancipation. This seaside glacé straw hat is adorned with a whole stuffed parrot and dyed ostrich plumes.

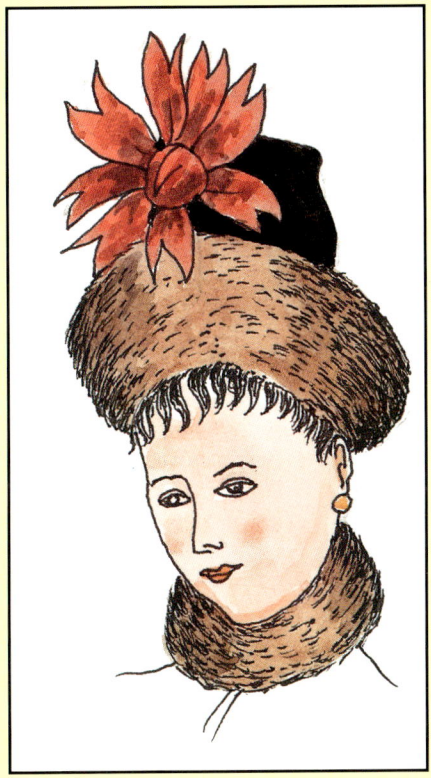

A velvet hat with a deep fur brim (with collar to match), given piquancy with a great silk bow.

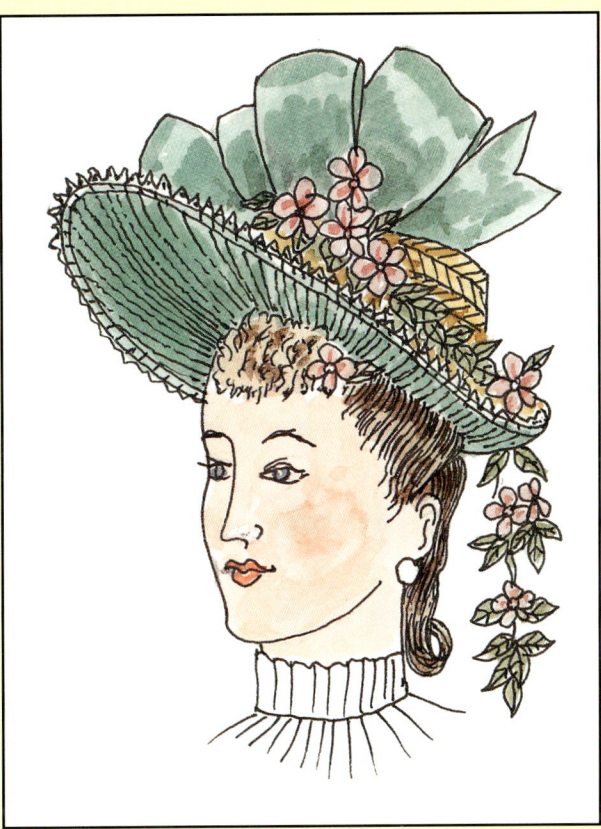

Very much for a girl or a young woman, a charming seaside straw hat lined with pleated silk and dripping with artificial flowers and leaves.

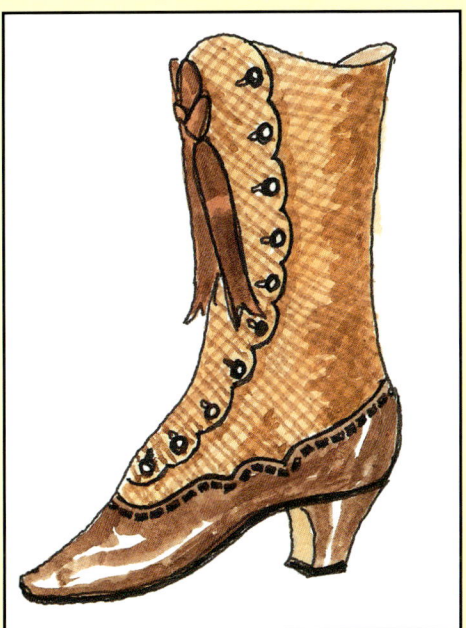

This calf boot has a tweed upper.

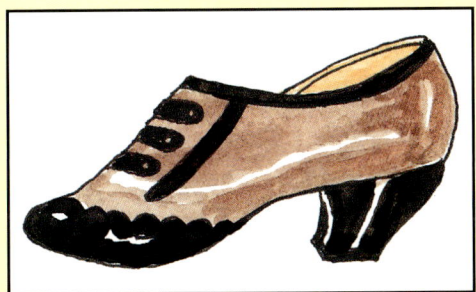

A patent leather and calf walking shoe.

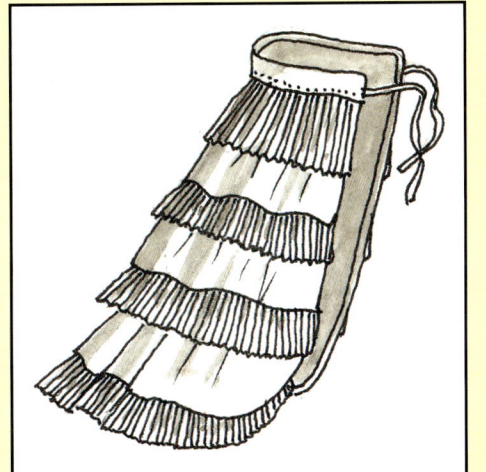

For those who wore the new, reduced, bustle shape, a "dress improver" was a necessity. This example, called the *Mignonette* consists of a horsehair foundation covered with cotton.

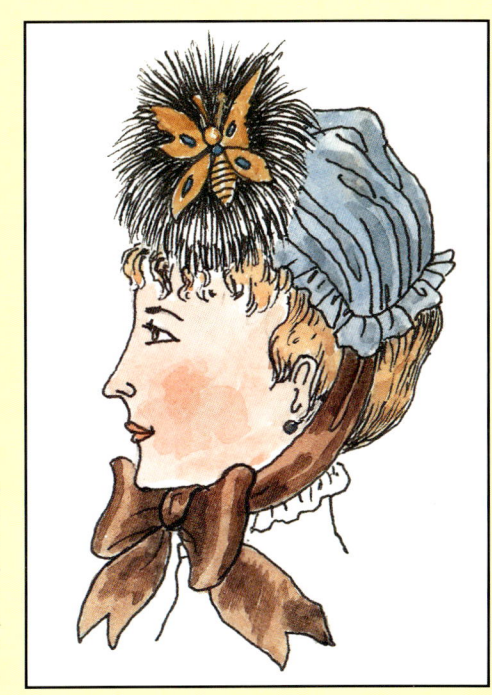

If rather old-fashioned, bonnets were still considered more "correct" than hats, especially by older women. However, this mob-cap of a bonnet is wittily enlivened with feathers and a gilt and enamel butterfly brooch.

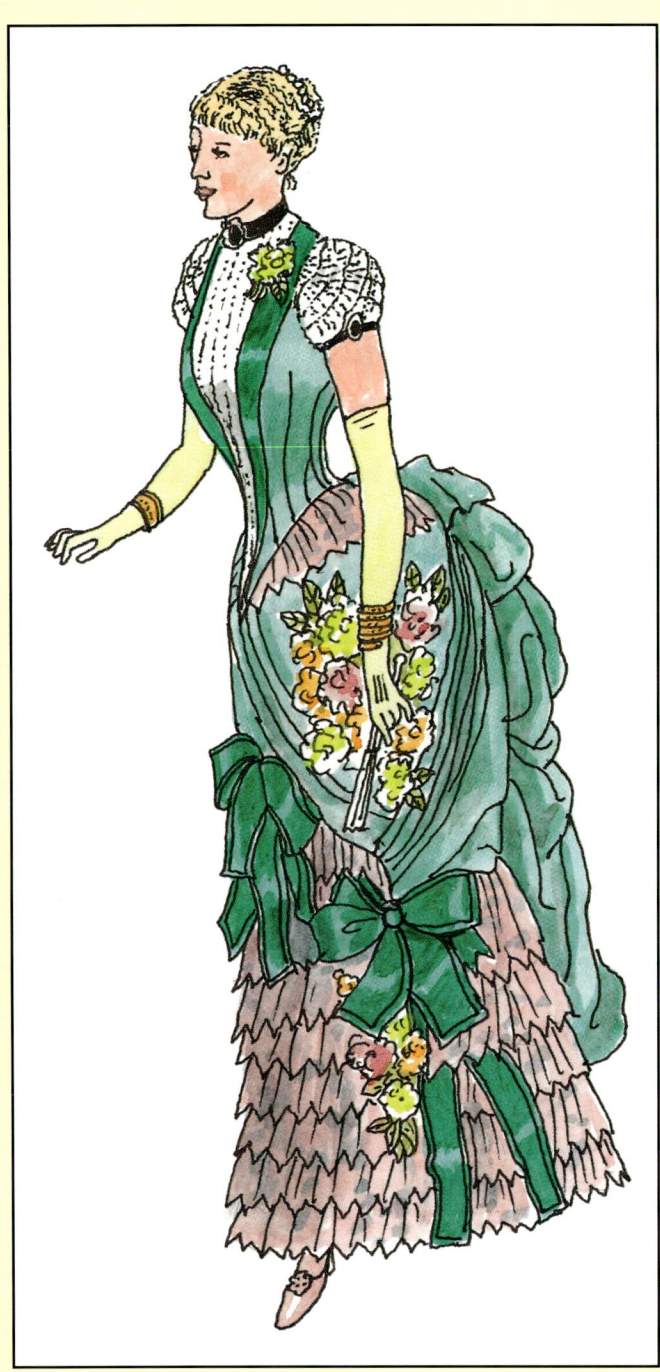

1880-1883 Evening Wear

    Overtrimmed evening dresses usually followed the "crinolette" line. The neckline was high and closed, or open but filled-in with a frilled chemise, which matched the short sleeves, as shown here.

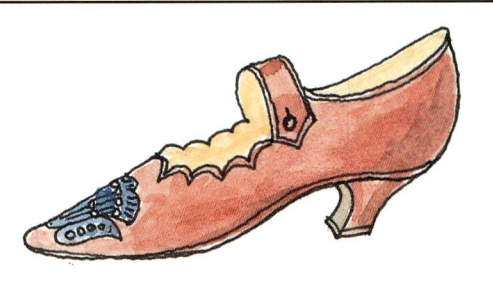

A silk strapped shoe with a beaded toe.

Probably a present for a wife or a fiancée, this flexible silver "ribbon" necklace tied in a True Lover's knot and finished with a heart-shaped locket.

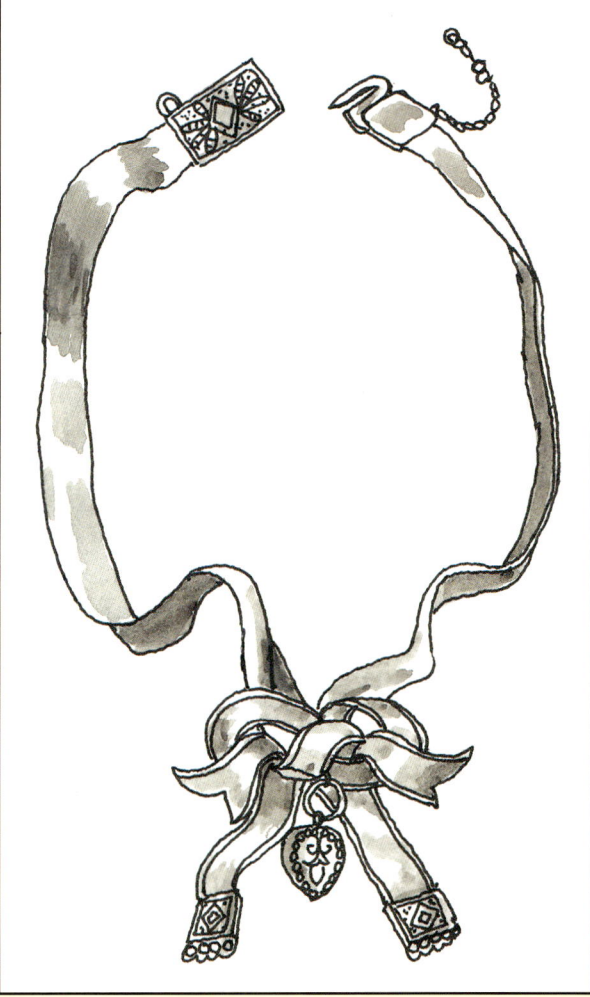

A conventional, hand-painted fan; the necklace carries a gold and sapphire pendant.

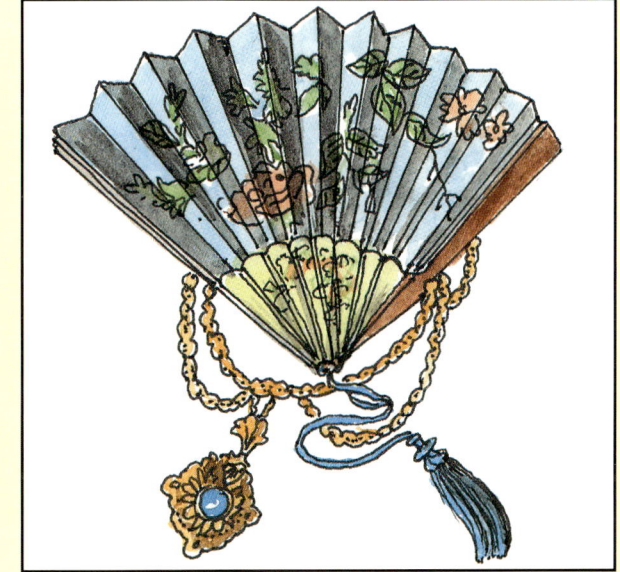

For those who followed the current European and American Aesthetic Movement, which worshiped anything Japanese, this paper fan, painted with a cherry blossom, and with bamboo sticks, was very fashionable.

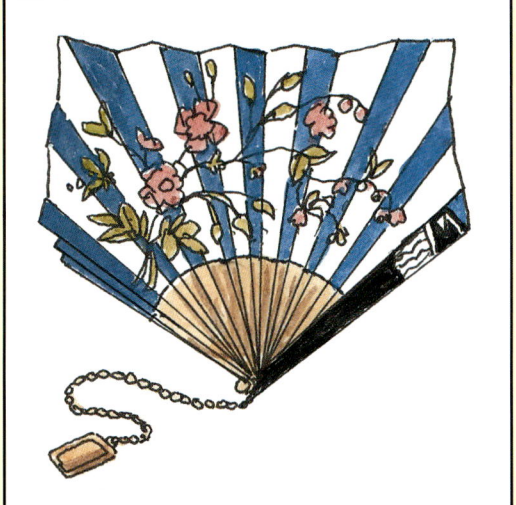

Given that women are supposed to be repelled by small reptiles and insects, it is surprising how popular jewelry in the form of such creatures was during the nineteenth century. This realistic lizard is encrusted in diamonds, emeralds, and rubies.

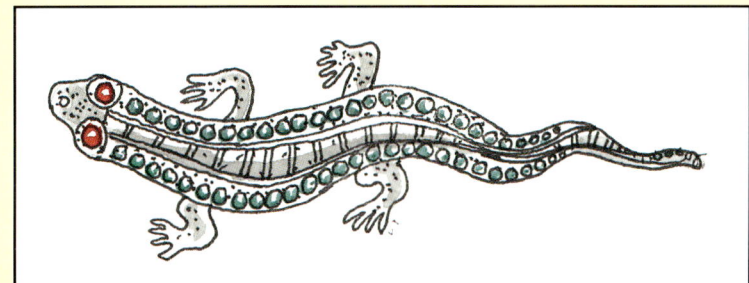

45

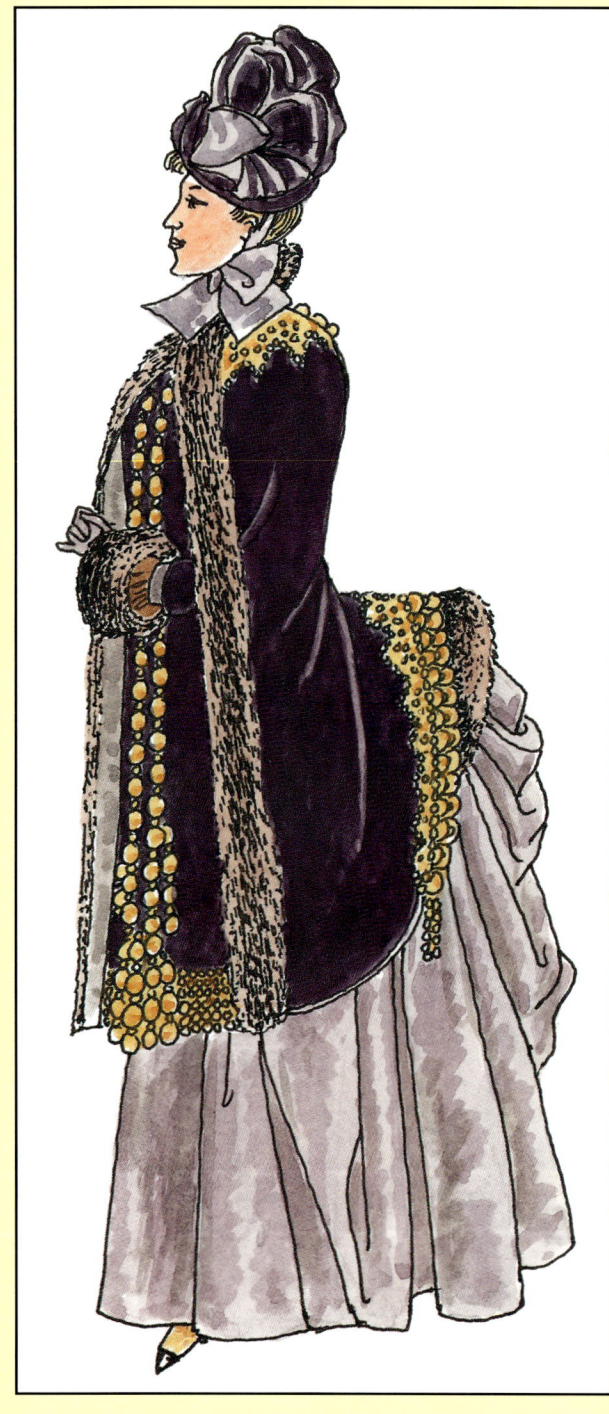

1883-1888 Day Wear

The second bustle is shown here. It thrust dresses out at the back into a horizonal line or shelf. At its most extreme, this bustle prompted the contemporary jibe that it could carry a "good-sized tea-tray." Dresses were either all-in-one or divided into bodice and skirt. Trimming was sparser but richer, with bands of embroidery and fur. This was particularly evident in a velvet winter mantle, as seen here; summer mantles were made in striped and spotted, lighter materials. Necklines on dresses remained high, sleeves tight but ending at mid-arm with deep underfrills.

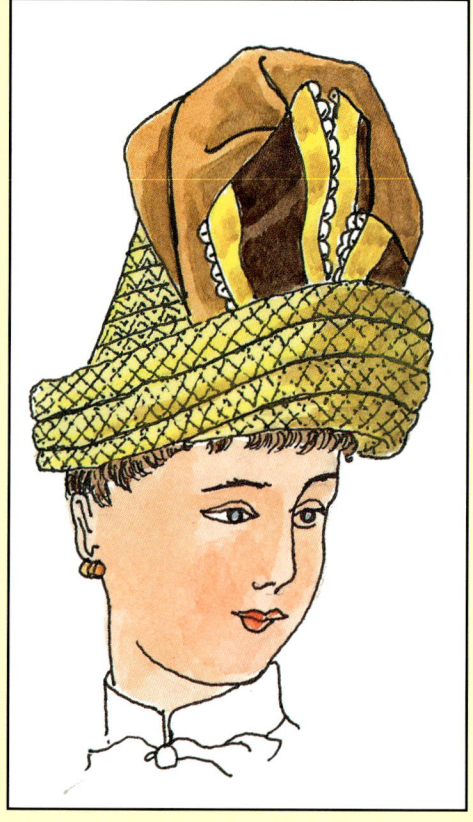

As the second nineteenth-century bustle protruded even further than the first, hats also rose higher, with all the trimming projected upward. In checkered straw this inverted flower-pot-shape hat with a turban brim is adorned with a bunch of velvet and a lace-edged silk ribbon.

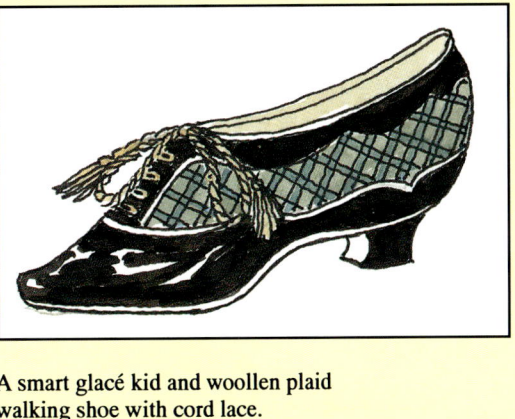

A smart glacé kid and woollen plaid walking shoe with cord lace.

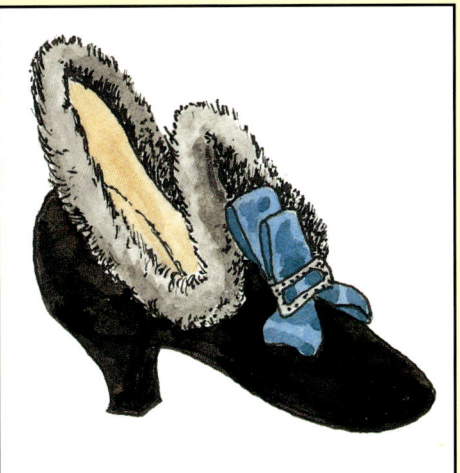

This carriage boot for winter is made warm with fur and made pretty with a silk bow and paste buckle.

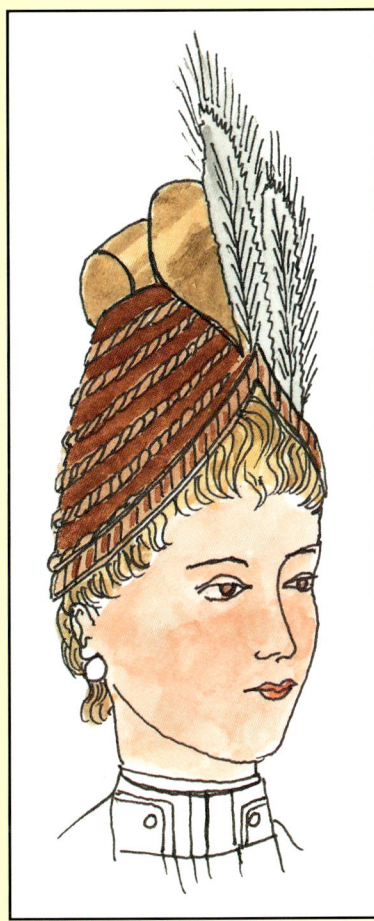

A felt and corded "Sable" toque, its height accentuated with ribbons and feathers.

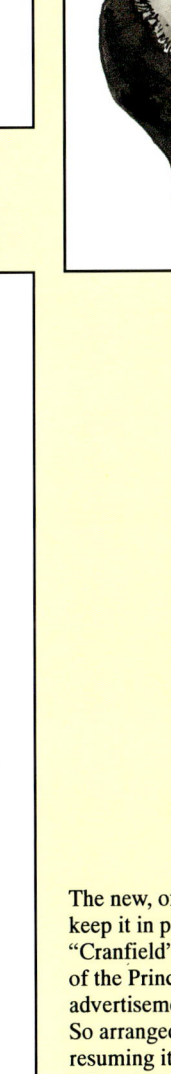

An extremely elegant felt tall hat, adorned with ribbons and remnants of birds.

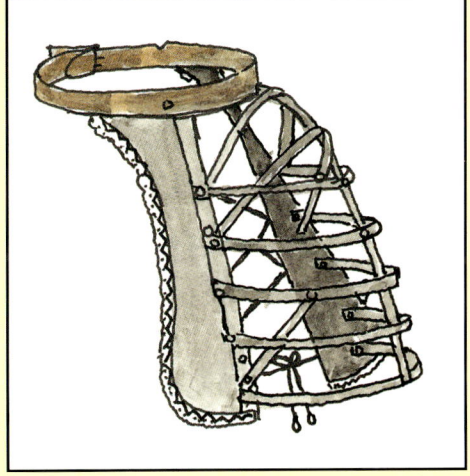

The new, often enormous, bustle-shaped dress required strong "dress improvers" to keep it in place. One such item was this steel and canvas version called the "Cranfield" or "Lily Langtry" - the latter after the actress Lily Langtry, a mistress of the Prince of Wales, later King Edward VII. The wording of the contemporary advertisement is worth giving in full to provide the period flavor: "For the million. So arranged as to spring up when the wearer is sitting or lying down. The Bustle resuming its proper position when rising. Size can be altered by means of an adjustable cord. Light, cool, easy to wear, never gets out of order, and is the correct Parisian shape. Best Bustle to fit a dress over. The only Bustle made to fit any lady and every dress. 8-inch depth, including band 11-inch. What more could a fashionable woman want?" What, indeed?

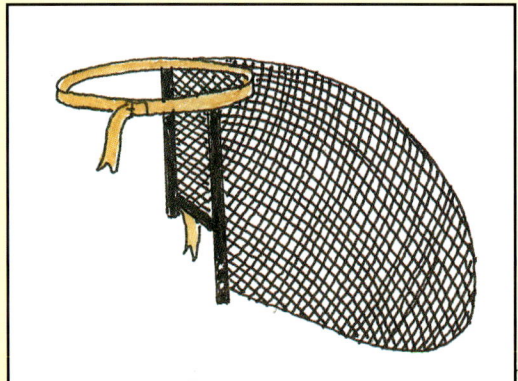

Made by the American Braided Company of London this bustle, made of the finest silver wire, was described as being "Light, Flexible, Strong, Durable, Perfect" and "Recommended by Physicians as being less heating to the spine than any others."

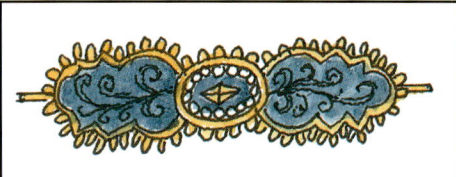

A bar brooch in gold and enamel. Such brooches were popular throughout the century.

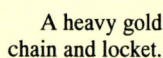

A heavy gold chain and locket.

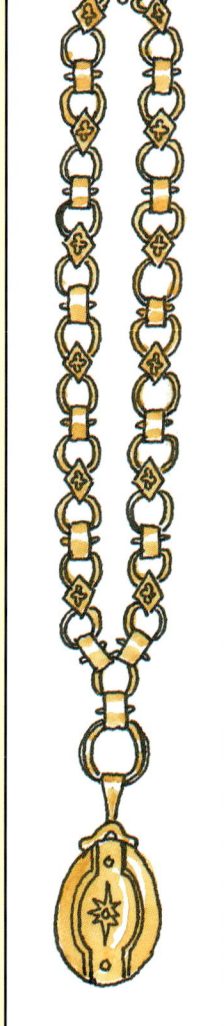

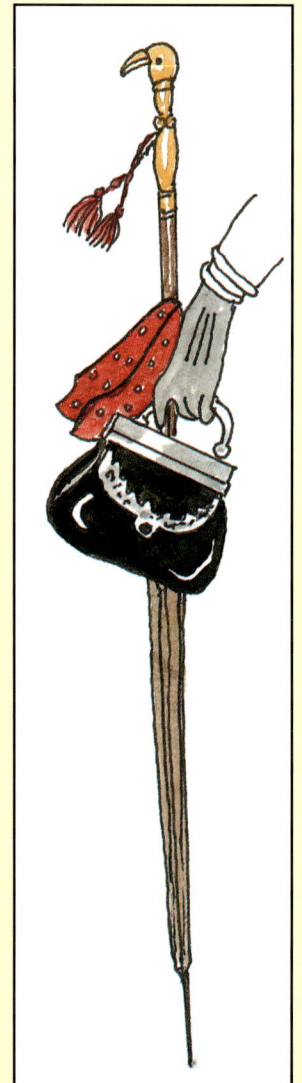

A woman traveling by train, horse drawn omnibus, or handsome cab must carry a serviceable leather, metal-framed handbag and an umbrella, this example with a bird-shaped handle.

It was still fashionable for ladies to wear fancy aprons at home, such as this one in lace-edged silk.

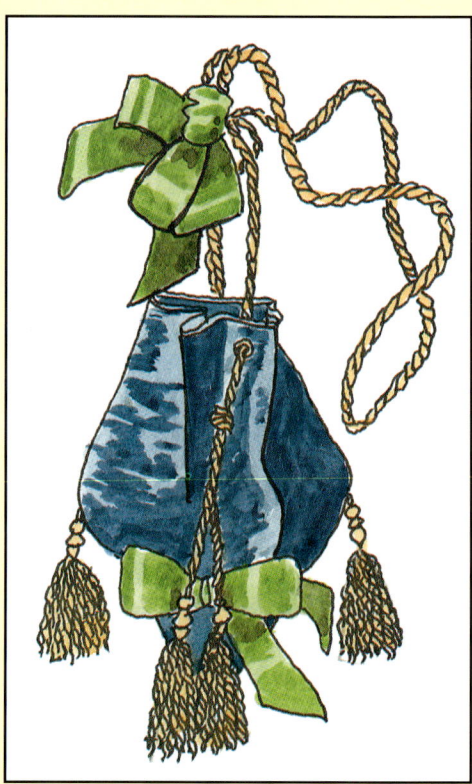

An excessively decorated grosgrain "at-home" bag in which, at most, a lady carried a handkerchief, smelling salts, and perhaps some sewing materials.

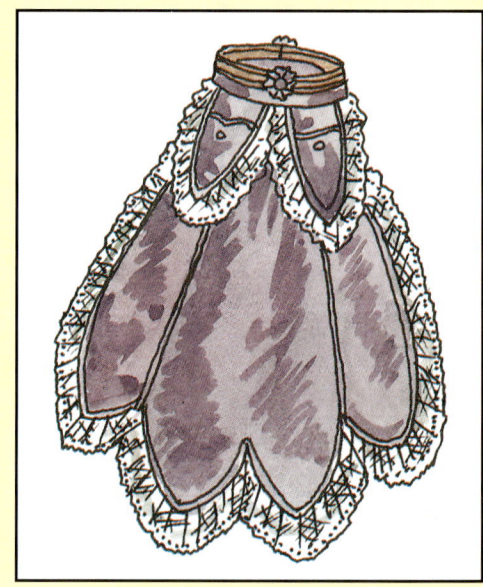

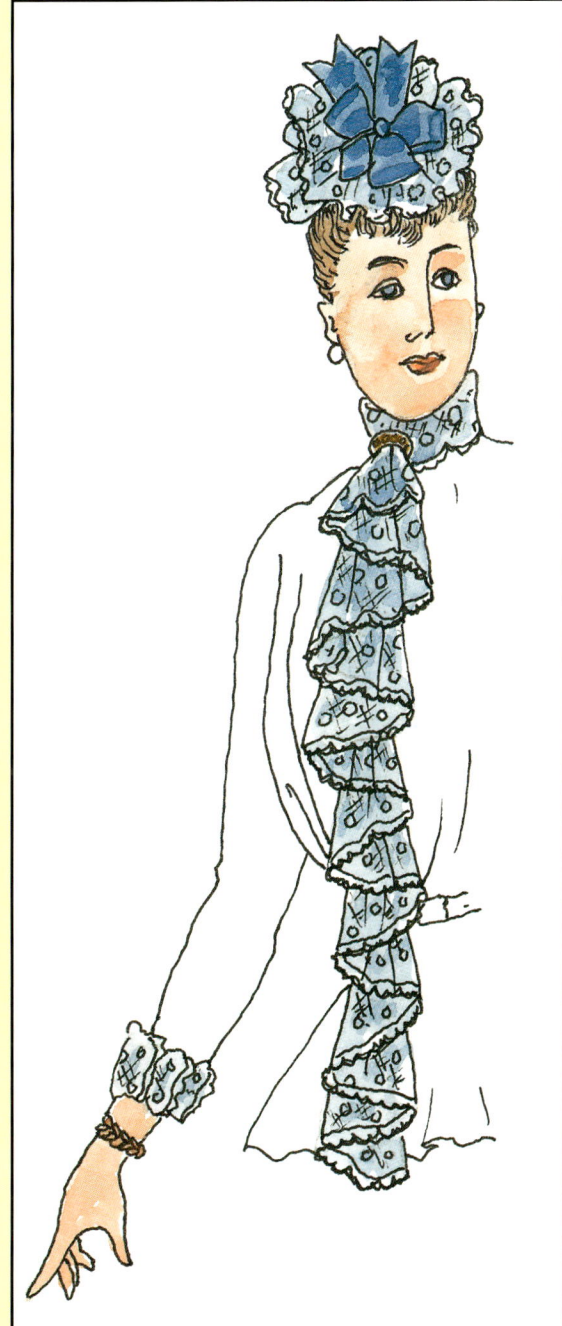

By this date, only matrons wore indoor caps during the day, except for breakfast and with tea-gowns, when such a matching dyed-lace cap, extra-long jabot, and cuffs, were considered necessary.

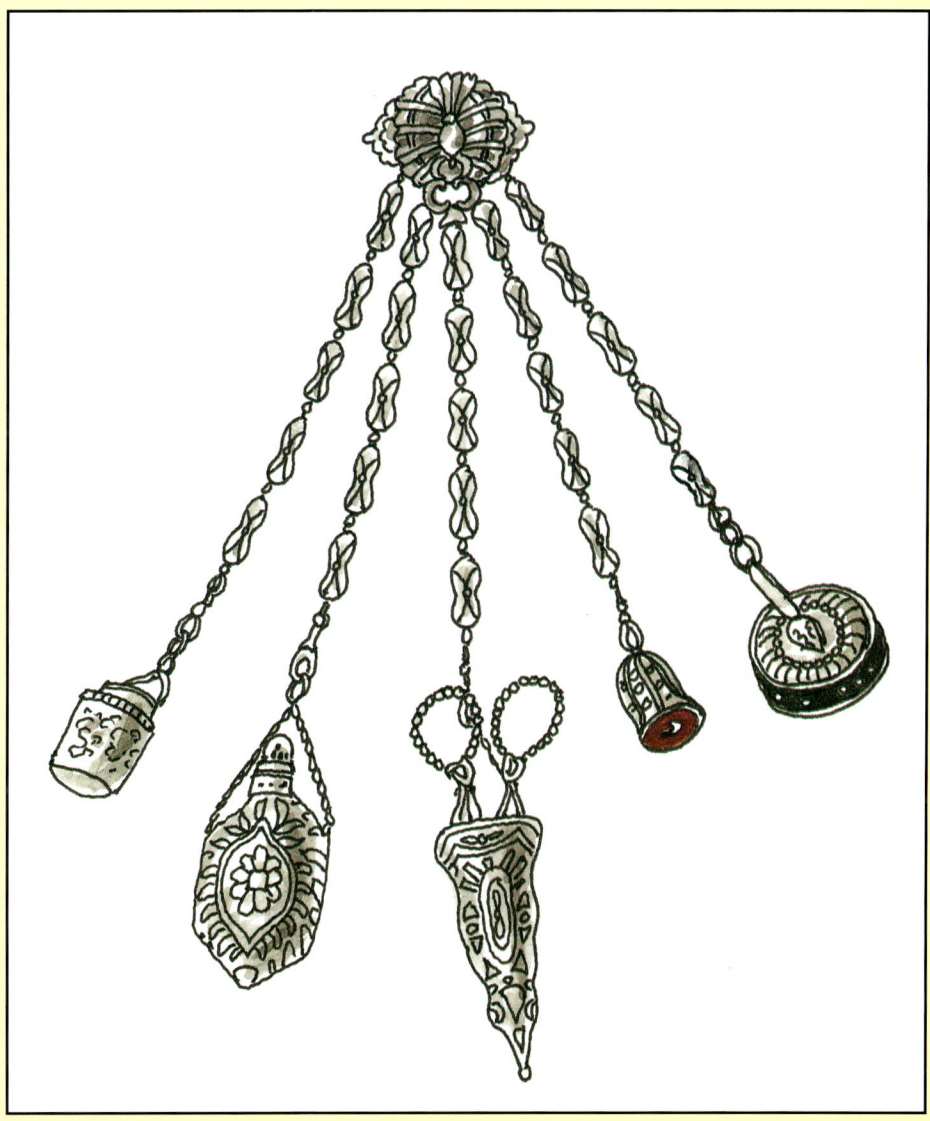

A silver chatelaine. For a number of centuries the "Mistress of the House," which is what a chatelaine means, often carried such an assemblage of chains, on a belt hook, bearing personal and household impedimenta. *Left to right:* a thimble in a bucket; a scent bottle; a pair of scissors in a holder; a seal, and a pincushion.

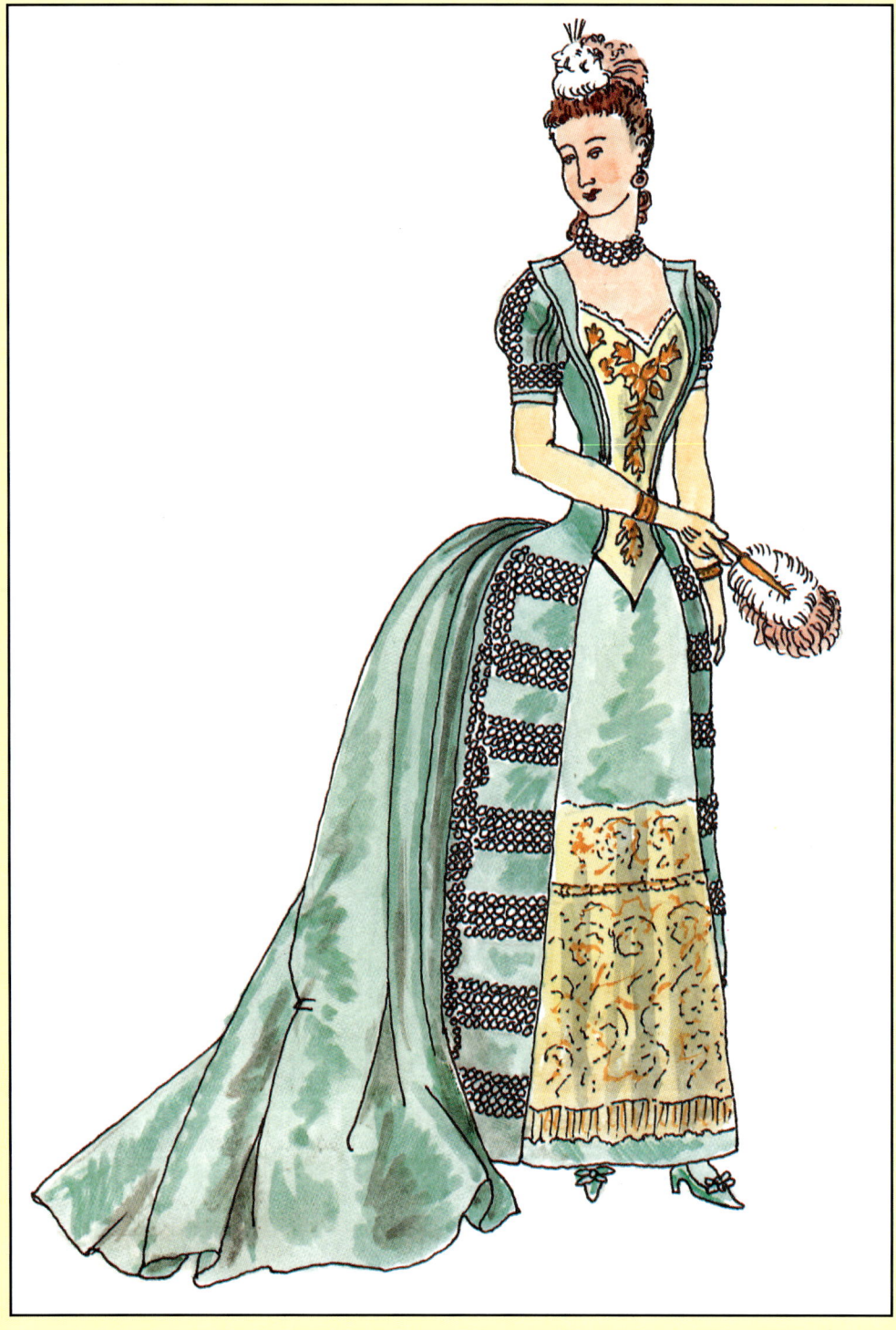

1883-1888 Evening Wear

Deep-bustled evening dresses were heavily trained, with elaborately-decorated corsages and sleeves. Skirts were often open at the front to reveal a lace-trimmed underskirt. Other dresses were made of lighter materials with less trimming and no trains.

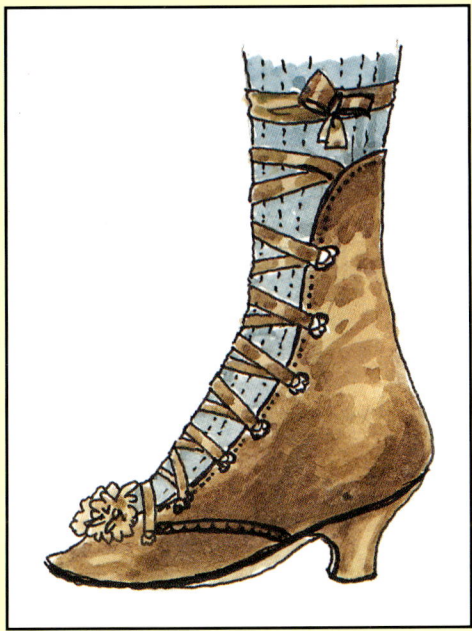

Because evening dresses revealed the entire foot, shoemakers could be adventurous in their designs, as in this kid shoe with cross-over ribbon lacing. Plain or patterned colored silk stockings also were fashionable.

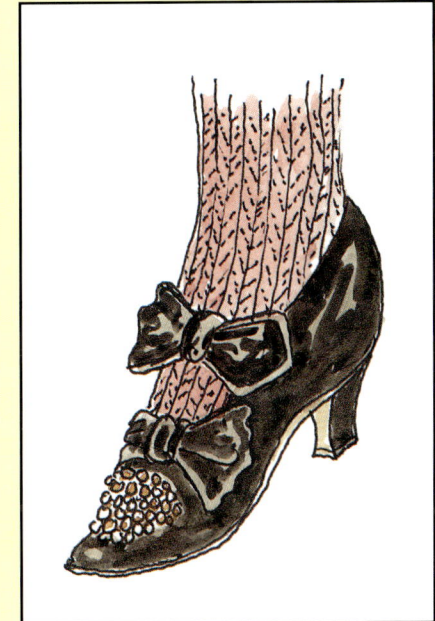

Almost as grand: glacé kid with jewels on the toe.

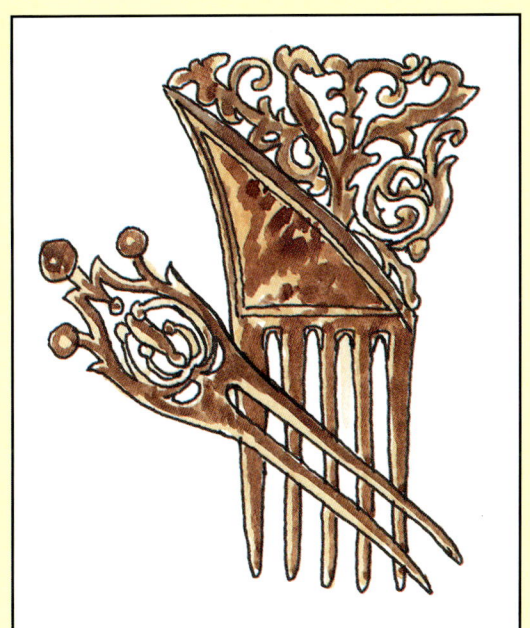

Real or imitation tortoiseshell combs were used to hold up piled hair or to fasten a headdress.

Another example of what one would not expect a woman to wear: a snail brooch, in diamonds, rubies, and emeralds.

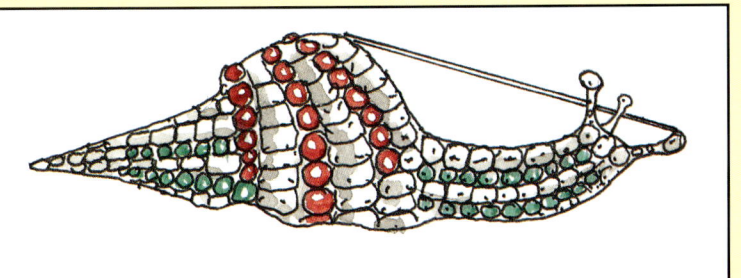

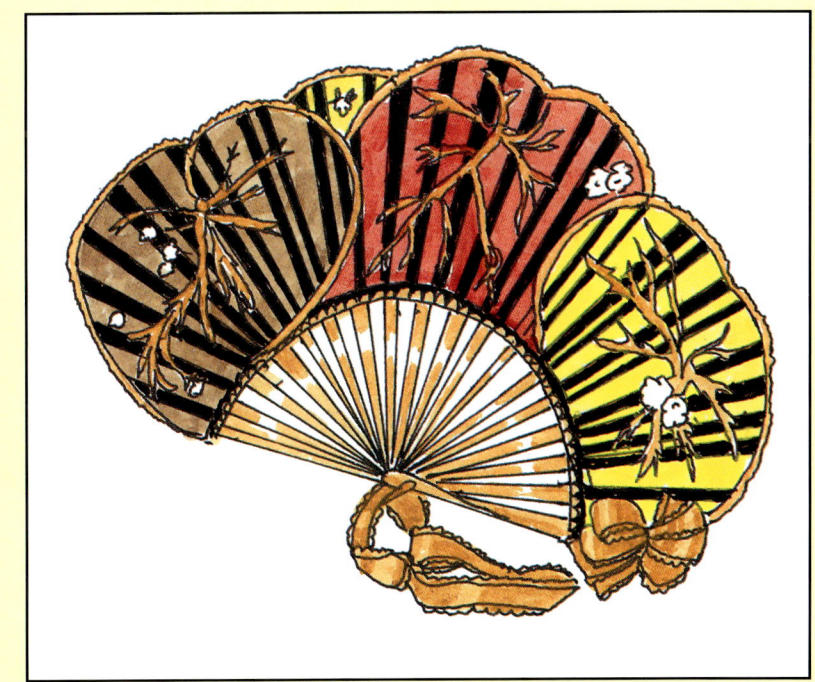

Painted paper or silk Japanese-style fans were still popular.

51

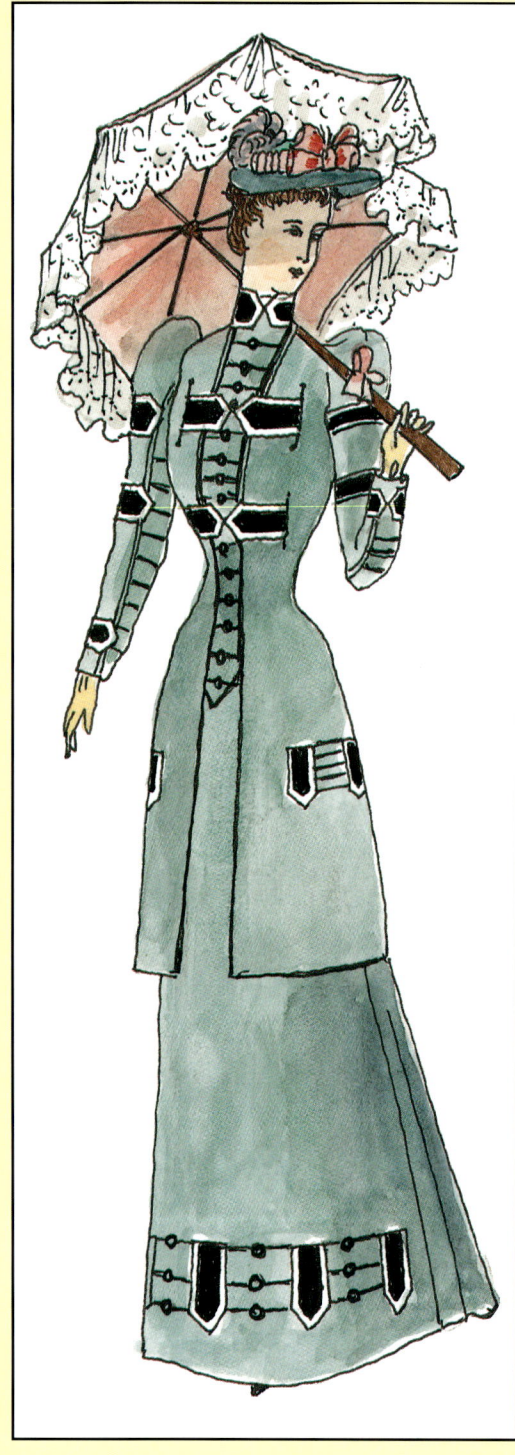

1888-1892 Day Wear

The second bustle was quite soon replaced by a new slimmed-down, narrow silhouette. The fashion had a certain "mannishness" about it; the first British tailor-made coat and skirt is shown here, which was to have a long life. The style immediately influenced American fashion, as it eventually did Parisian fashion. This change had much to do with the emergence of the "New Woman," who saw herself as a much freer person: riding a bicycle, rowing, playing tennis, climbing mountains, and most of all, taking a job. It was fashionable to look healthy and tall in a long jacket (often open to show a vest) and a slim skirt with trimming kept to a severe minimum. However, for all her attempt at being "new," a woman could still carry a lacy parasol!

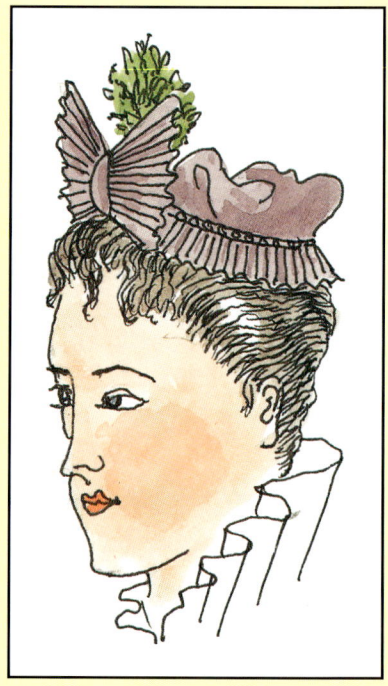

With the disappearance of the bustle, women's hats and bonnets could be so small as to make a contemporary observer remark: "as if they were intended for a doll." Hence this singularly tiny silk hat perched on top of the head.

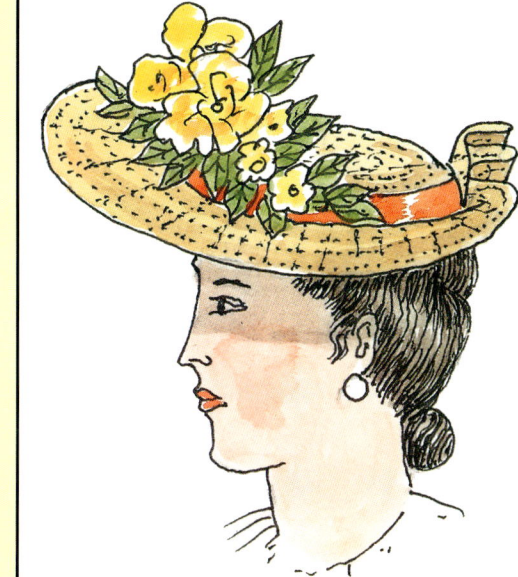

Summer hats tended to be larger, such as this straw flower- and leaf-bedecked example.

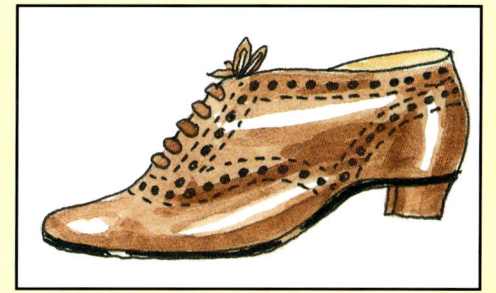

Sturdy, punched, and stitched leather shoe, possibly for country wear.

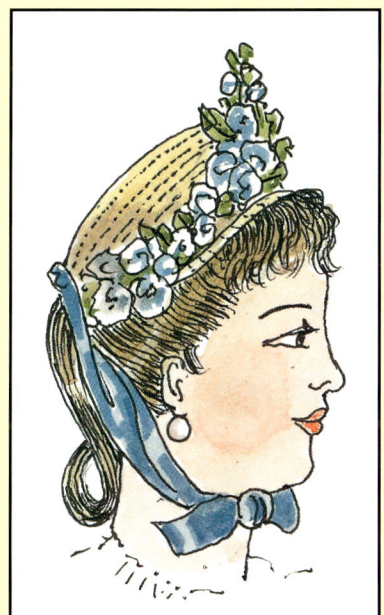

A small straw bonnet tied firmly under the chin; otherwise it might have fallen off.

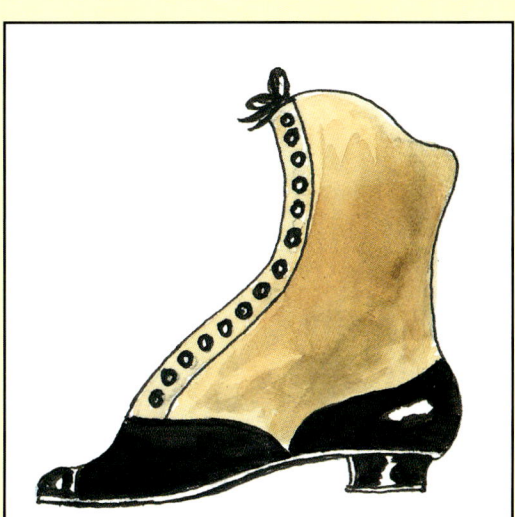

A man's style patent leather and cloth buttoned boot with a bow to give it a touch of femininity.

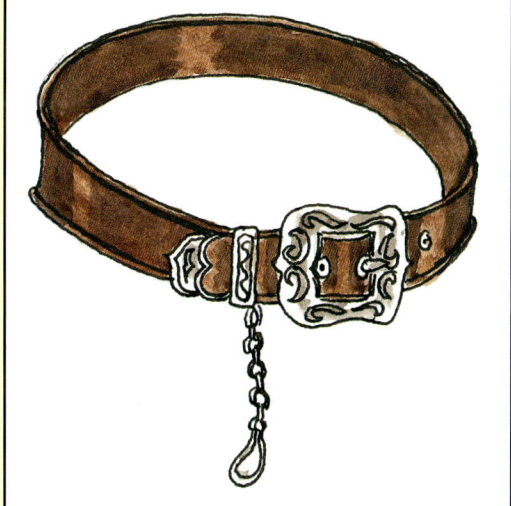

The new fashion for daytime blouses worn with gored skirts meant that belts became all-important: a leather example with a silver buckle and attachments.

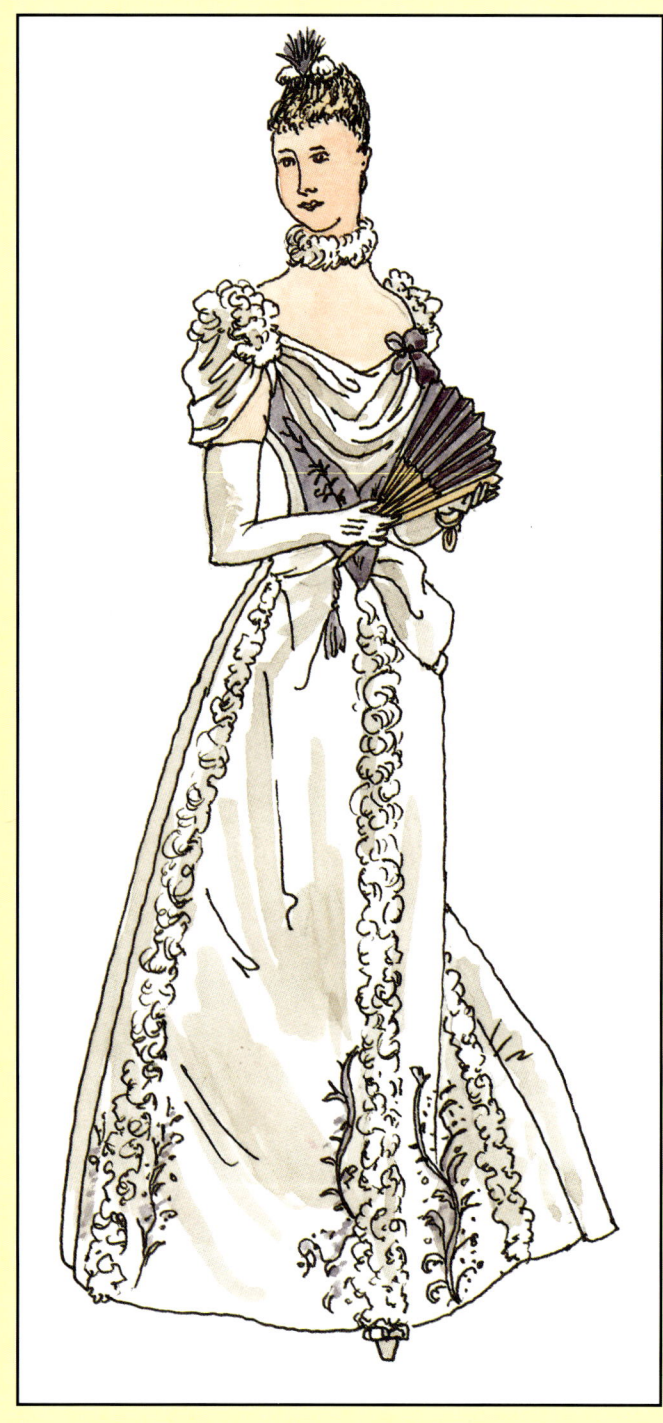

1888-1892 Evening Wear

Even the "New Woman" did not or could not lose her femininity in the ballroom. Although narrower than before, dresses still had trains. The low, deep bodice was pointed and festooned with swags of silk and bunches of lace, matching the low-slung short sleeves. Elaborate trimming on skirts had by no means vanished, either.

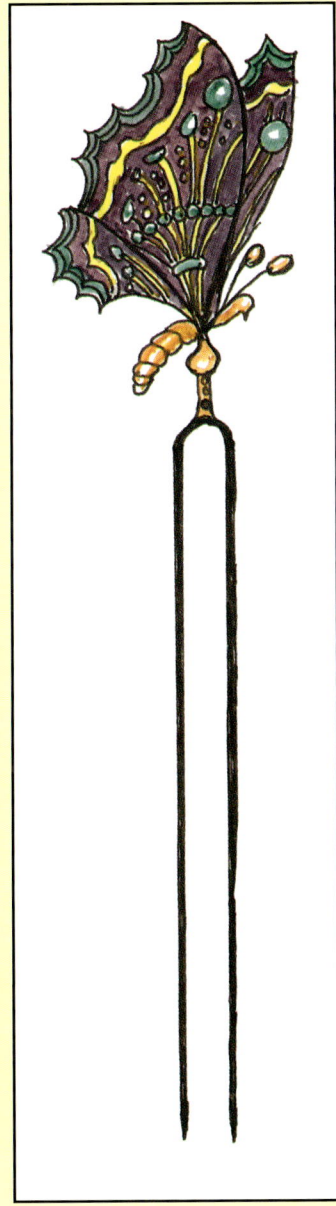

An enameled and jeweled butterfly hair ornament.

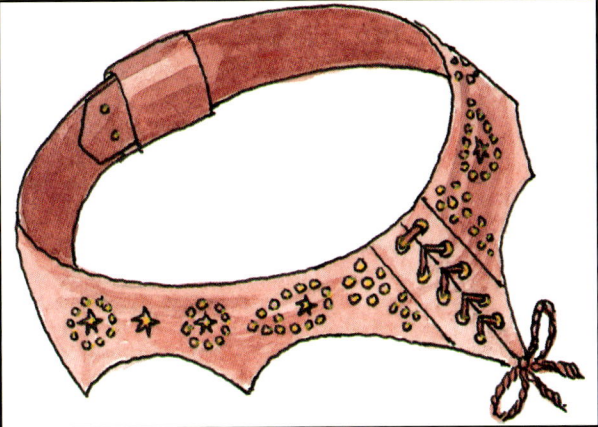

Some evening dresses were belted; hence, this rather corset-like one.

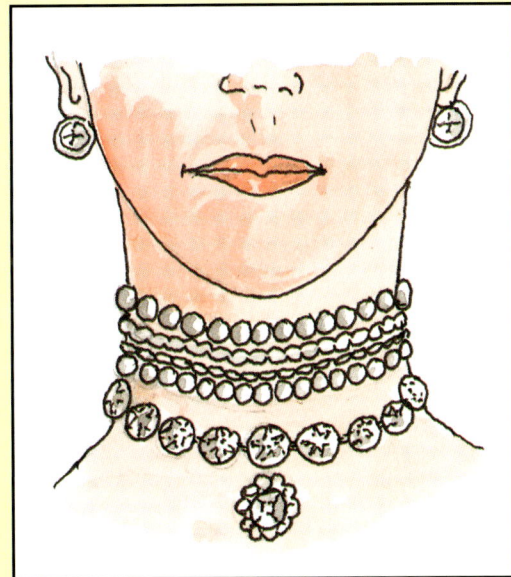

A pearl and diamond choker. This style of necklace is said to have been created by Princess Alexandra after she married the Prince of Wales in 1863, to conceal a scar on her neck. As she was not only royal, but also beautiful and a leader of fashion, society ladies were quick to follow her example.

A silk "Dorothy" bag adds to the evening accessories of gloves, heavy bracelet, and tiny ostrich-feather fan.

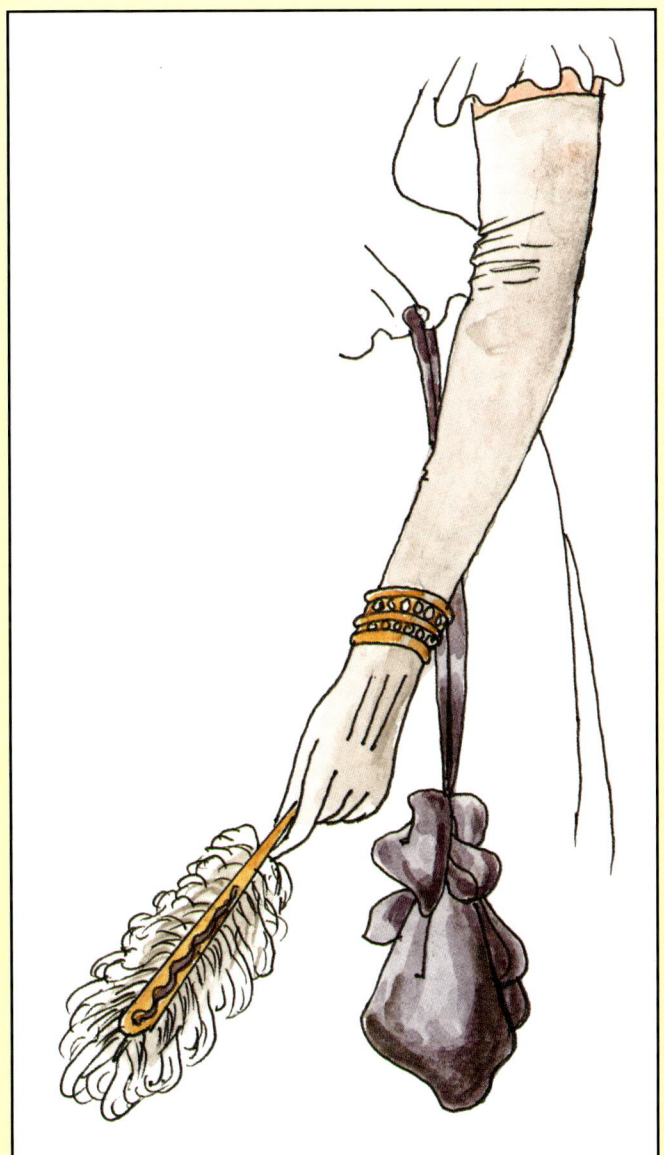

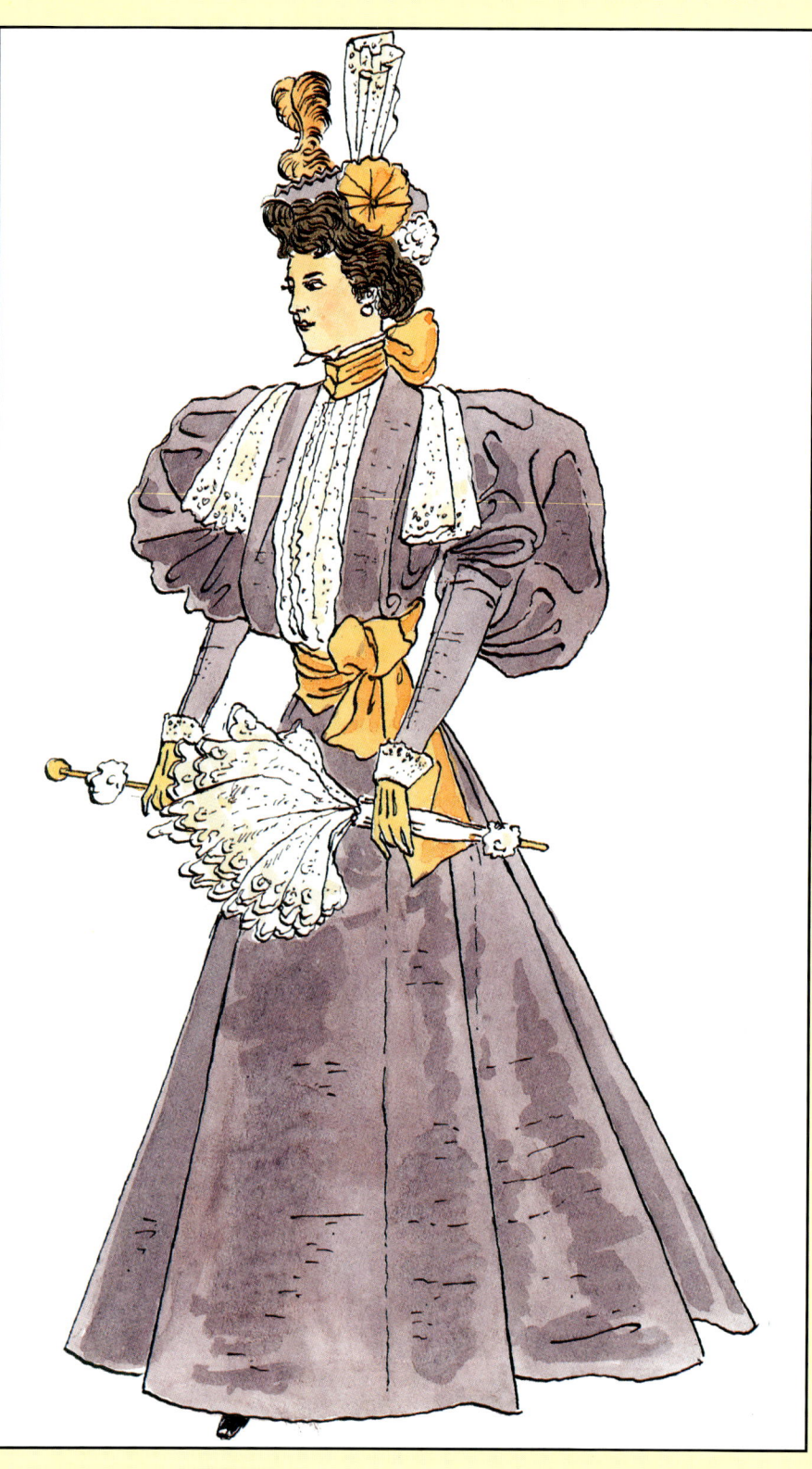

1892-1897 Day Wear

The "New Woman" had not disappeared, but fashion decreed that (except for sports) women should look more feminine again, if with a rather aggressive air. This style was mostly brought about by the introduction of the gigot or leg-of-mutton sleeve which reached maximum width between 1895 and 1897. Bodices had a pronounced full, slightly drooping bustline. Fuller, bell-like skirts were achieved not with pleating, as before—except at the back—but with goring at the front, which was to become a feature of dresses well into the next century. Some dresses were richly embroidered, especially on vest-like bodices with wide revers. Waists were belted or swathed with wide ribbons. Short, velvet or brocade capes, heavily trimmed with braid or jet, came into fashion in approximately 1893.

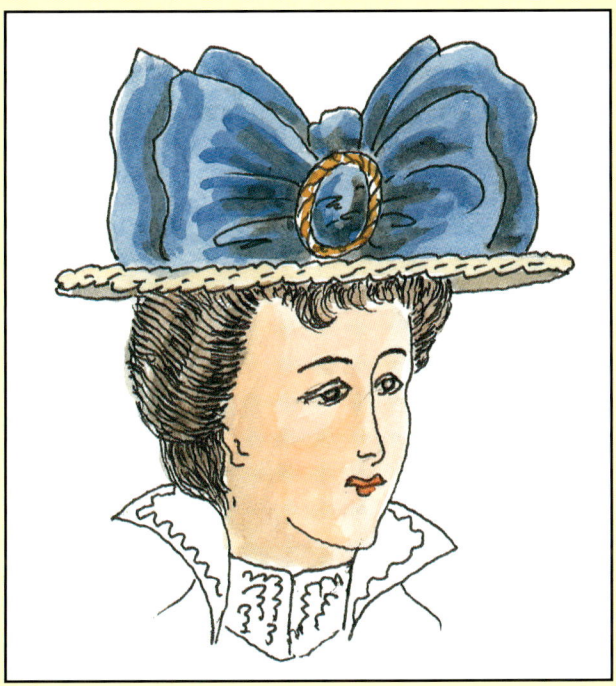

To compliment the trend toward femininity and aggressiveness, hats tended to be larger and more highly decorated. This straw is given height, width, and importance with a gilt-buckled silk bow.

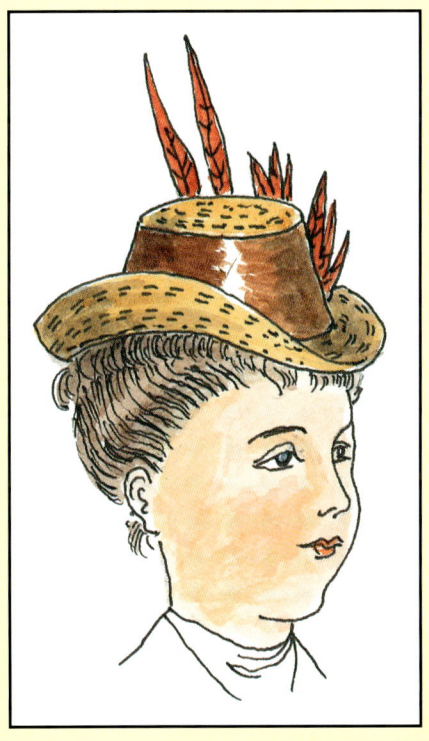

The "New Woman" in a man's straw homburg, rendered feminine with a few feathers.

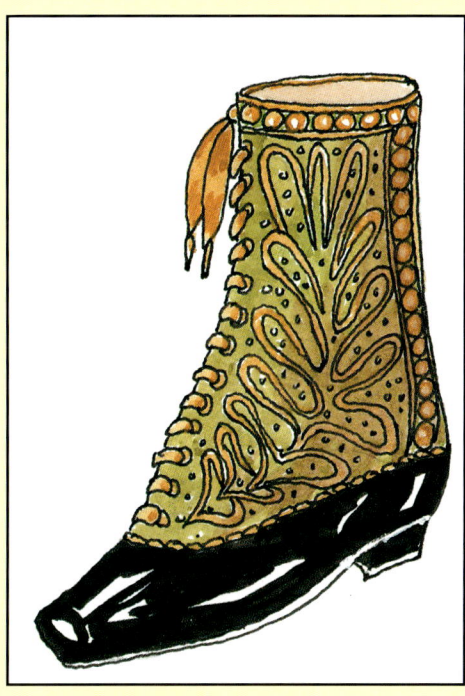

A patent leather boot, its cloth upper excessively decorated with braid, beads, and buttons.

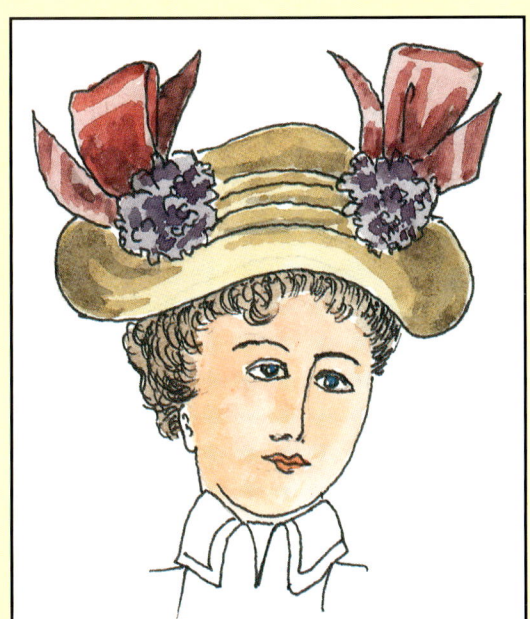

A ridged felt with rabbit ear-like decoration.

An elegant calf walking shoe.

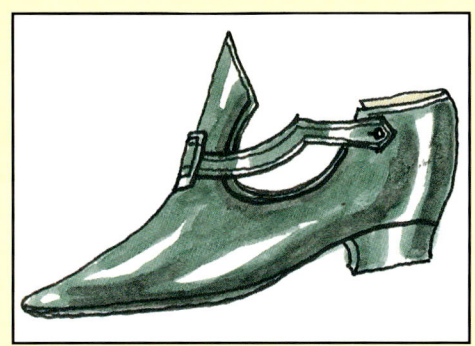

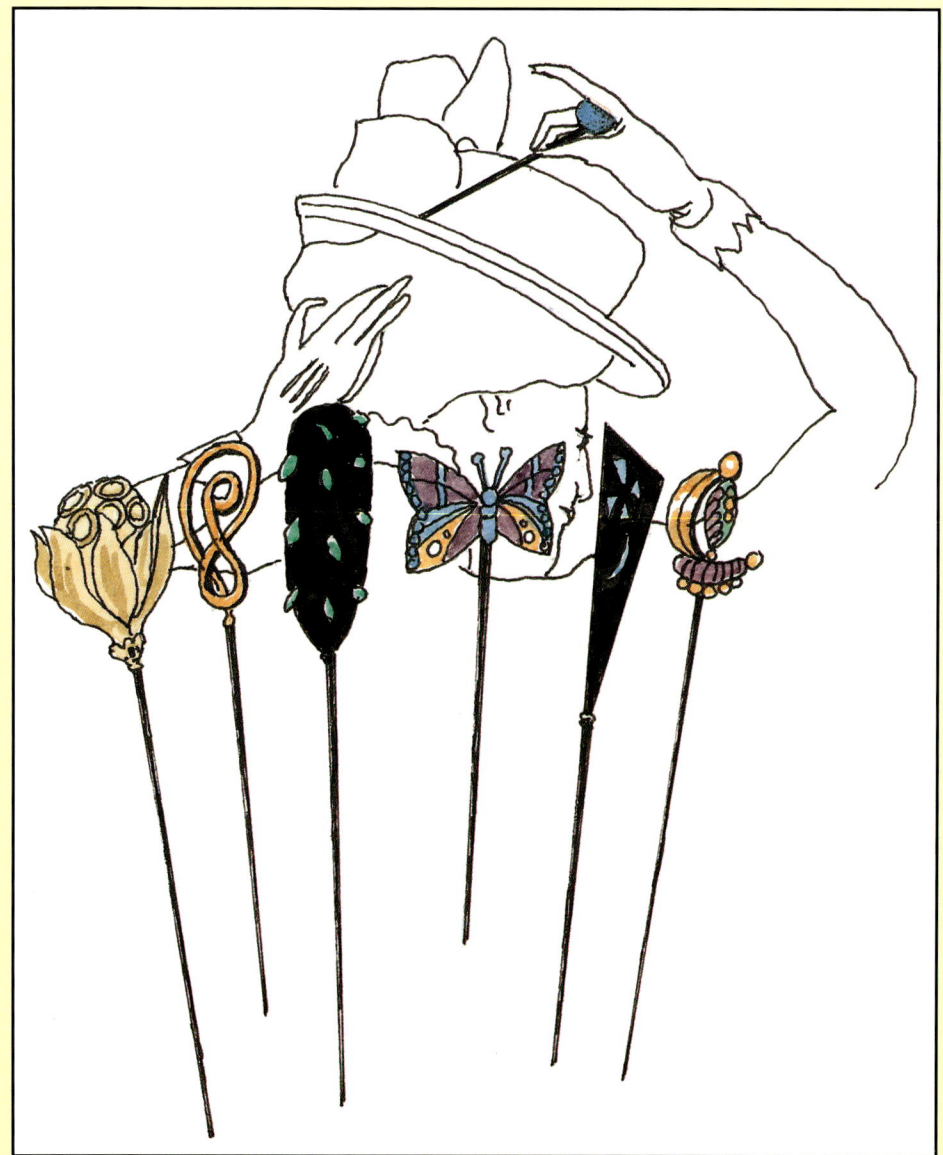

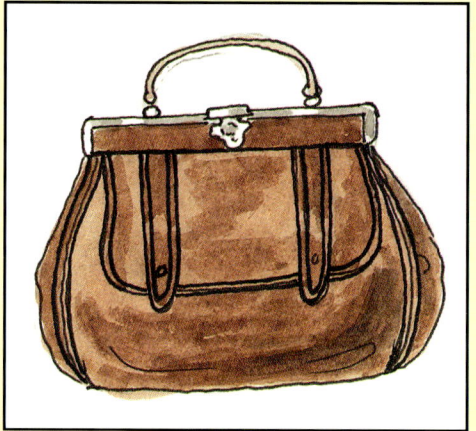

A strong leather traveling bag, the kind of which played so large a part in Oscar Wilde's play *The Importance of Being Earnest,* which opened in London in January 1895.

Hat pins had, of course, been in style for a long time and would continue to be so, but here seems to as good a point as any to show a few of the variations. *Left to right:* a waxed and gilded flower; an Art Nouveau gold twist; padded velvet sewn with glass beads; an enameled butterfly, an enameled triangle, and a gold and enameled sword.

As with so many parasols, a frill of the material was used to decorate the handle.

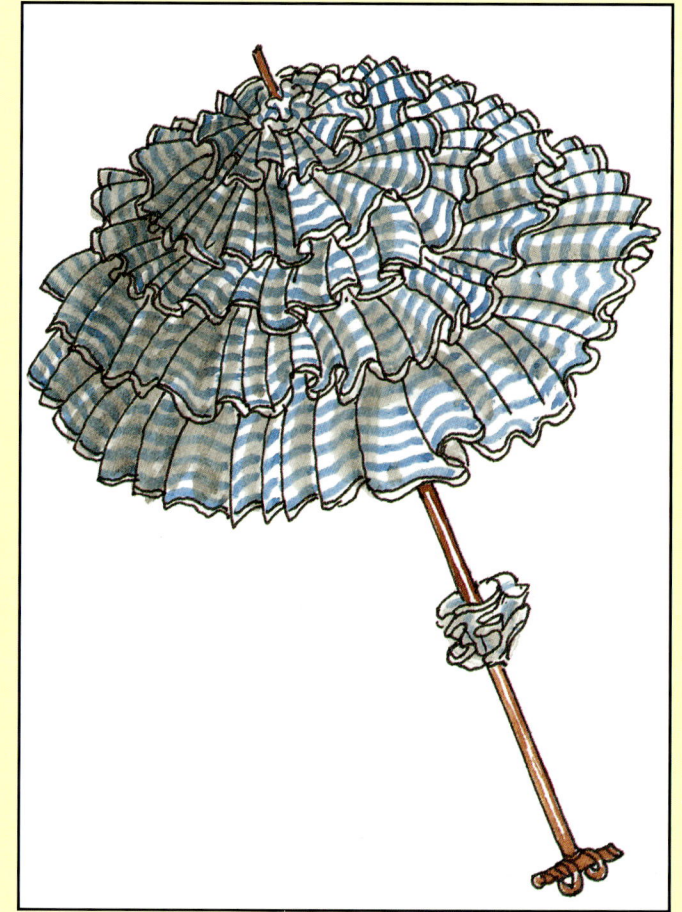

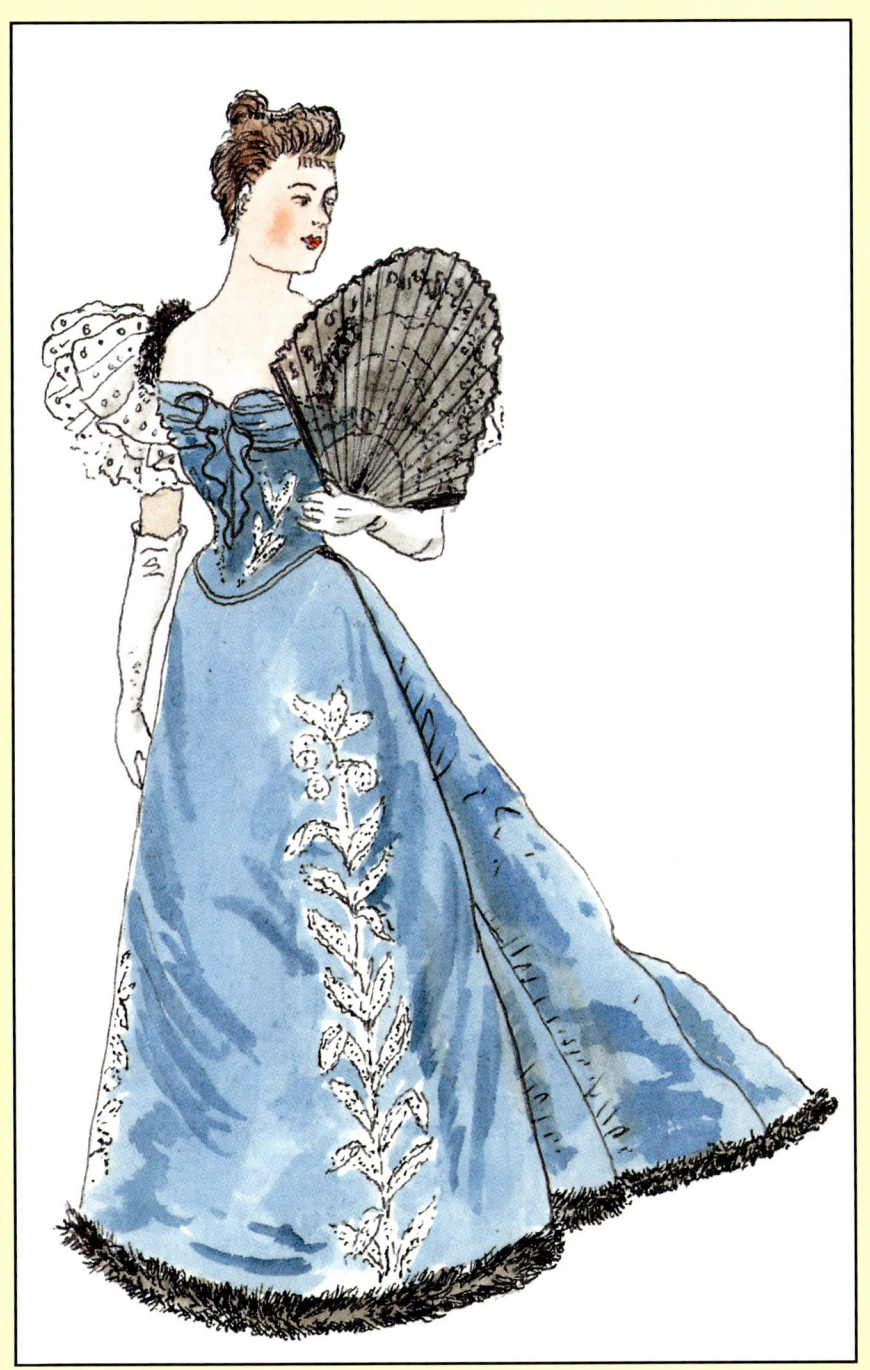

1892-1897 Evening Wear

Short, ultra-wide, often lace-covered gigot or leg-of-mutton sleeves nearly pushed men away. Full, trained, and front-gored dresses were richly decorated along the gores with embroidery, sequins, lace, or ribbons. Colors could be violent, such as crimson with yellow, but eau-de-nile and pale blue were the most fashionable colors after 1897.

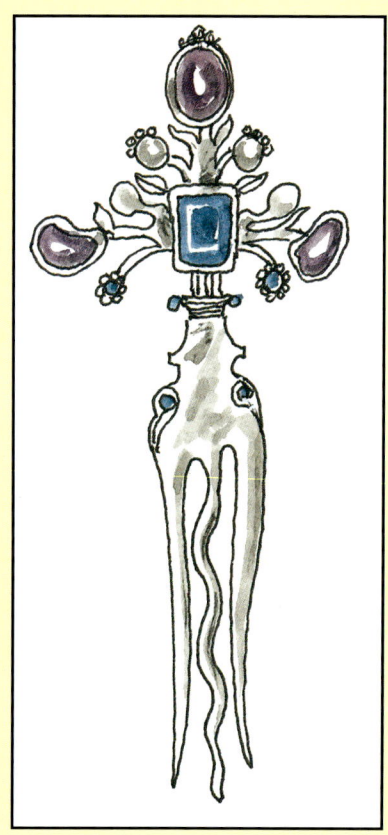

A silver, gem, and pearl encrusted comb.

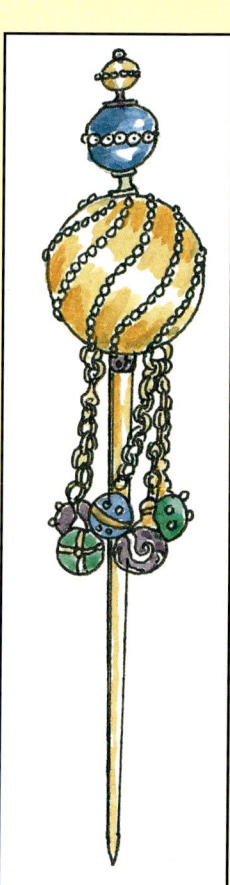

An evening hairpin: gilded, jeweled, and enameled.

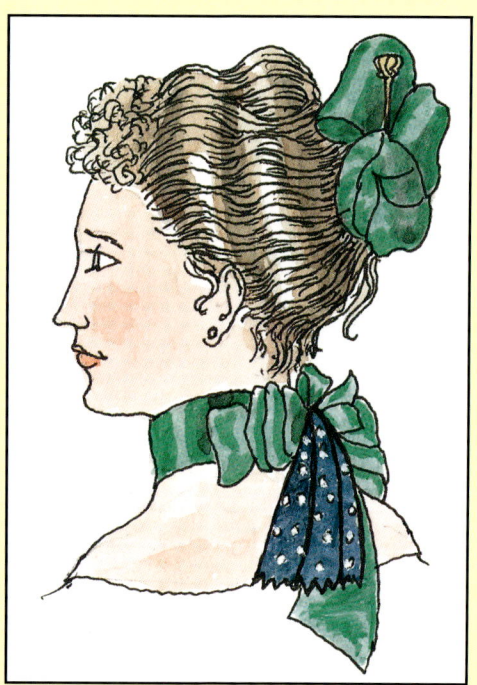

The "bun" on top of this evening coiffure is accented by a silk ribbon bow secured by a jeweled pin; a matching bow around the neck is embellished with a pleat of sequin-studded chiffon.

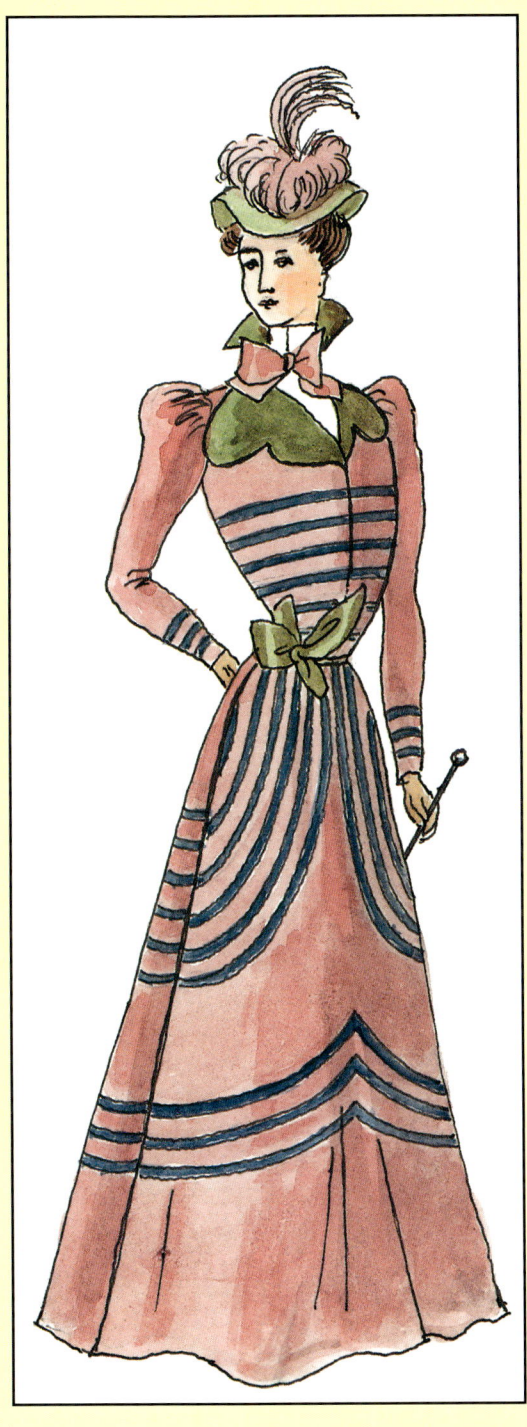

1897-1902 Day Wear

This period saw a sudden return to early "90s severity, but with sleeves puffed at the shoulders, an even more pronounced bustline, and large lapels, with often a sash at the waist as a softener. Trimming usually consisted of braid. For those women who still wanted to look feminine, there was a discreet use of lace and frills. A man's collar and flowing bow necktie were considered very smart.

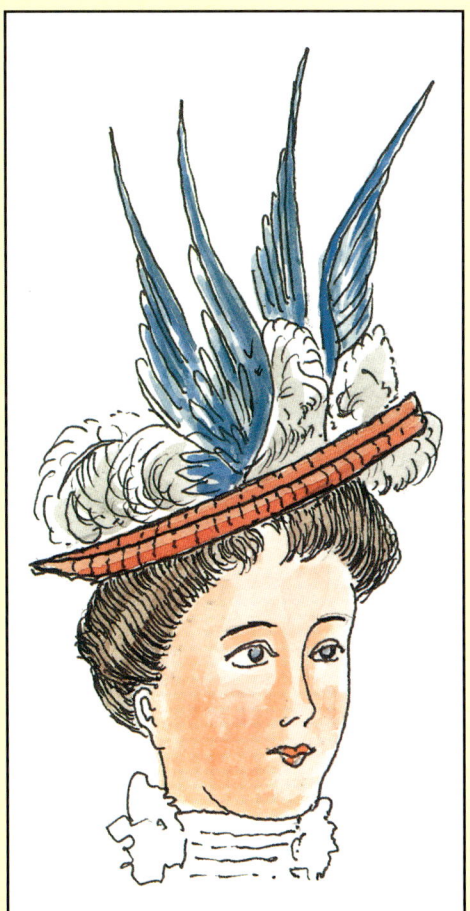

When dress shoulders lost their width, hats suddenly gained height: one of fashion's periodical foibles. This saucily tilted straw hat is "elevated" with feathers and wings. In 1897, a shocked British critic noted that "some twenty to thirty million dead birds are imported annually to supply the demands of the murderous millinery trade." In the following year, hats had practically supplanted bonnets, causing one commentator to ask: "Where is the popular bonnet? It seems to have fallen into limbo of forgotten things in spite of patronage by Royalty." Until her death in 1901, Queen Victoria always wore a bonnet or a widow's cap after 1861.

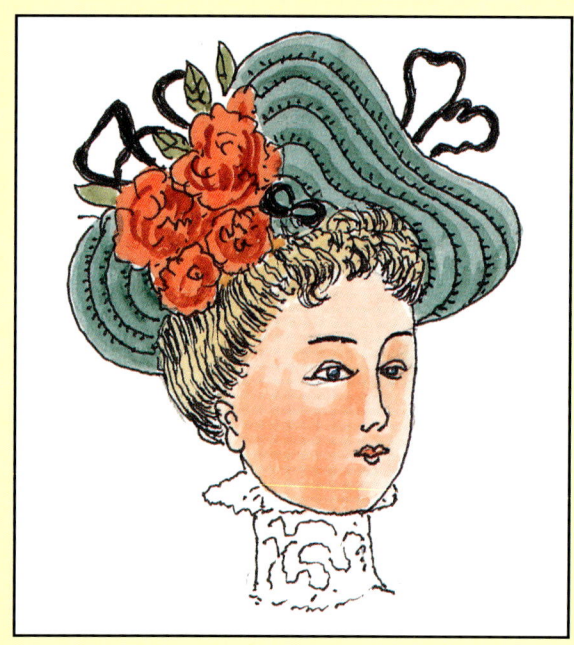

A well-off-the-face padded and ruched silk hat, the loops made of ribbon stiffened with wire.

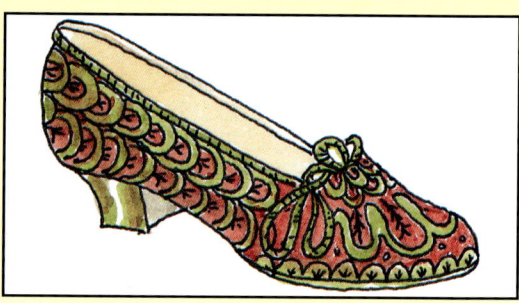

A house shoe thick with braid, embroidery, and cords.

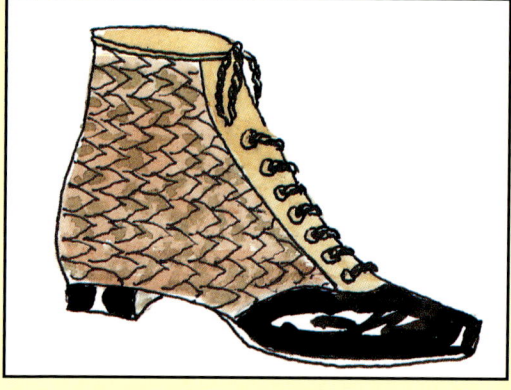

An elegant patent leather, cloth, and snakeskin boot.

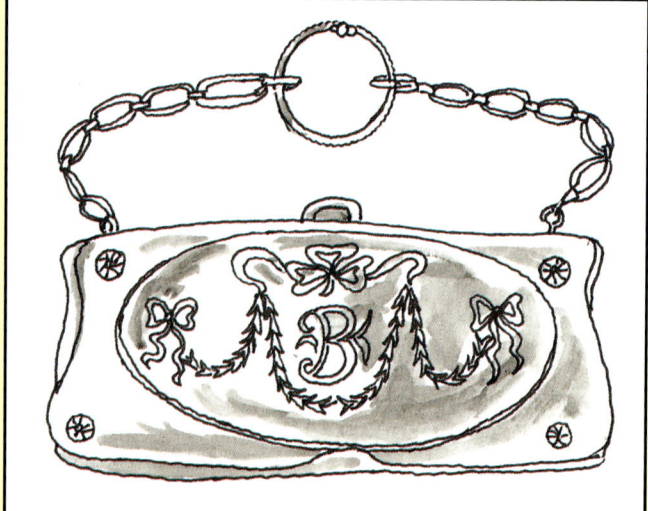

A little silver finger-purse; the rococo design carried out in repoussé work.

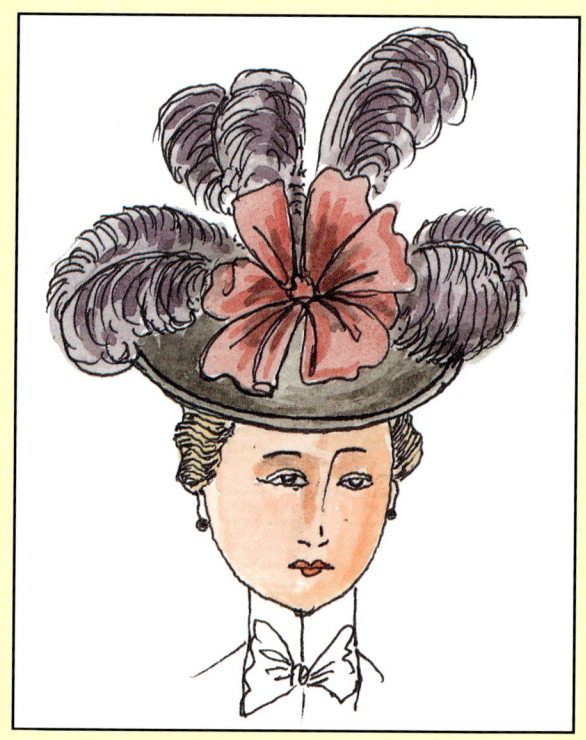

A hat which any society woman, caricatured in one of Oscar Wilde's plays, would have been proud to wear.

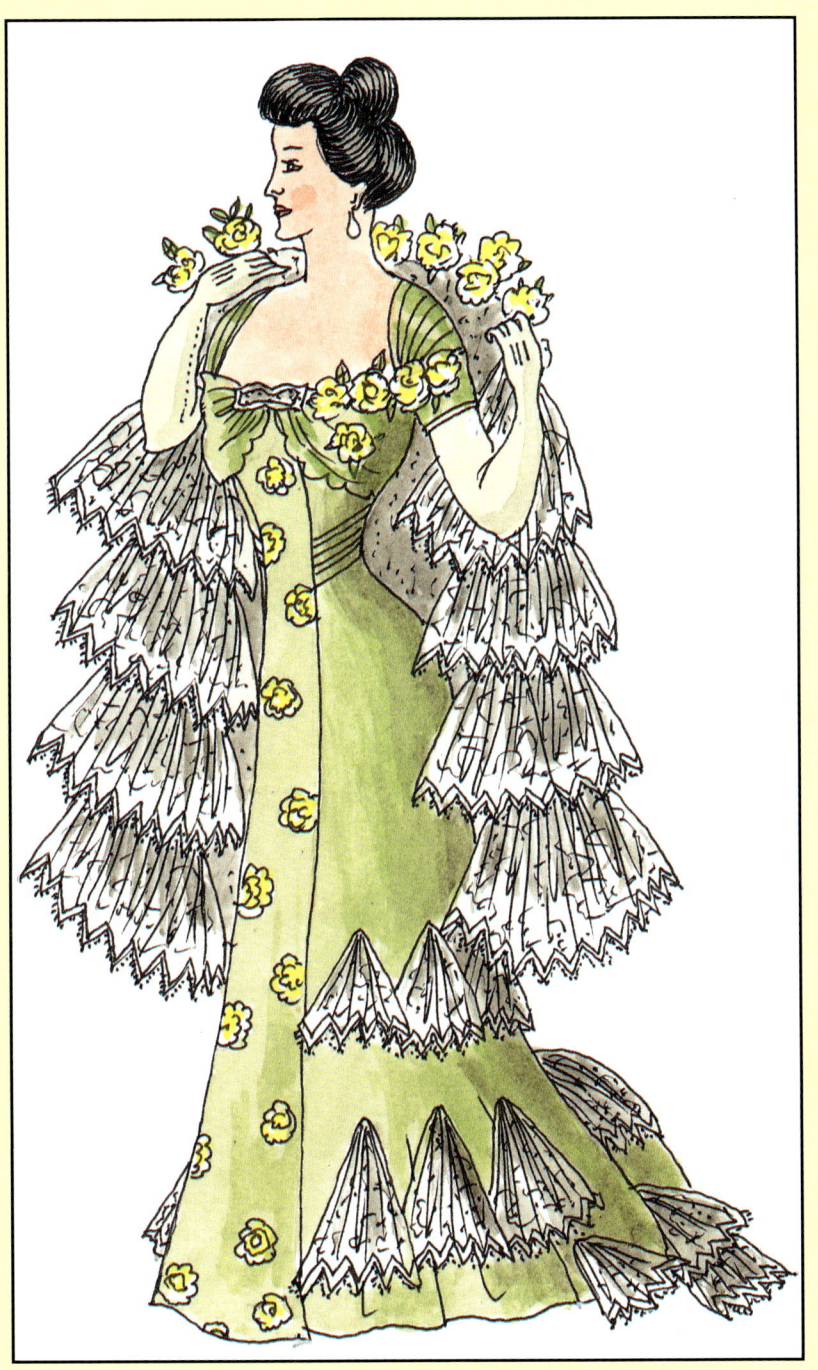

1897–1902 Evening Wear

Even if you were a "New Woman," you could not escape having to look ultra-feminine at a ball in a hip-hugging dress with a protruding, ever-decorated bustline and a trained skirt—all excessively adorned with bows, flowers, lace, and a silk-and-lace cape to match.

The fragile dragonfly appealed to Art Nouveau designers; on this brooch, it is made solid in enamel, diamonds, emeralds, and a ruby.

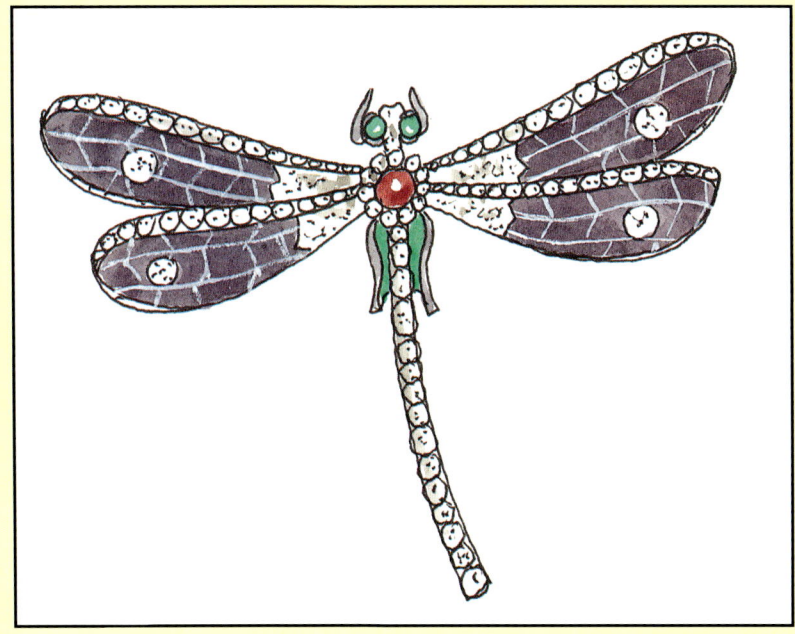

A delightfully flamboyant wired and sequinned muslin headdress, with a matching neck ruffle.

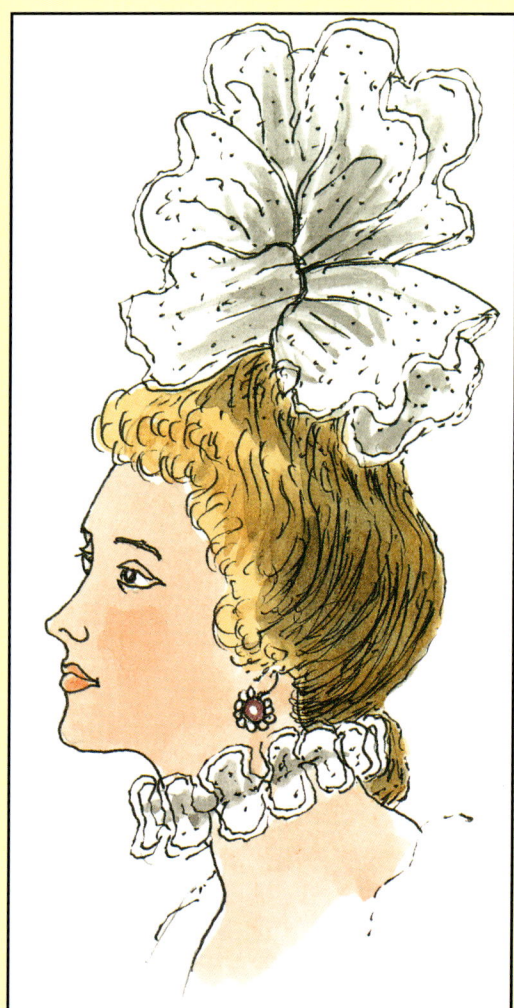

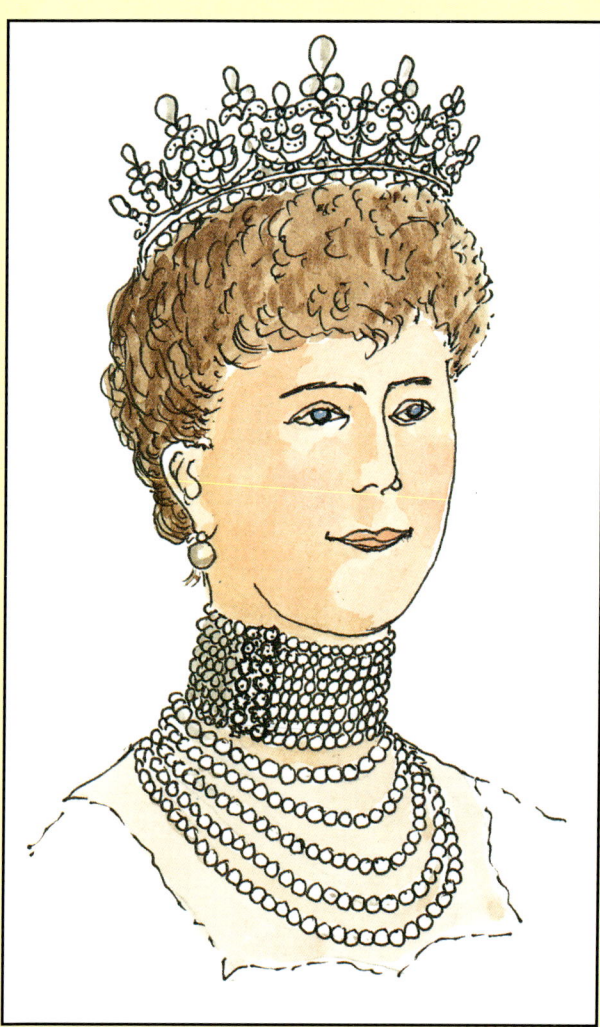

For grand occasions, royalty and the aristocracy donned diamond and pearl tiaras. Also here is a pearl choker, in which can be seen the open-work diamond clasp that kept the strings of pearls in place. Pearl or diamond necklaces added to the splendor, as did pearl earrings, traditionally fastened through pierced ears. The first screw-on earrings appeared in 1899.

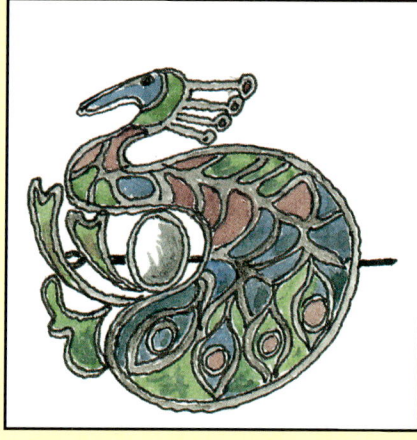

An Art Nouveau peacock brooch in enamel, with a pearl center.

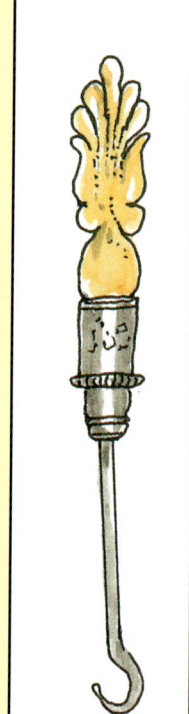

A small steel and carved-bone glove button hook. Such hooks were naturally much in use before, but even more so when, at this period, evening gloves could have up to 20 buttons.

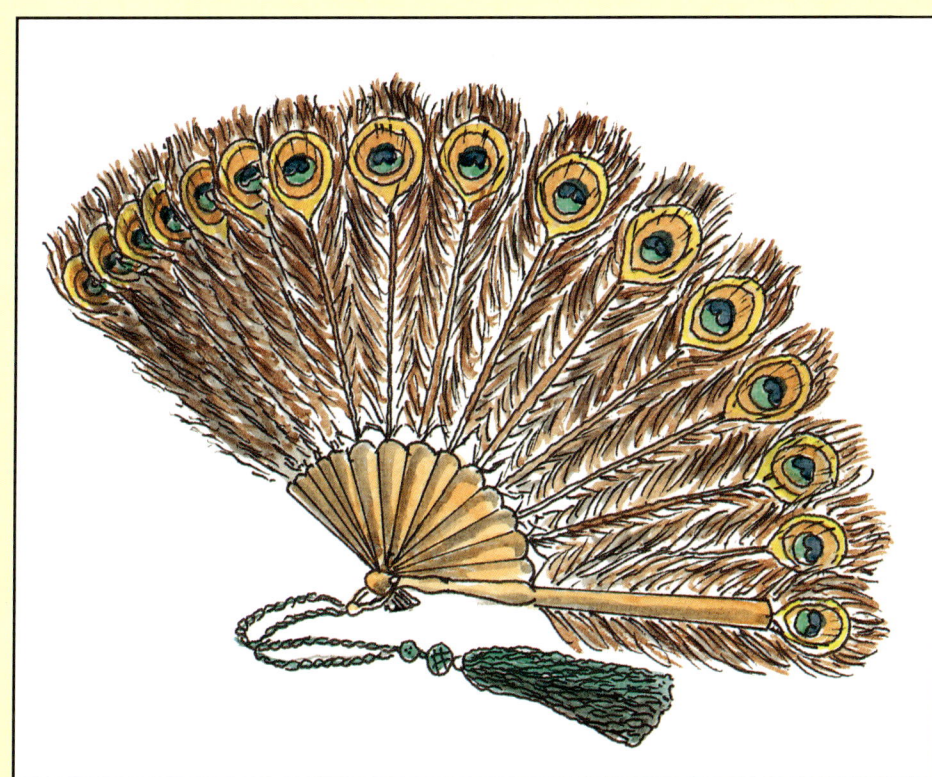

Real peacock-feather fans had been popular since about the 1870s, but because the bird was a symbol of the 1890-1910 Art Nouveau Movement, similar fans gained more popularity during this period.

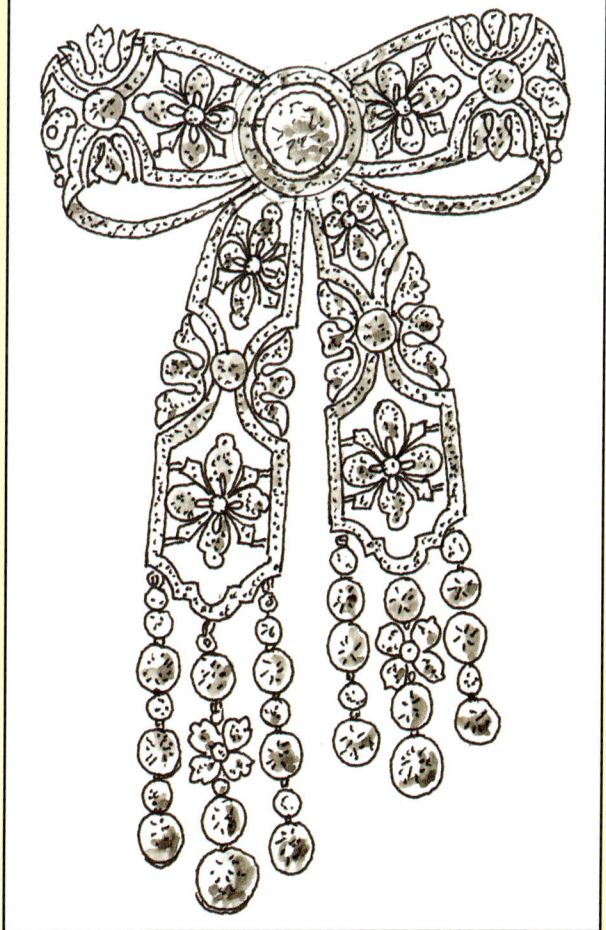

Diamond or paste bow-shaped jewelry dates from the eighteenth century; this very elaborate brooch or corsage ornament gave luxury to a very grand evening gown.

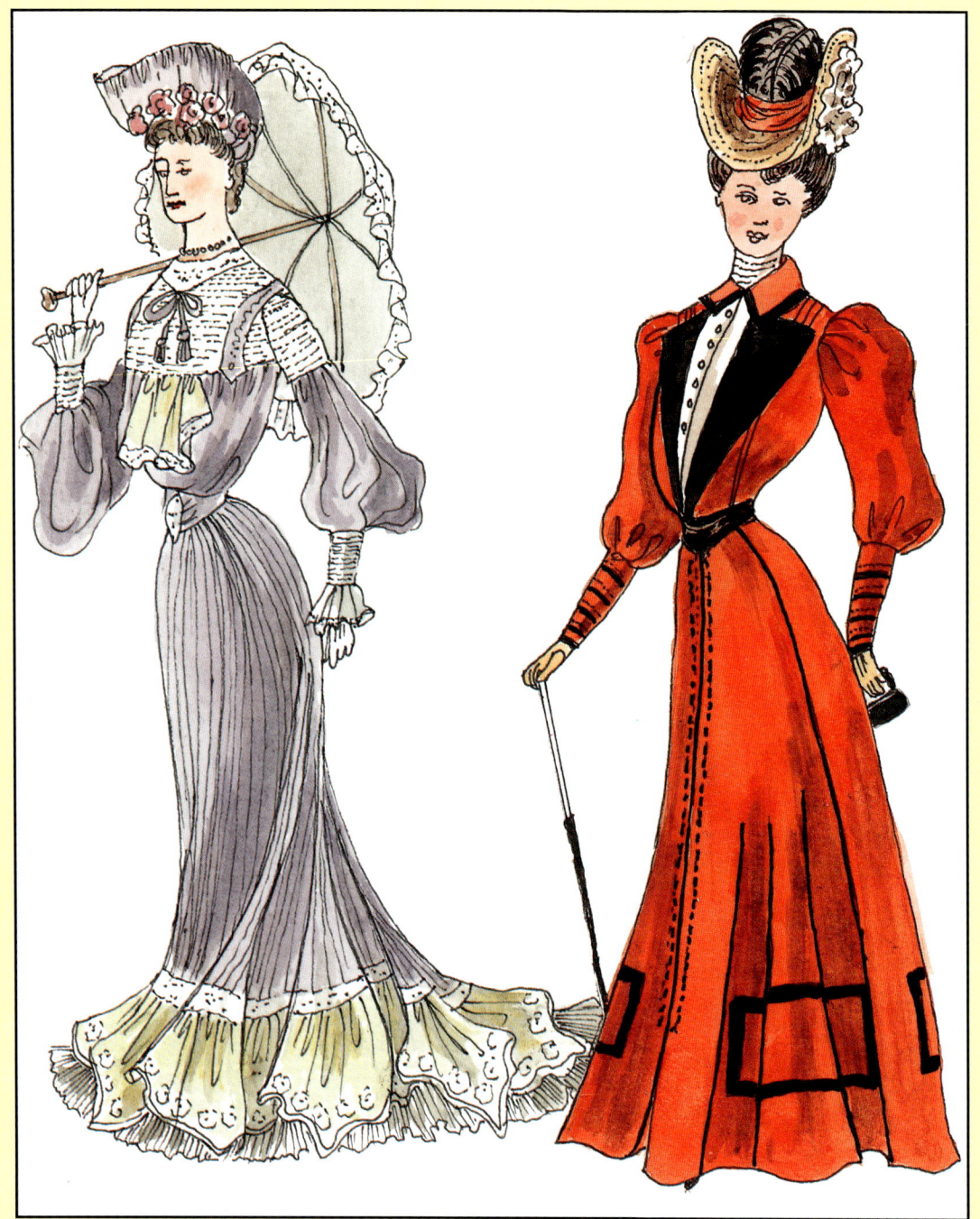

1902-1908 Day Wear

This was the period of the "Edwardian Summer" in Britain and "La Belle Epoque" in France. For this period of great luxury (for those who were well-off), the Americans seem to have no equivalent term, but along with women of other countries, rich American women flocked to Paris to buy the latest fashions, accompanied by dressmakers intent on creating copies for their less-affluent customers. America, however, could claim it as the era when mass-production exploded, goods sold in an ever-increasing number of department stores, and New York City was *the* shopping center.

Once again, fashion decreed that women be forced into an unnatural shape. The "S" bend, achieved by a corset which thrust the bustline out and down over a tiny waist and a protuberance at the rear. This line was also dubbed the "Gibson Girl" look, after American actress Camille Gibson, who popularized it.

For grand occasions, such as garden parties, the races, or society weddings, entire outfits (at left) were confections of soft silk or chiffon, with lace (often refurbished, valuable old lace) predominating, plus frills, furbelows, and long trains. Fashionable colors were white, violet, cream and pale green. In contrast, both for occasions and for everyday, simple tailor-mades (at right) with full upper sleeves, gored but not trained skirts, and a minimum of trimming, were equally smart.

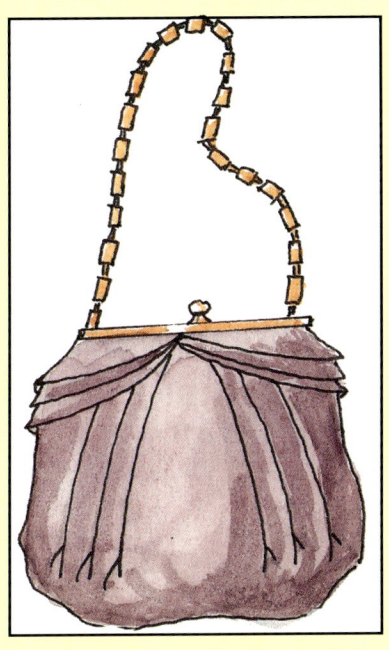

Handbags were either very small, as in the full-length figure, or large, in soft leather with gilt chains.

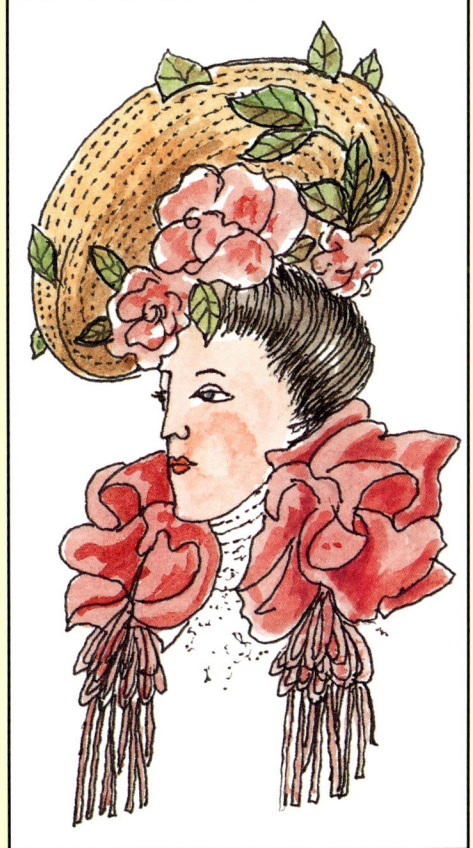

Another extravagant straw hat for summer.

During the brief "Edwardian Summer" of garden parties, Ascot and Henley Regatta, milliners excelled themselves with light-hearted creations such as this straw hat which must have been secured by a multitude of pins. Its silk roses are echoed in the ornate chiffon and ribboned boa.

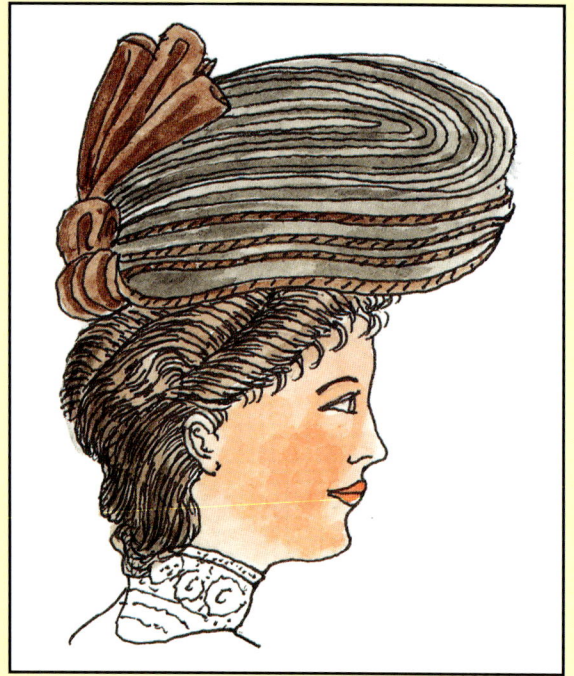

This type of ribbed and corded silk hat was critically called a "cake tin" or a "pie."

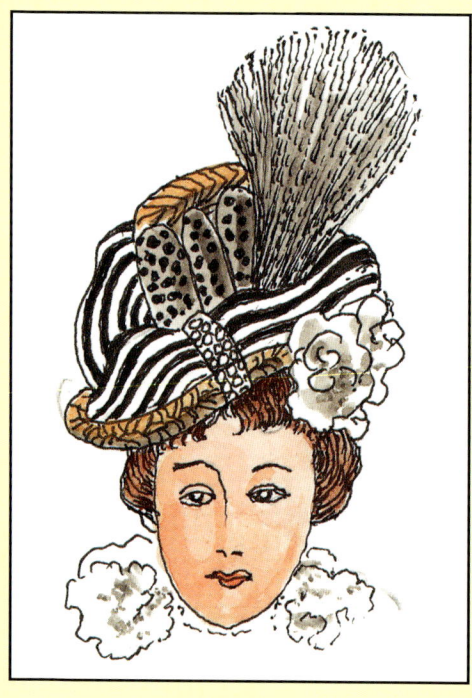

Toques were fashionable, such as this very elaborate creation with all kinds of materials and contrasting trimmings.

With the invention of the motorcar in 1896, women took to being driven around with great avidity. Because the cars were open, a new kind of hat in leather, felt or tweed, was created, tied on with a chiffon or gauze veil, which could be as much as 3/4 yards wide and 2 yards long.

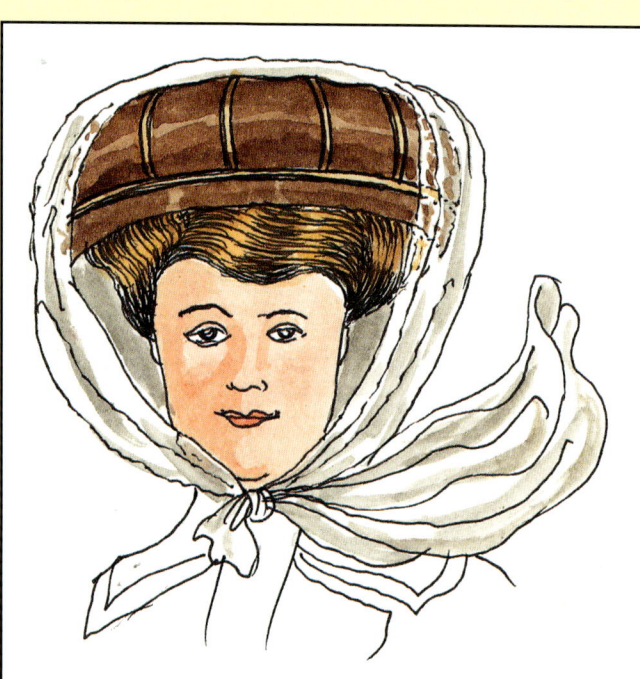

A straw boater hat was worn chiefly at the seaside or for tennis.

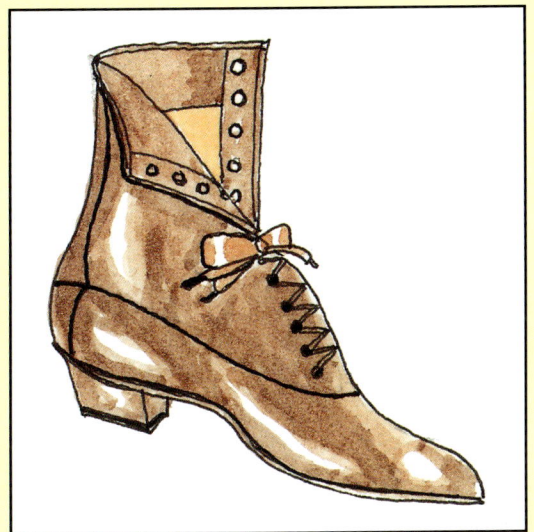

This leather boot has a fashionable Cuban heel.

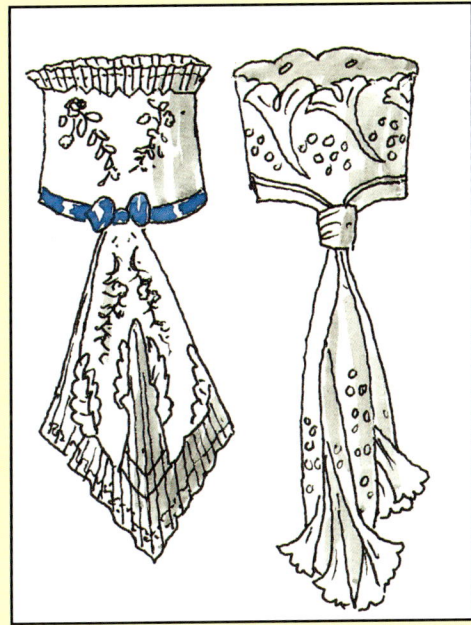

Two of the many kinds of separate embroidered linen, muslin, *broderie Anglaise,* or lace jabots, worn with equally ornate blouses.

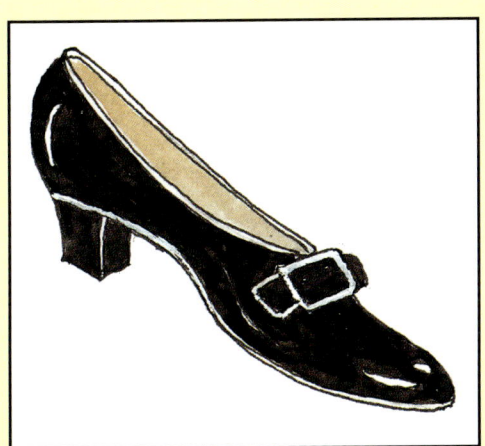

A patent leather shoe with a buckle.

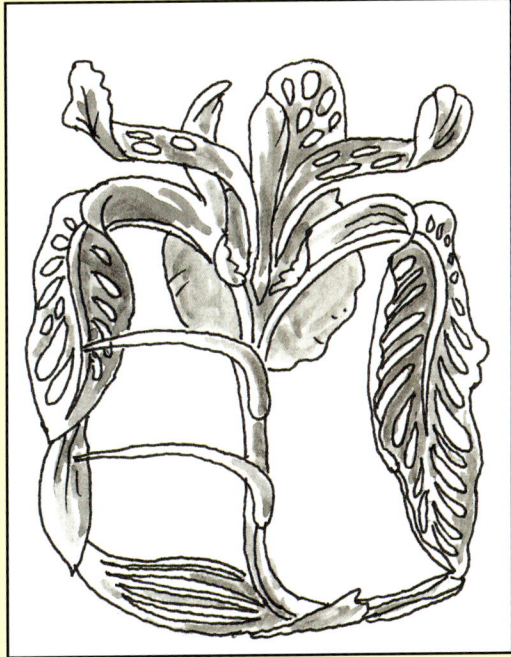

The fashion-dictated "S" bend could only be achieved by wearing an armor-like, unhealthy corset; even so, this corset was made out of patterned material and bedecked with ribbons and lace.

A silver Art Nouveau belt buckle.

69

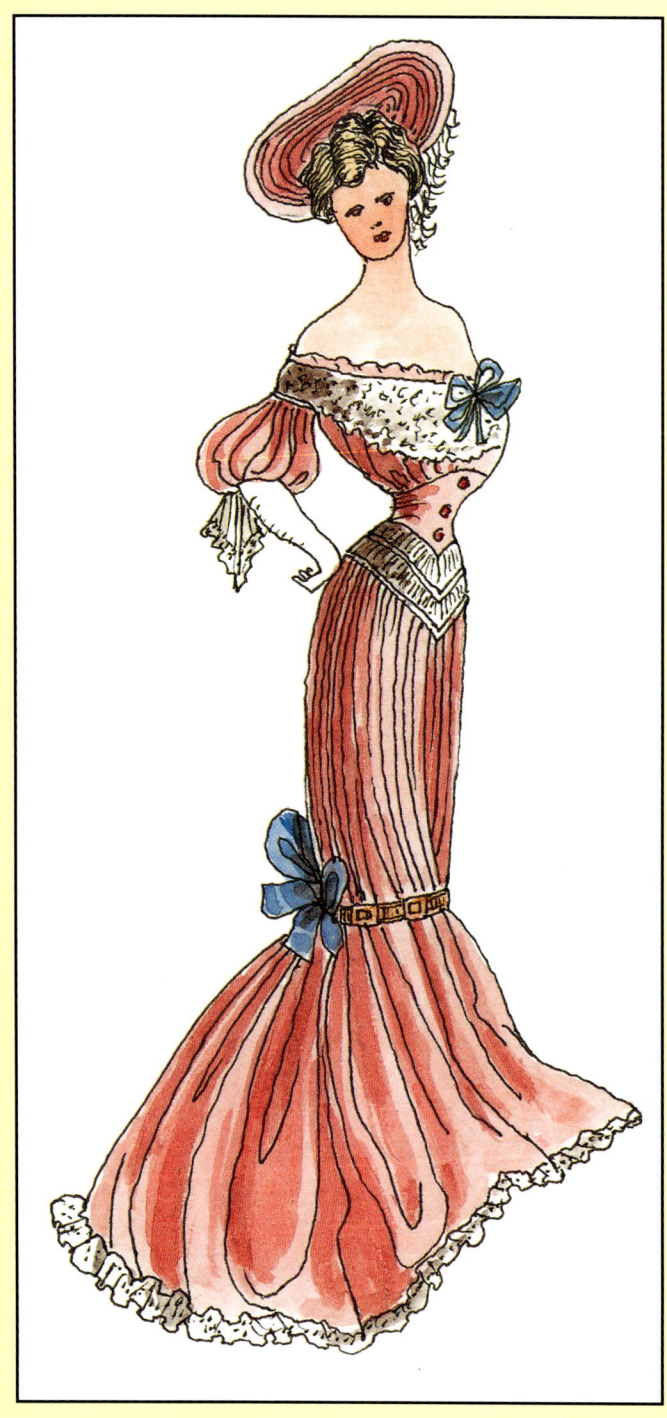

1902-1908 Evening Wear

The "Gibson Girl" look was even more evident in the ballroom. Dresses had pouter-pigeoned décolletage nearly falling off the shoulders, and the bustline was bedecked with lace, ribbon, and jewels; the waist was very small and pleated skirts were tight to the knees where they spread out into wide, frilled and laced, fan-shaped trains. Although white, black, or both together, were fashionable, as the "garden party" look, colors were also soft and delicate. Following French fashions, huge hats were worn in restaurants and in the theater.

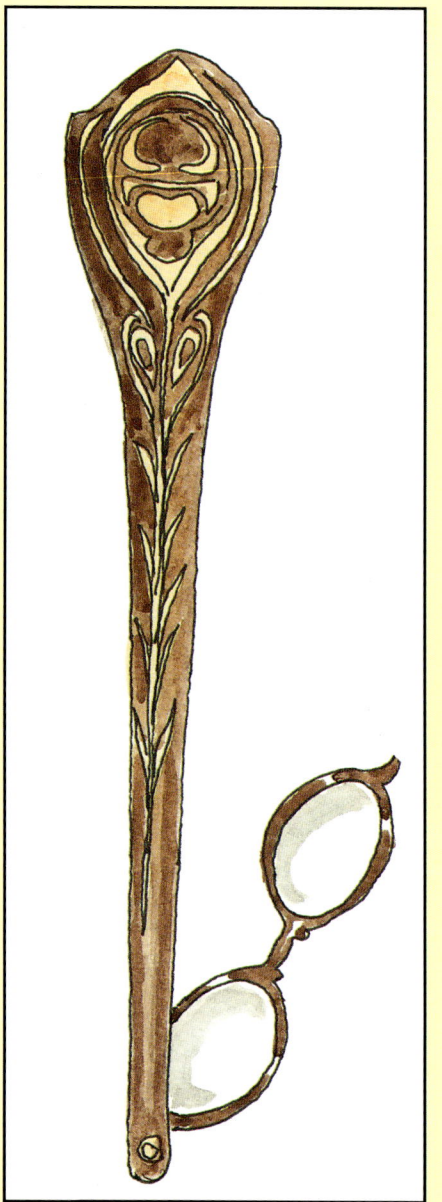

A pair of lorgnettes; the wooden case shaped and carved in Art Nouveau style.

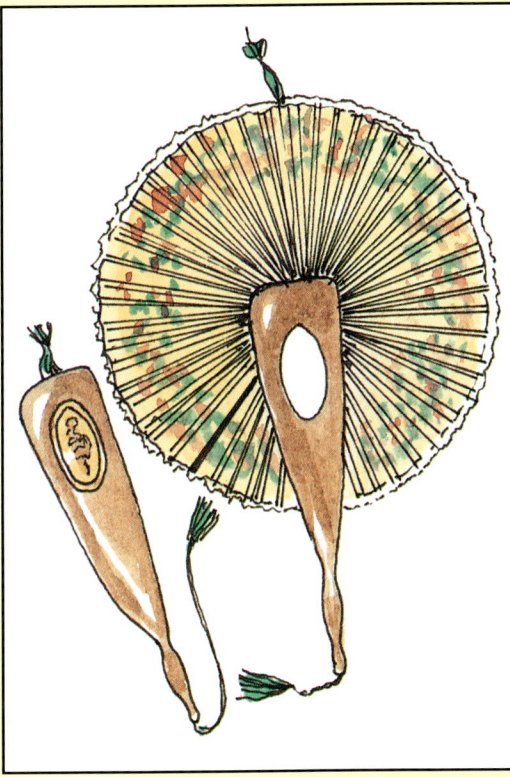

Conventional fans were made of sequinned lace, feathers, or painted silk, but a novelty was this "souvenir" fan. The olive wood "guard" holds a pleated, lace-edged "leaf" which is extended by pulling the top tassel and returned to its "guard" by pulling the lower one. One side of the "guard" is decorated with marquetry, the other with a mirror.

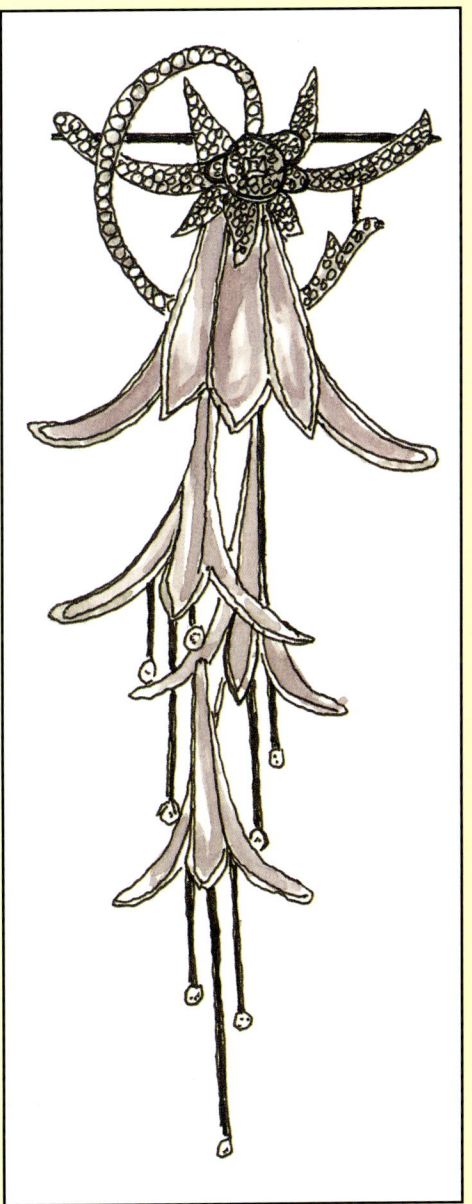

A particularly lovely fuchsia-shaped brooch in diamonds and translucent enamel.

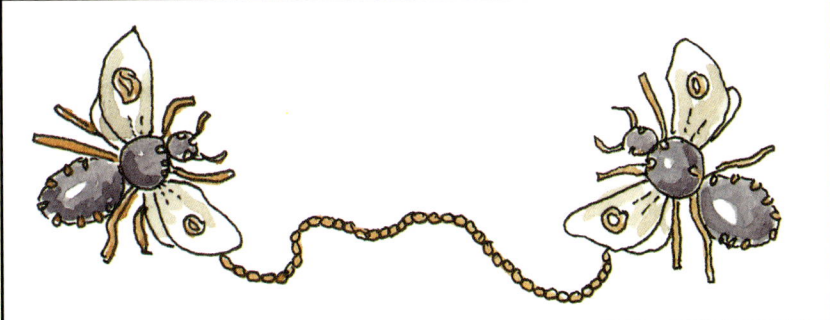

An evening cloak-fastener: two gold, amethyst, and enamel butterflies linked by a gilt chain.

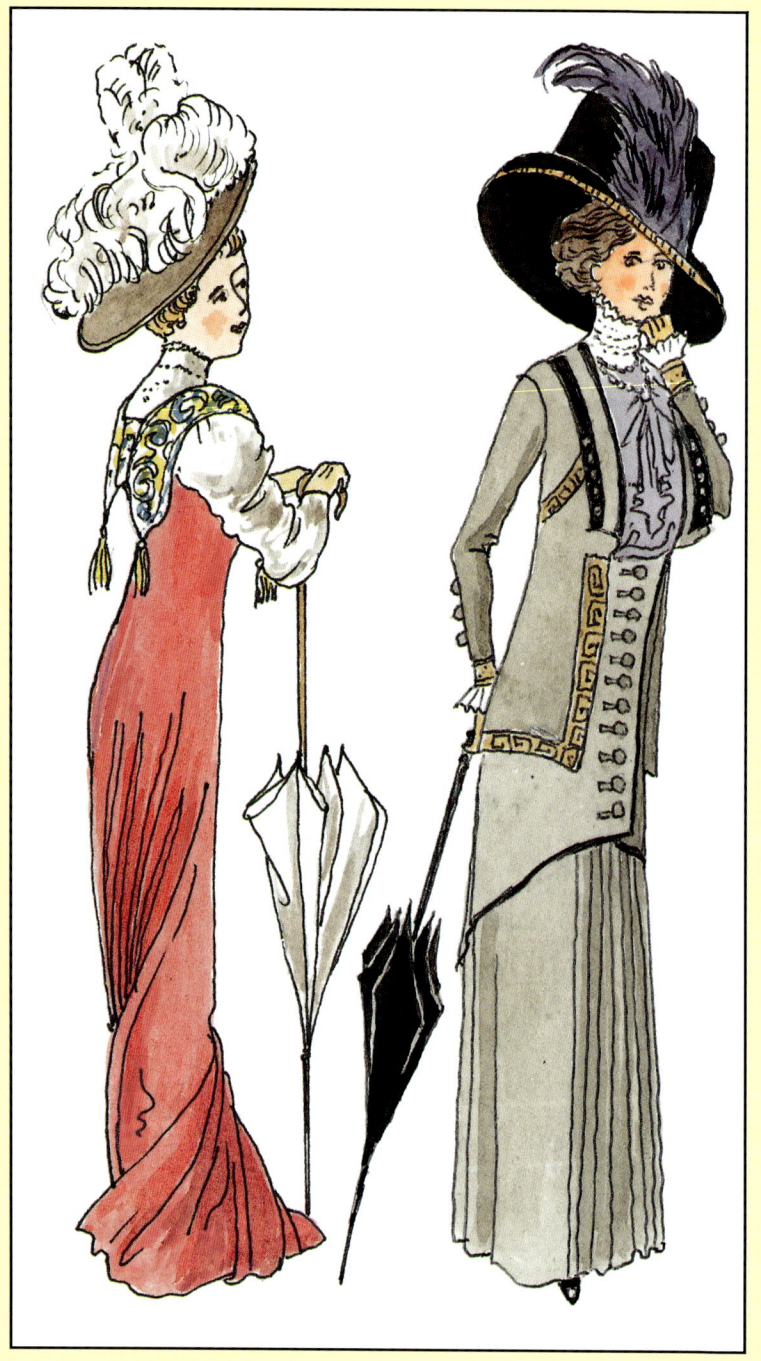

1908-1911 Day Wear

Another startling change occurred in this period—a fashion revolution in fact. In 1908, the French couturier Paul Poiret decreed that the figure-distorting "S" bend be abandoned and that women should return to their natural shape. He is credited with dismissing the corset altogether, but even his new silhouette required some support. The ultra-smart "feminine" woman (at left) wore a train on her narrow dress with its sparse but rich trimming. Tailor-mades (at right), still fashionable for all types of women, were equally narrow but with no trains and with simple trimming. The only garment in the old style was the lace or silk, frilled blouse with its high, boned collar. Huge hats literally dominated this period.

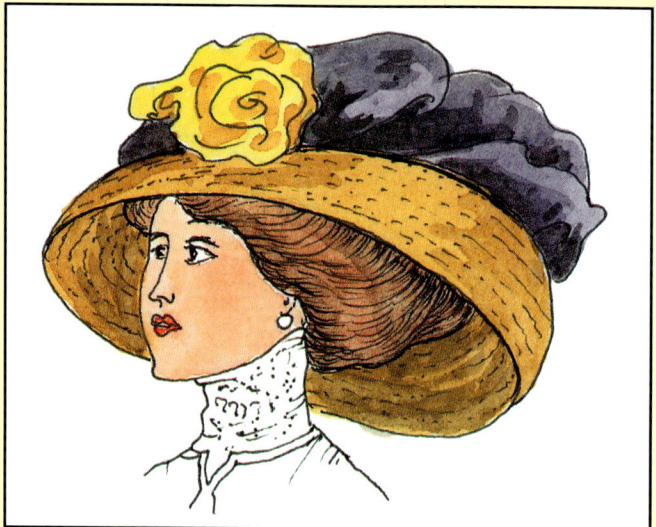

An overwhelming straw hat piled high with a mountain of silk.

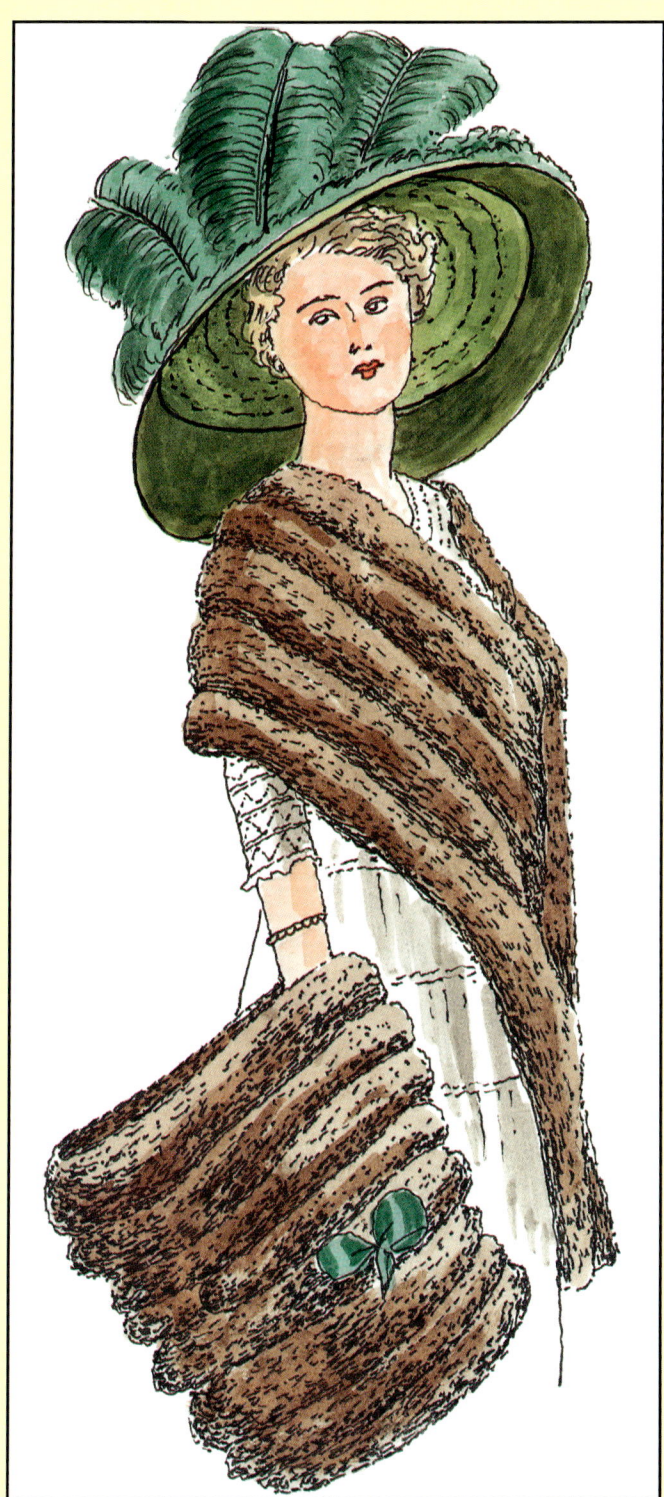

"Merry Widow" or "My Fair Lady" hats overwhelmed the new narrow figures, making women look like heavy-headed flowers on thin stalks. This "cartwheel" felt and stitched silk creation certainly swamps the wearer. Fur stoles, in sable, chinchilla, or skunk, were very fashionable and worn with large matching muffs.

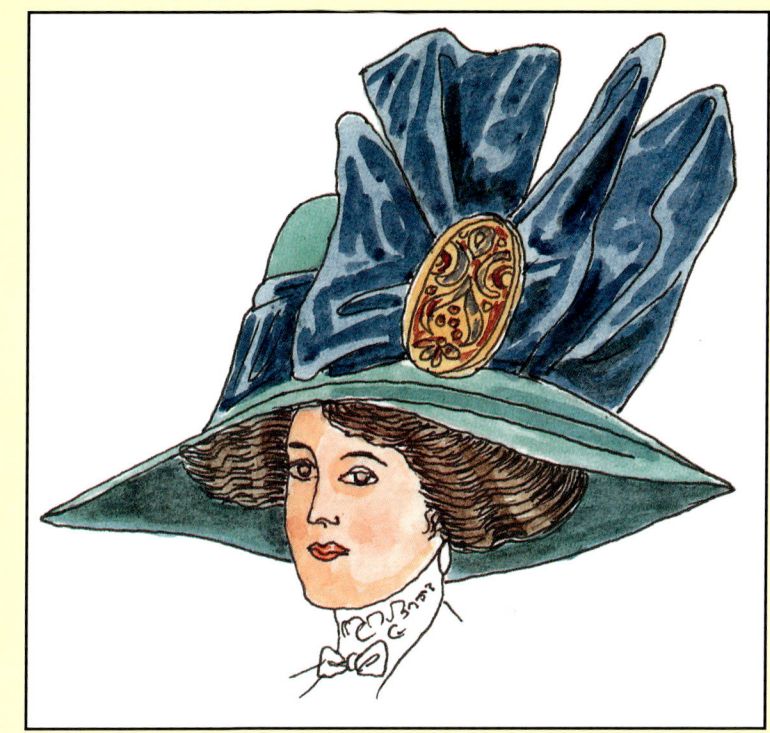

Felt and ribbon hat, secured by a gilt and enamel brooch.

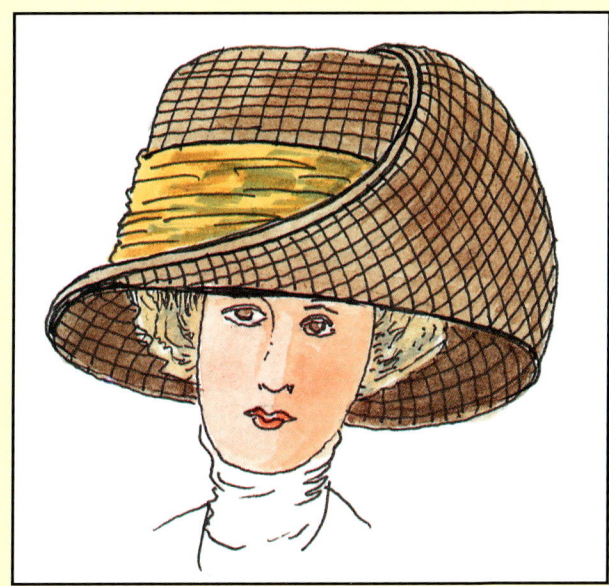

Stitched silk and silk ribbon make up this creation.

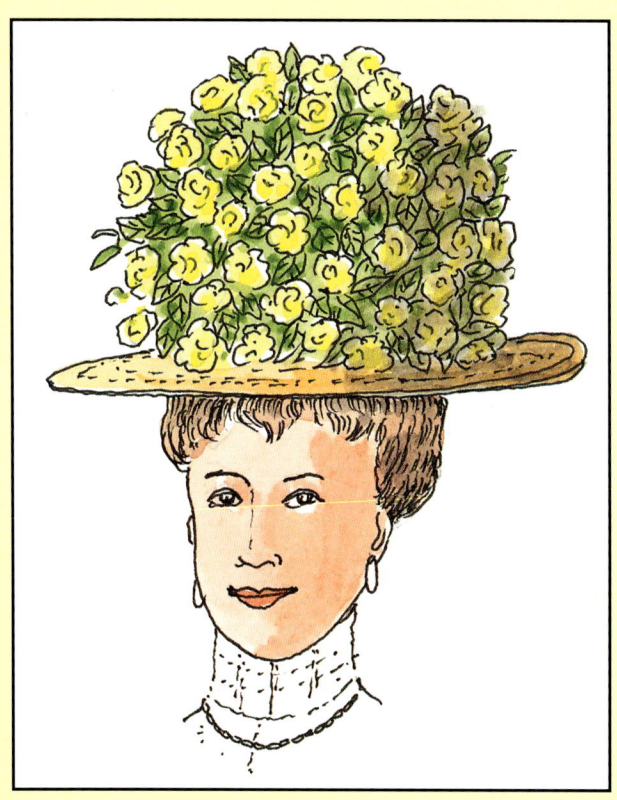

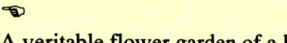
A veritable flower garden of a hat.

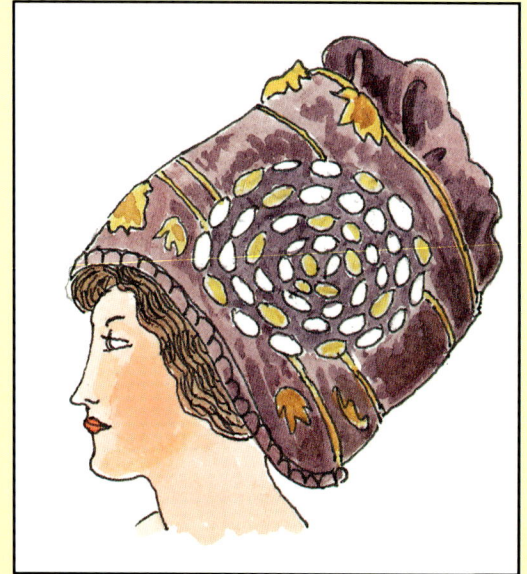

Boots still prevailed; this one in punched and stitched leather.

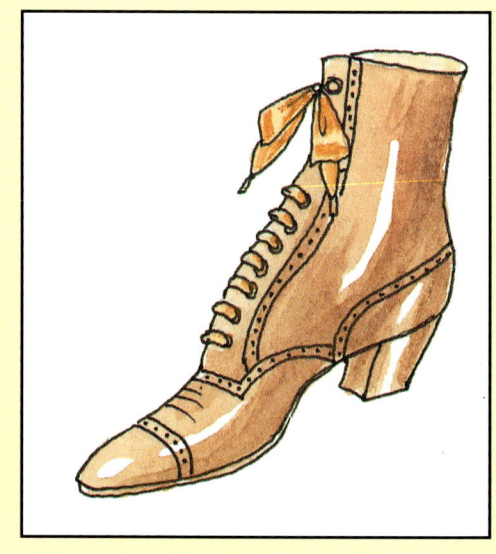

Probably worn in a restaurant or at the theater, a silk turban, liberally sewn with gold embroidery, ornaments, and beads.

Much-folded velvet hat fastened together with a barbaric hammered-metal and semiprecious jeweled clasp.

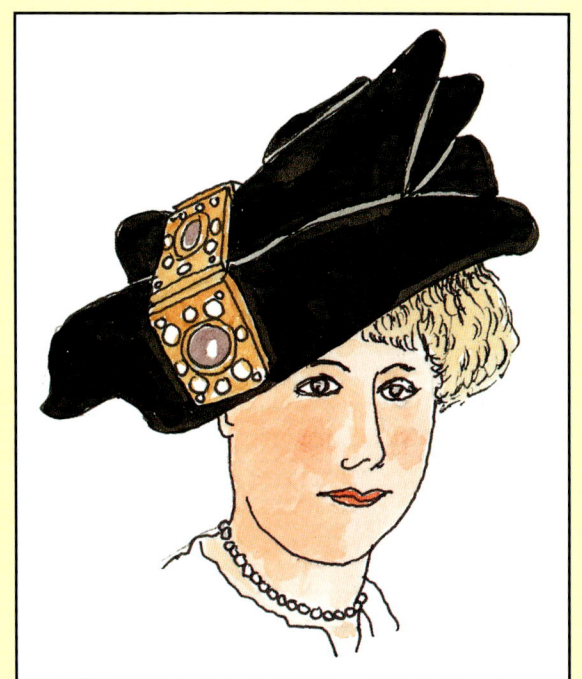

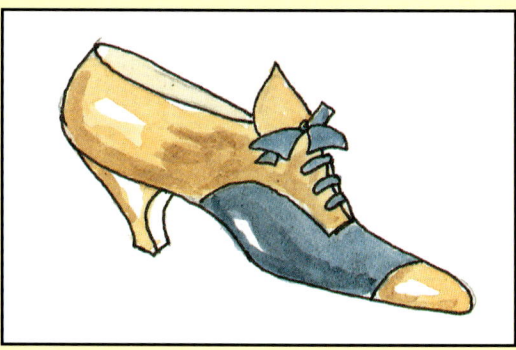

Two-colored leather shoes with louis heels were popular

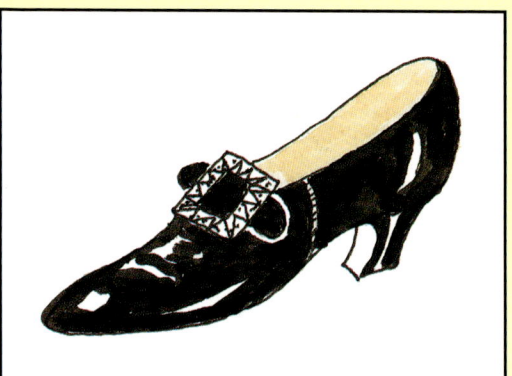

Extra-large paste or metal buckle on a man's style patent leather shoe.

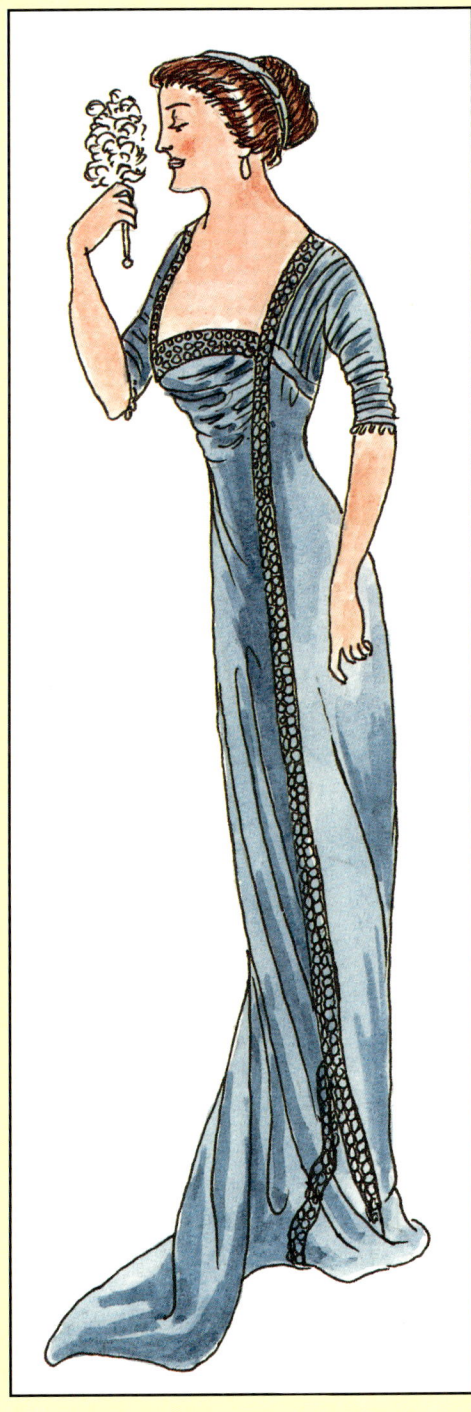

1908-1911 Evening Wear

For evening, women must have been relieved to abandon the "S" bend for a svelte but still trained dress, which could be simply or richly trimmed with braid or embroidery, although lace had not completely been abandoned as a trimming.

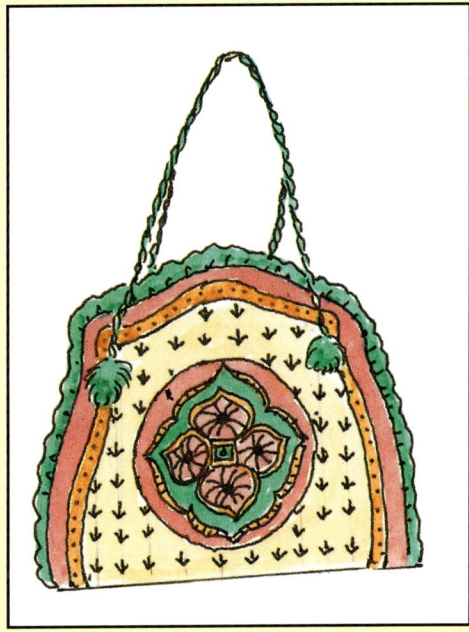

This ornate evening bag, at the time called surprisingly "simple and graceful," is a welter of satin, taffeta, embroidery, cords, and tassels.

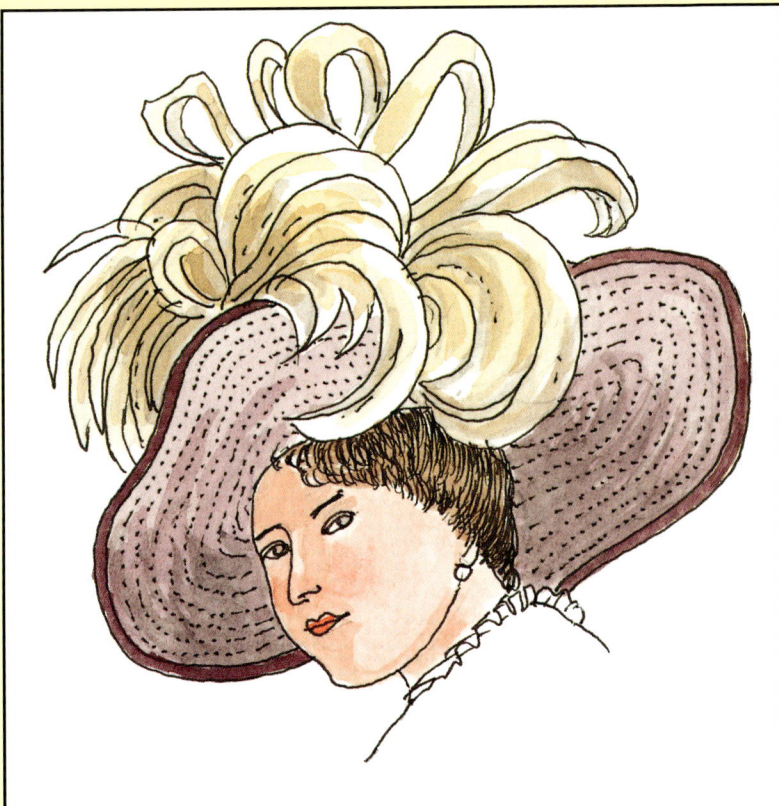

Still following the European fashion, large, often feathered, hats were worn in London and New York restaurants. At the theater they provoked the annoyance of anyone sitting behind the wearer. A contemporary cartoon showed a man complaining. "I've paid ten guineas for my seat and I want to see the stage." To which the lady replies: "And I've paid ten guineas for my hat, and I want to be seen."

75

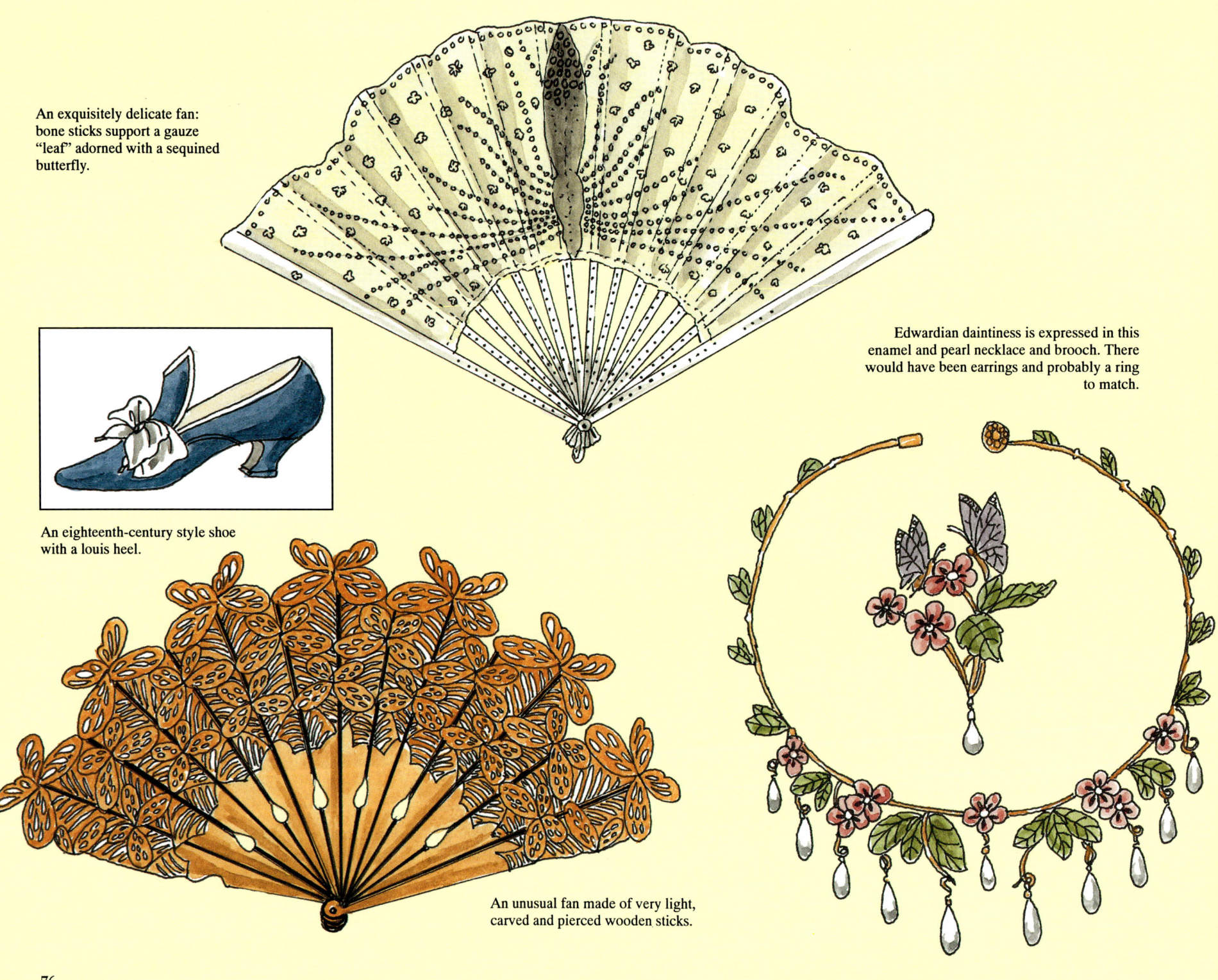

An exquisitely delicate fan: bone sticks support a gauze "leaf" adorned with a sequined butterfly.

An eighteenth-century style shoe with a louis heel.

Edwardian daintiness is expressed in this enamel and pearl necklace and brooch. There would have been earrings and probably a ring to match.

An unusual fan made of very light, carved and pierced wooden sticks.

1911-1915 Day Wear

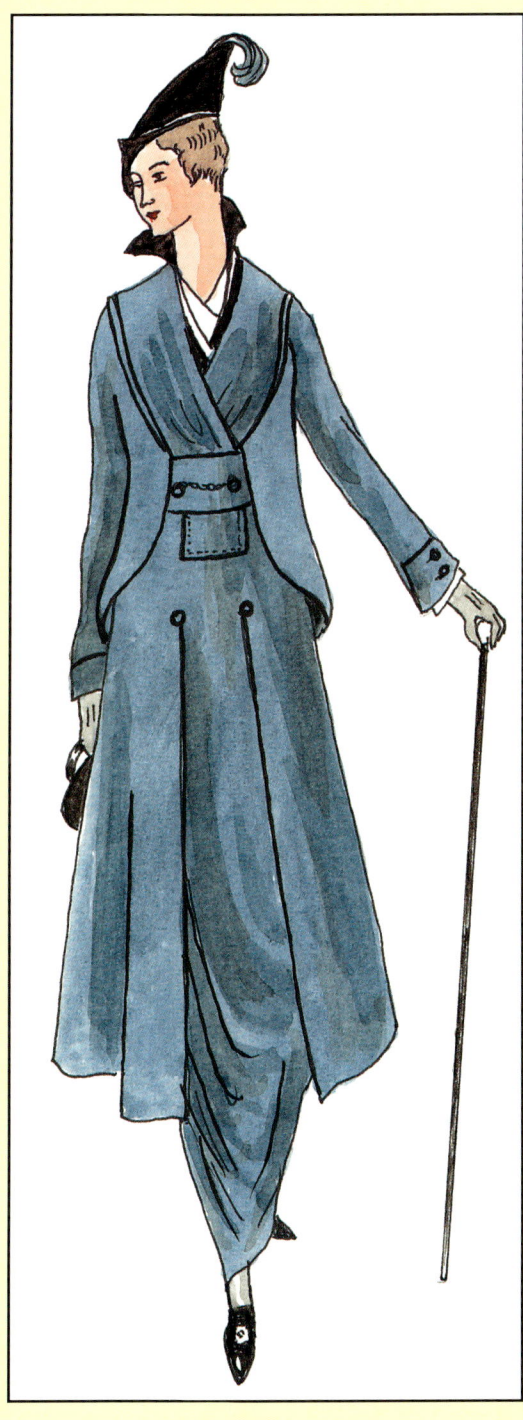

During this period, fashion was notable for its variety, with Poiret's influence still strongly felt. The bustline was at its natural level as was the waist, which was defined by a sash, band, or peplum. Skirts showed the ankles and could be swept up to the hips in two tiers. So tight around the ankles was the "harem" or "hobble" skirt (condemned by the Pope) that walking was difficult, but this was a fashion for only the few. The look was slim and elegant or rather bulky. Trimming was minimal with fur edging for winter. Materials included serge, sprigged, or striped silks and muslin for summer. Colors were both bright and subdued.

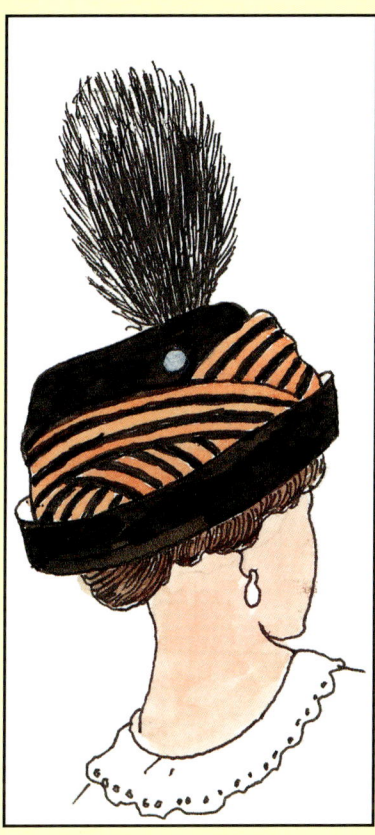

This trim little felt toque bound with silk ribbon (which, incidentally, matched the dress), with the addition of a brush-like aigrette.

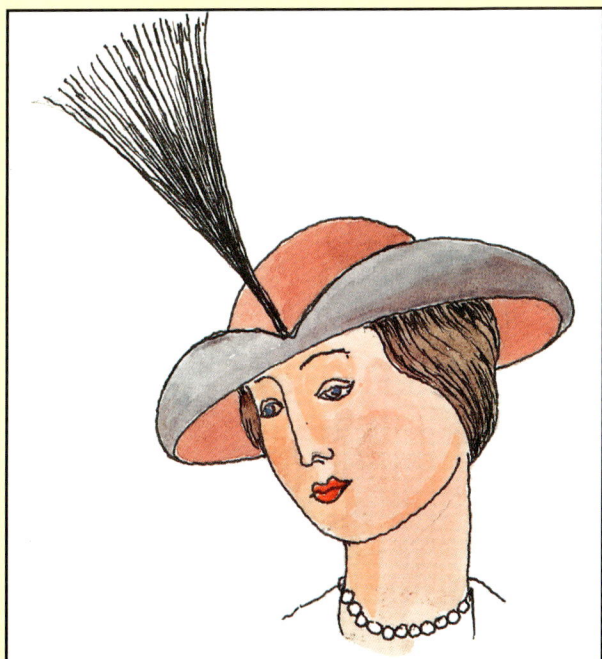

A stiffened velour hat made less simple with an aigrette.

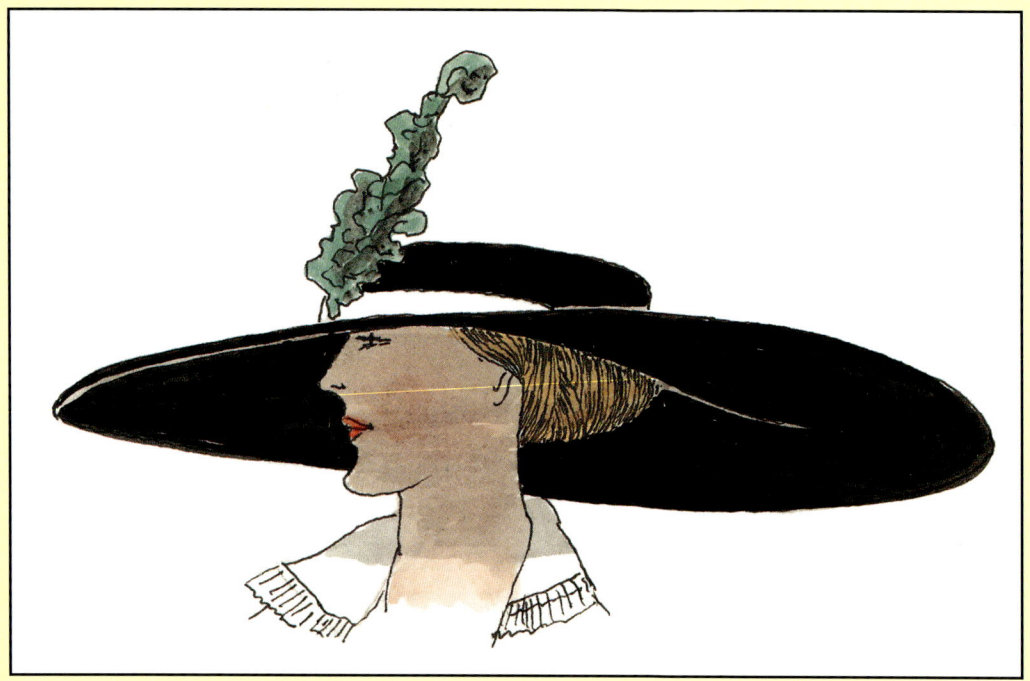

A shallow velvet "cartwheel" hat, sparked with a long feather.

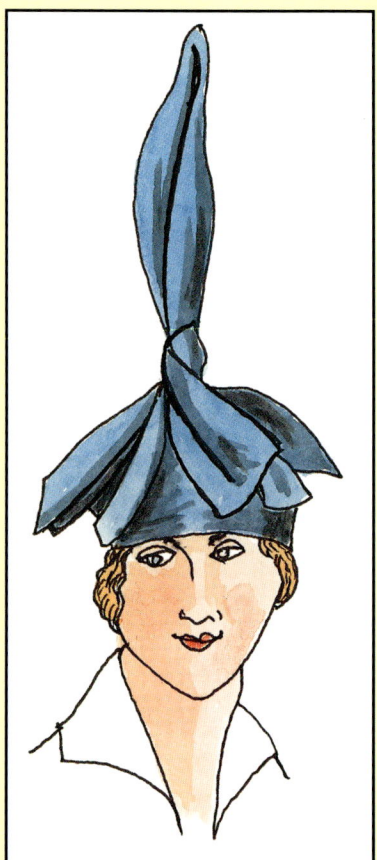

An exclamation mark of a hat: a velvet pillbox surmounted by wired twists.

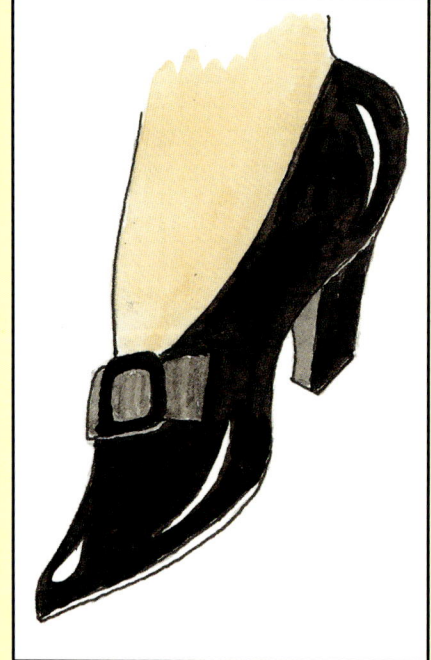

Bowed and buckled patent leather shoes were more visible when worn with the new tight, ankle-revealing skirts, especially if they were of the "hobble" variety.

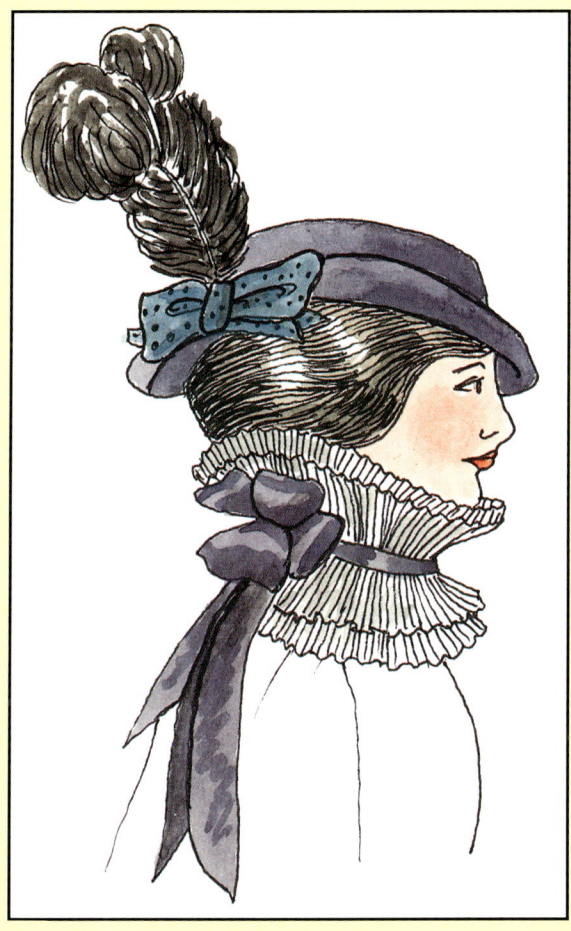

A mannish felt hat softened by a bow and ostrich feathers. Frilled, ribbon-secured, starched silk ruffs were very fashionable.

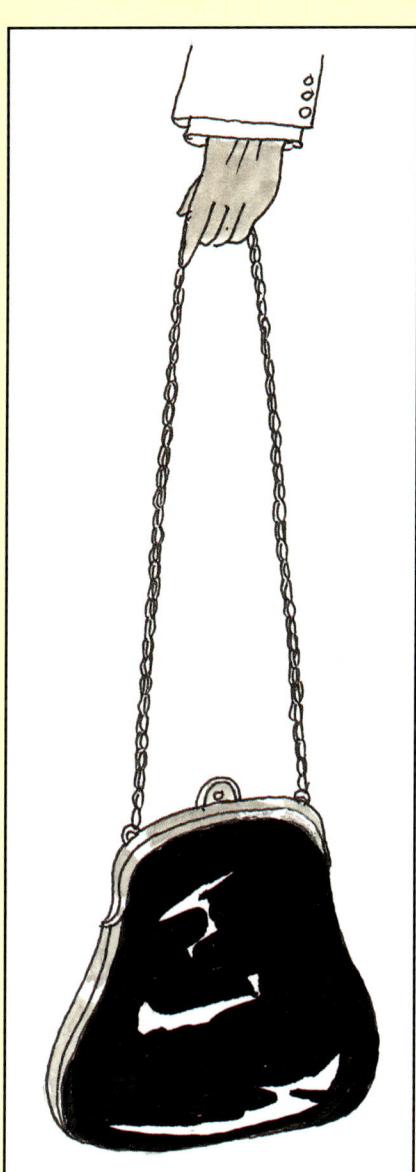

Huge leather handbags on long chains were very much in fashion. They could prove heavy and cumbersome, which was a gift to cartoonists.

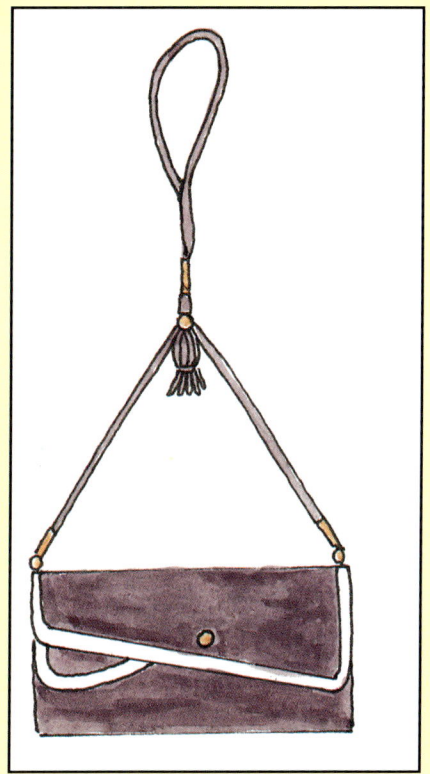

Smart and simple leather handbag.

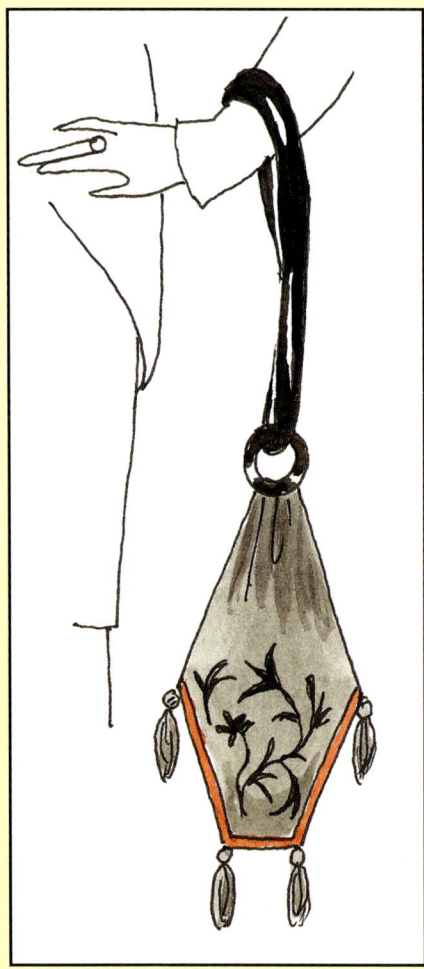

Rarely have handbags been so diverse as during this period: here, a tasseled and embroidered silk example.

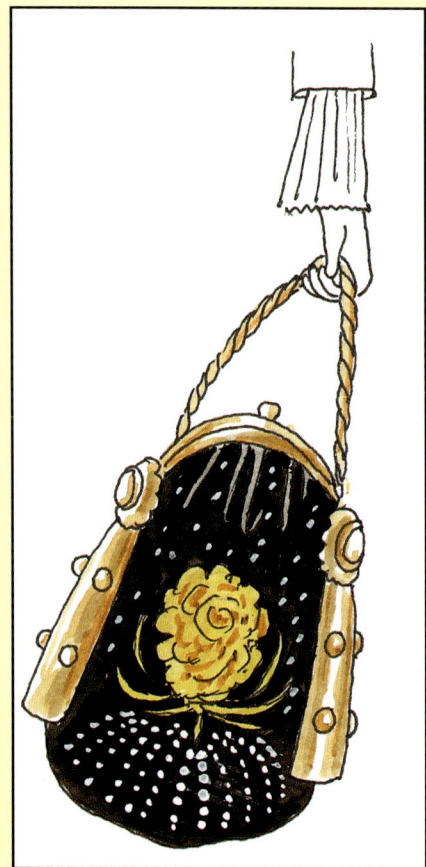

A particularly ornate handbag: made of velvet, embroidered, beaded, with a silk rose, it is mounted on a very complicated gilt frame.

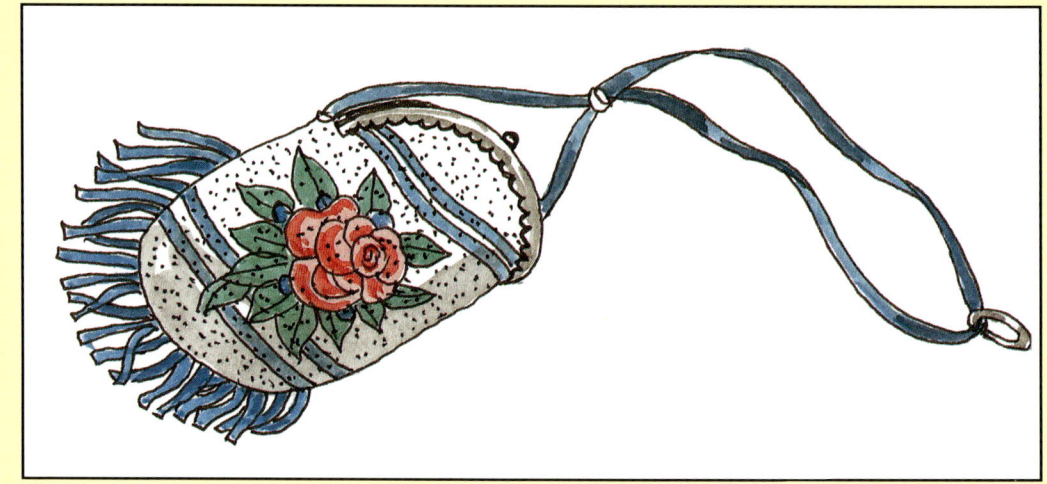

Heavily beaded handbag with a silk fringe.

1911-1915 Evening Wear

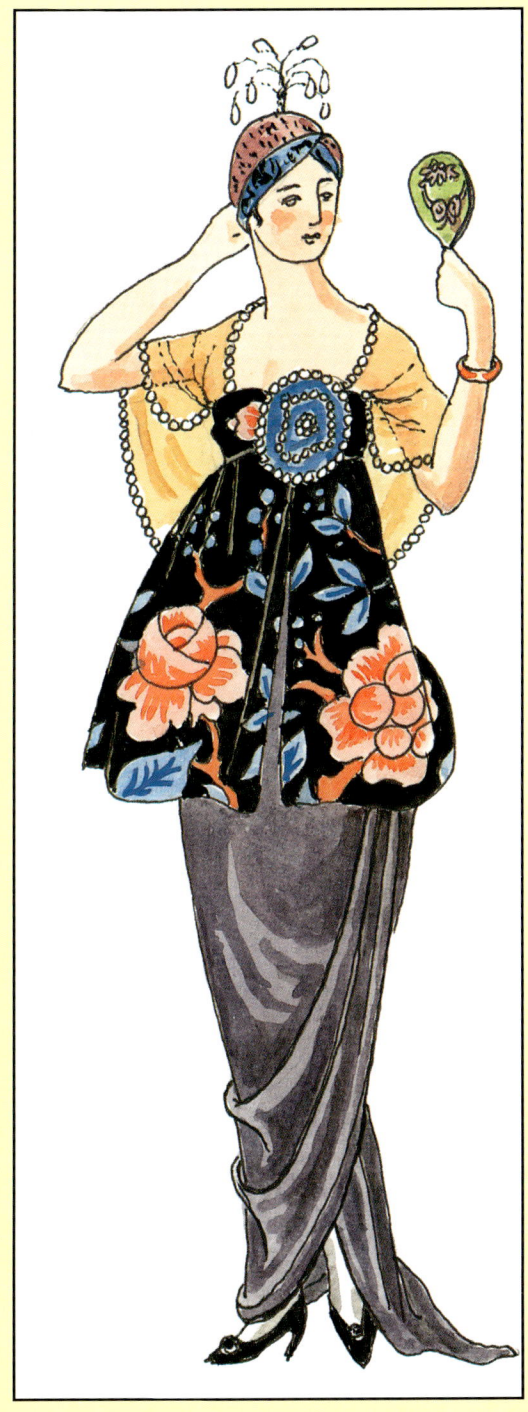

It was in evening wear that Poiret's influence was most strongly felt, with some of the most outlandish dinner and ball gowns ever known. Poiret particularly favored utmost simplicity with his "Greek" French Empire or British Regency dresses: narrow, low-necked and short-sleeved columns of muslin, topped by turbans. Turbans were also featured as the result of another evening fashion influence, that of the Russian Ballet which, with its rich sets, costumes in highly patterned materials, and violent, clashing colors, had shocked the cultural and fashion world when it first appeared in Paris in 1909 and in London in 1911. The ballet's "barbaric" and "eastern" costumes inspired some bizarre creations, as seen here: trained skirts topped by "Turkish" tunics in contrasting fabrics and plain or elaborate patterns.

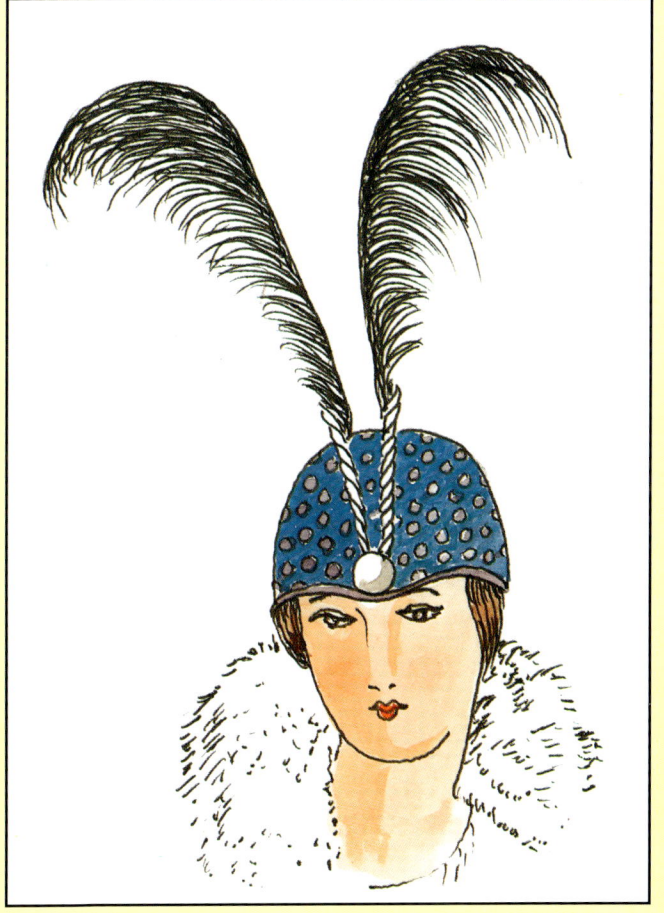

To compliment Russian Ballet-inspired evening dresses, turbans were much worn. Here, sequin-stitched velvet is surmounted by huge aigrettes and secured by a large bead.

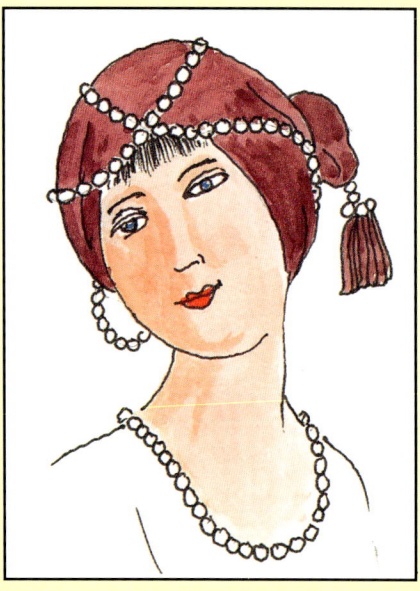

A simple satin turban bound with imitation pearls.

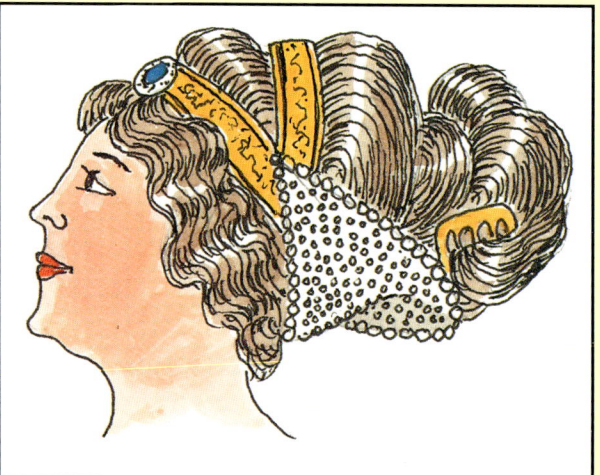

The "Grecian" look achieved with a gold braid, sequin-studded silk bandeau, and a gilt comb to secure the top-heavy coiffure.

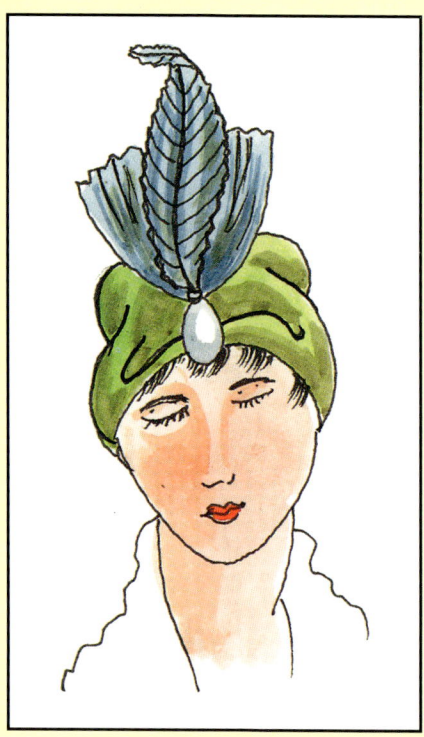

Feathers and a large "pearl" drop enliven a crushed-velvet turban.

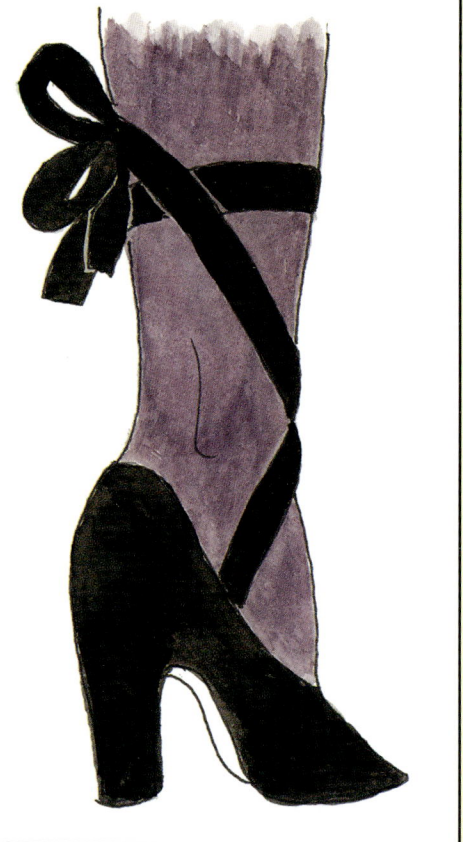

Draped evening skirts revealed yet more of a woman's foot, ankle, and leg. Hence this velvet shoe, secured by wide ribbons; colored stockings for evening were still the rage.

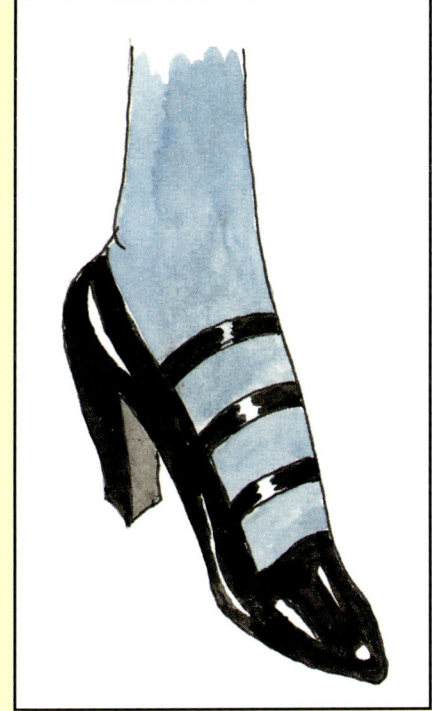

A simple patent-leather shoe made interesting with straps.

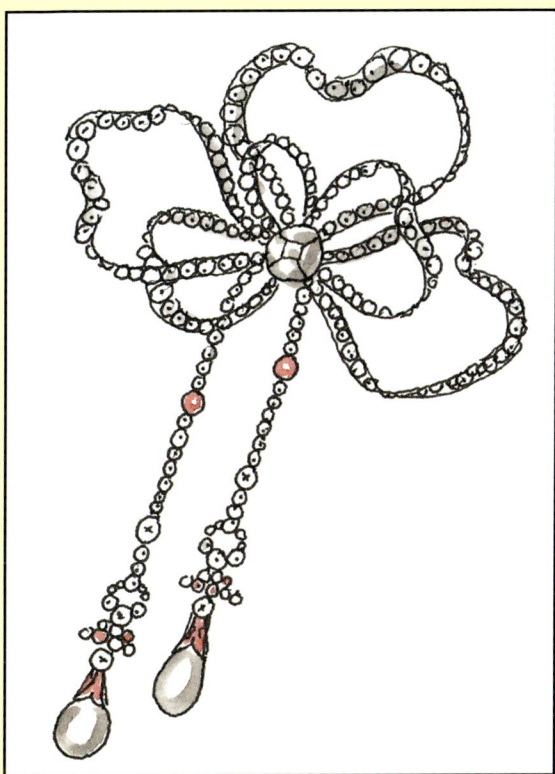

A conventional-minded woman would wear a traditional bow-shaped diamond brooch or corsage ornament; even so, in Edwardian taste, asymmetrical tied.

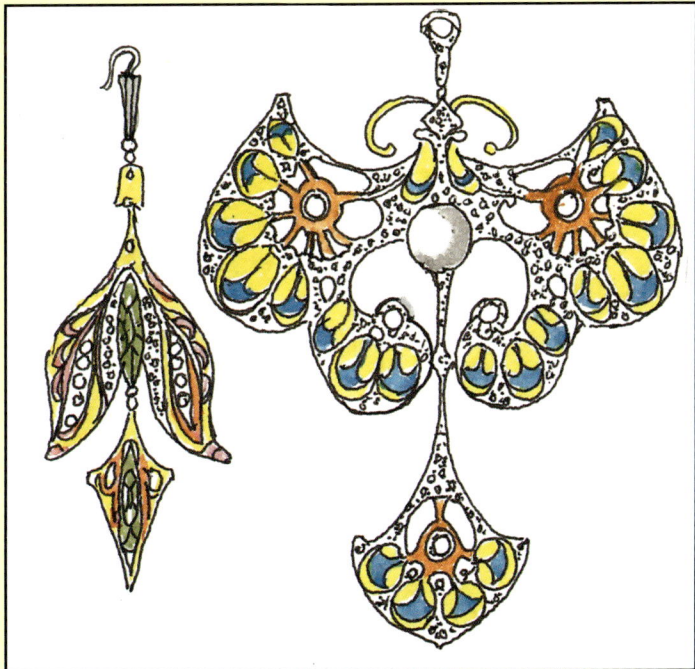

A Russian Ballet-influenced gold, enamel, diamond, and pearl earring and pendant.

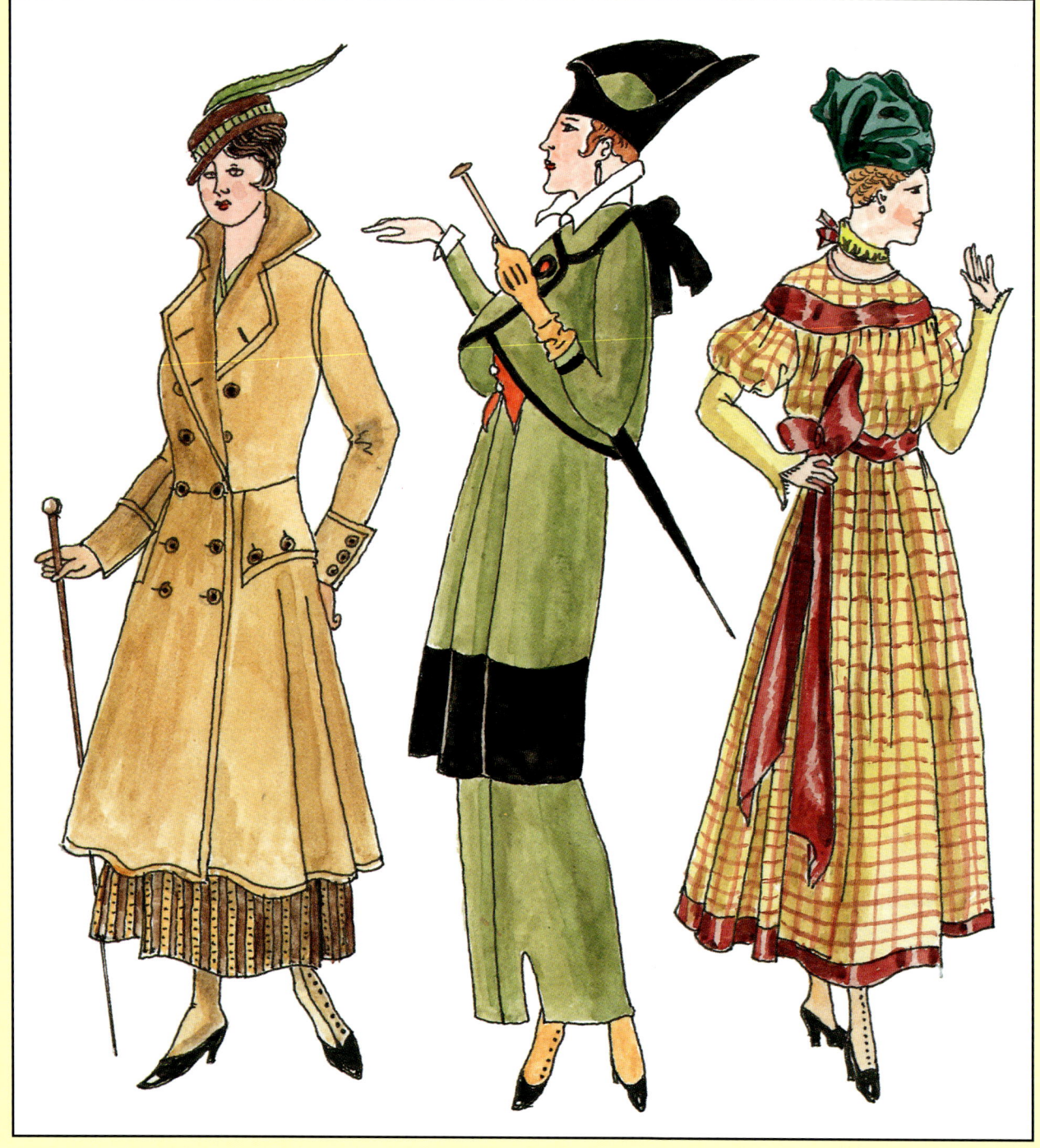

1915-1919 Day Wear

The First World War (1914-1918) did not affect fashion that greatly, especially because Paris, the fashion fountain-head, was unoccupied. British civilians suffered comparatively little and the Americans hardly at all. But, as shown in the three figures here, there were national differences for those women who wanted to look patriotic or not patriotic at all. The ankle-restricting skirts vanished and as British *Vogue* stated: "smartness no longer lay in 'slim economy of line'." This statement was not entirely true for French fashion, however.

The patriotic British woman (at left) is dressed in a simple coat and skirt in khaki, the color of military uniforms. The patriotic French woman (center) looks "warlike" in a simple coat and skirt but chic in the way in which only French women know how. The woman on the right is wearing the kind of French dress worn by those who carried on as if the War were not happening, although many British and American women also dressed in this manner to brighten up service men on leave.

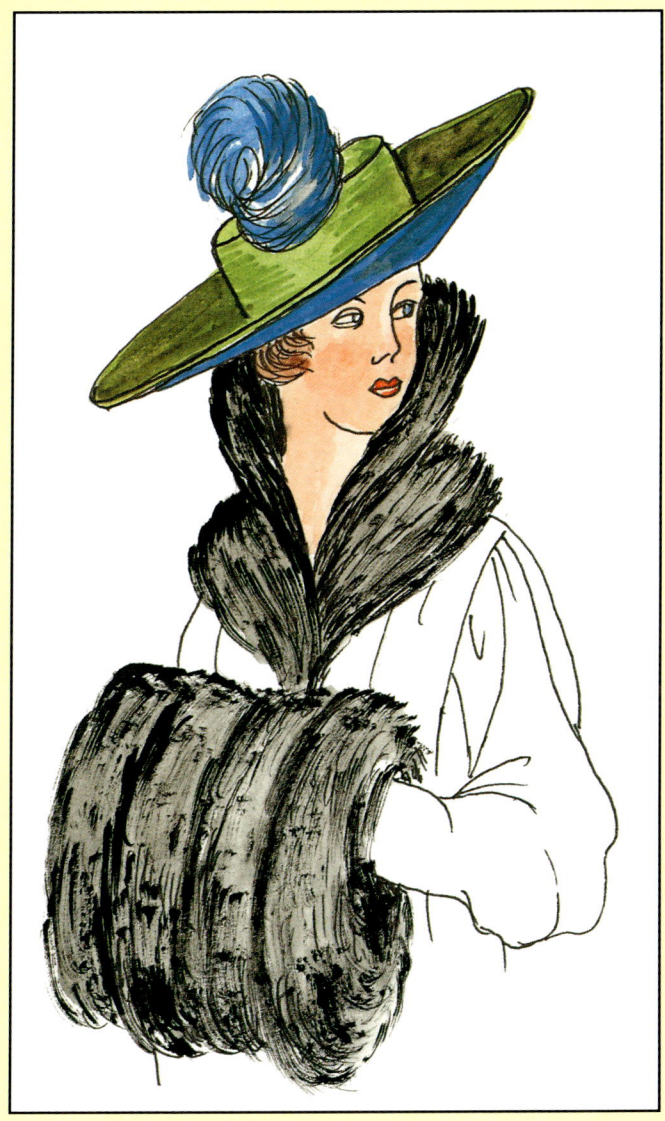

During the First World War, hats were varied and often eccentric. Perched at a fashionable angle, this silk hat is lined with velvet. In 1916 British *Vogue* showed "dainty accessories in fur for the immediate use of those who fancy them."

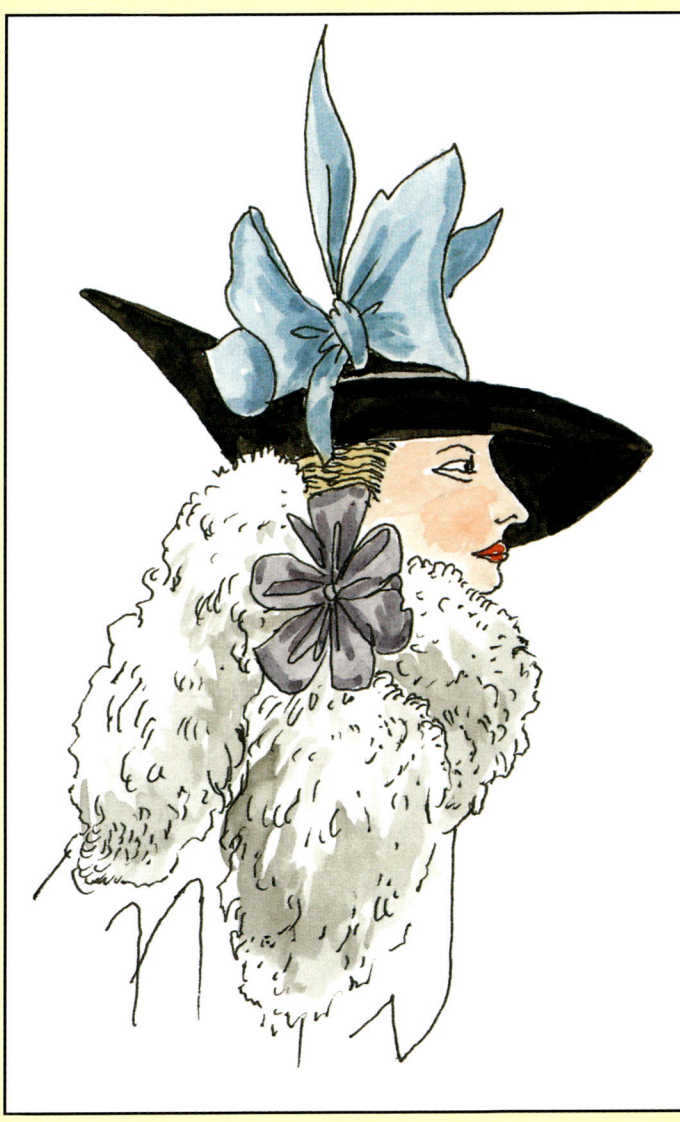

A huge silk bow gives style to a velvet hat, worn with an ostrich feather boa.

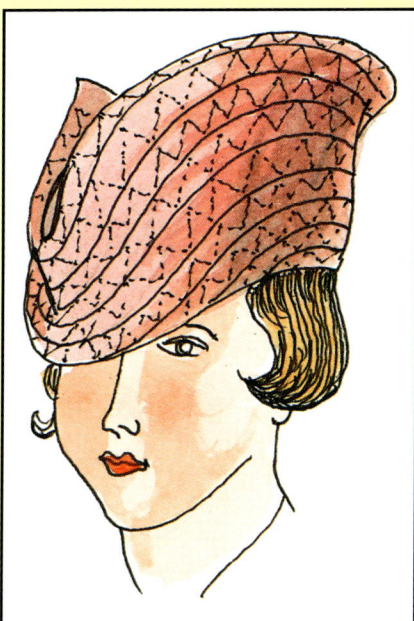

In contrast to wide or tall hats, little toques were also much worn; here, chenille and braid make up this tip-tilted example.

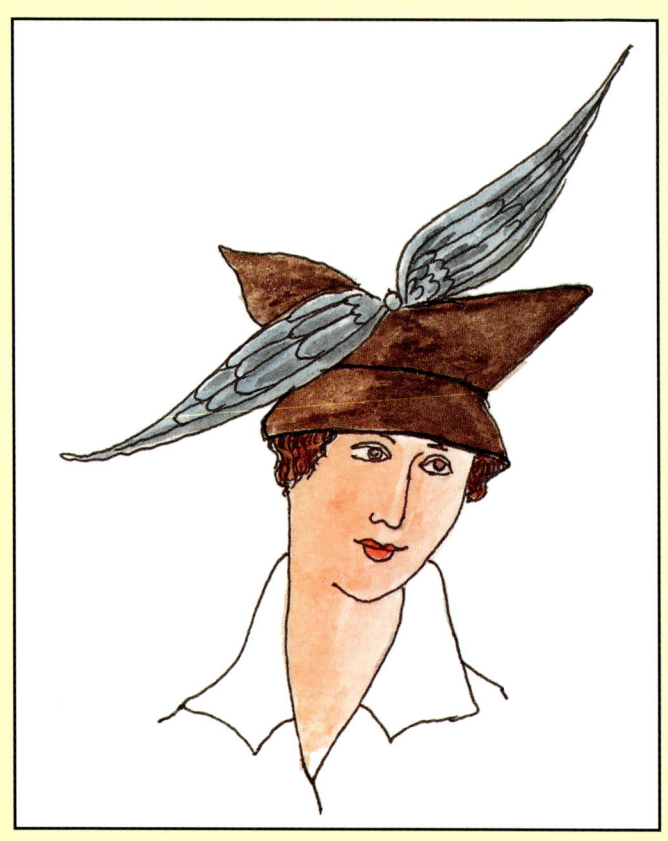

A pair of bird's wings "come to rest" on this peaked felt hat.

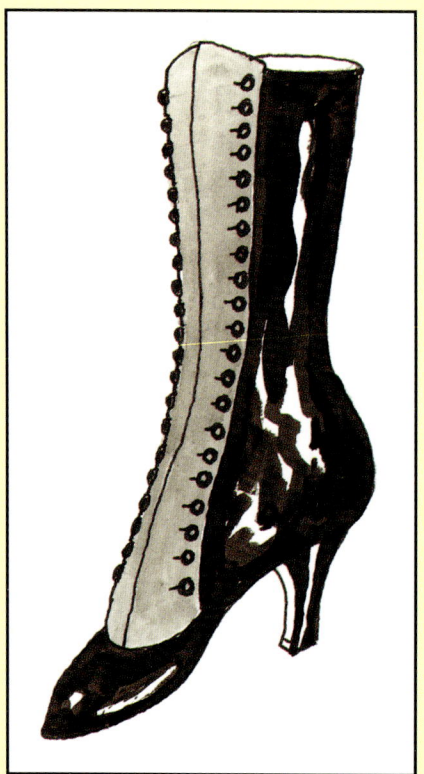

A patent-leather boot decorated and fastened with a multitude of buttons marching down the cloth front.

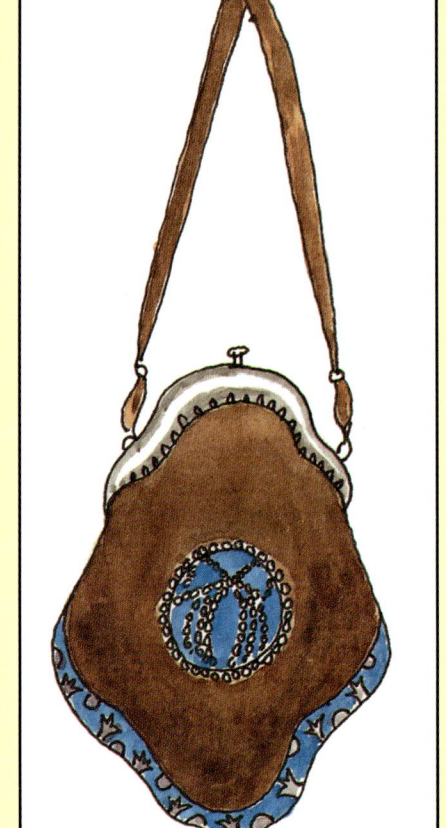

This suede handbag is garnished with bead-encrusted decoration.

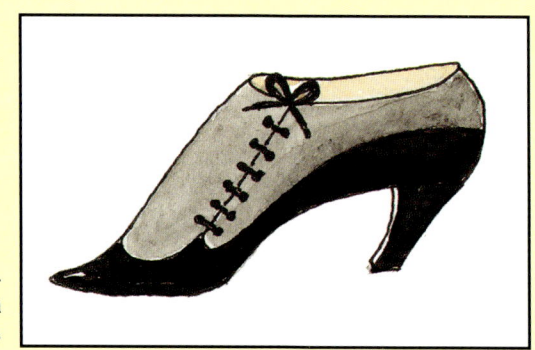

A dainty patent-leather and cloth shoe.

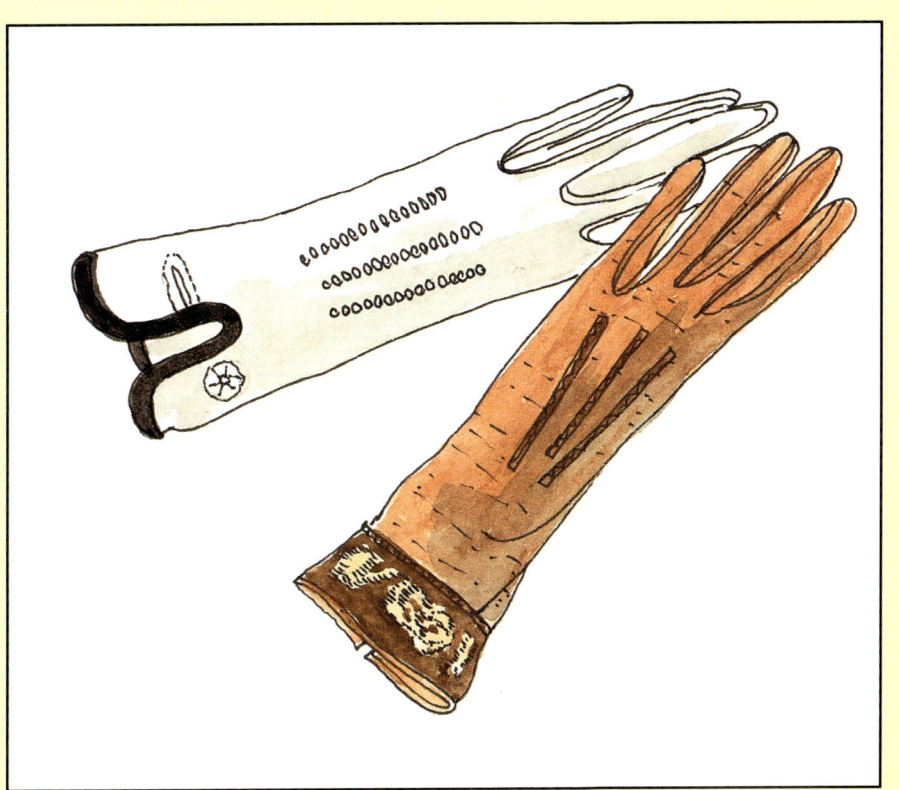

The white kid glove with silk edging is fastened by a crystal button; the fine kid glove has a machine-embroidered contrasting cuff.

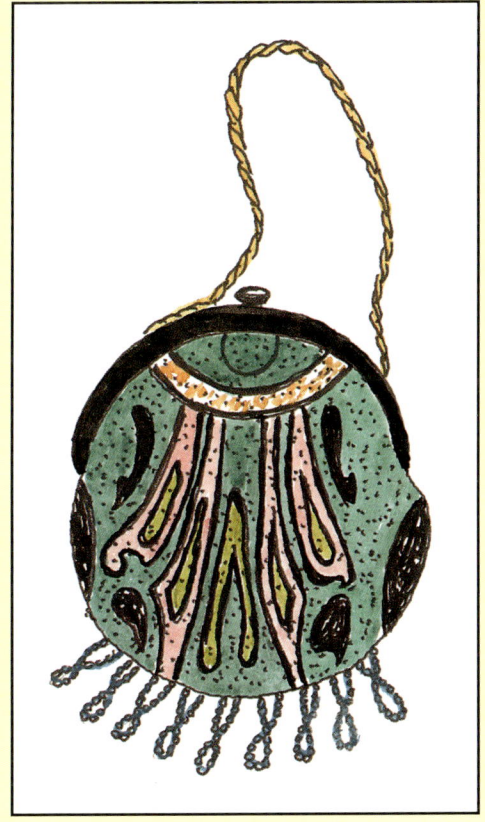

The ubiquitous beaded handbag, displaying the influence of the Russian Ballet.

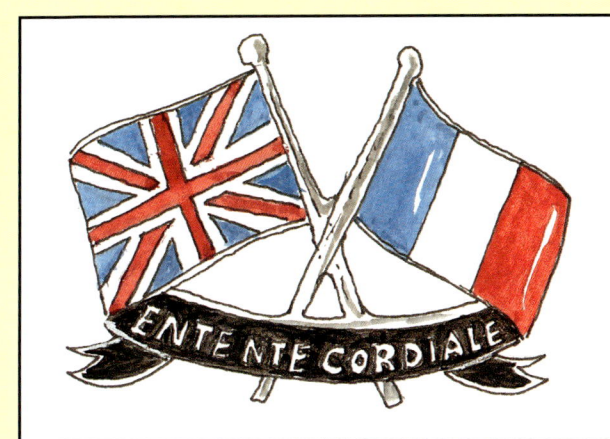

During the War, women could choose from a number of appropriate enameled brooches to show their patriotism. Other war-like subjects included the flags of allied nations, army crests, tanks, and submarines.

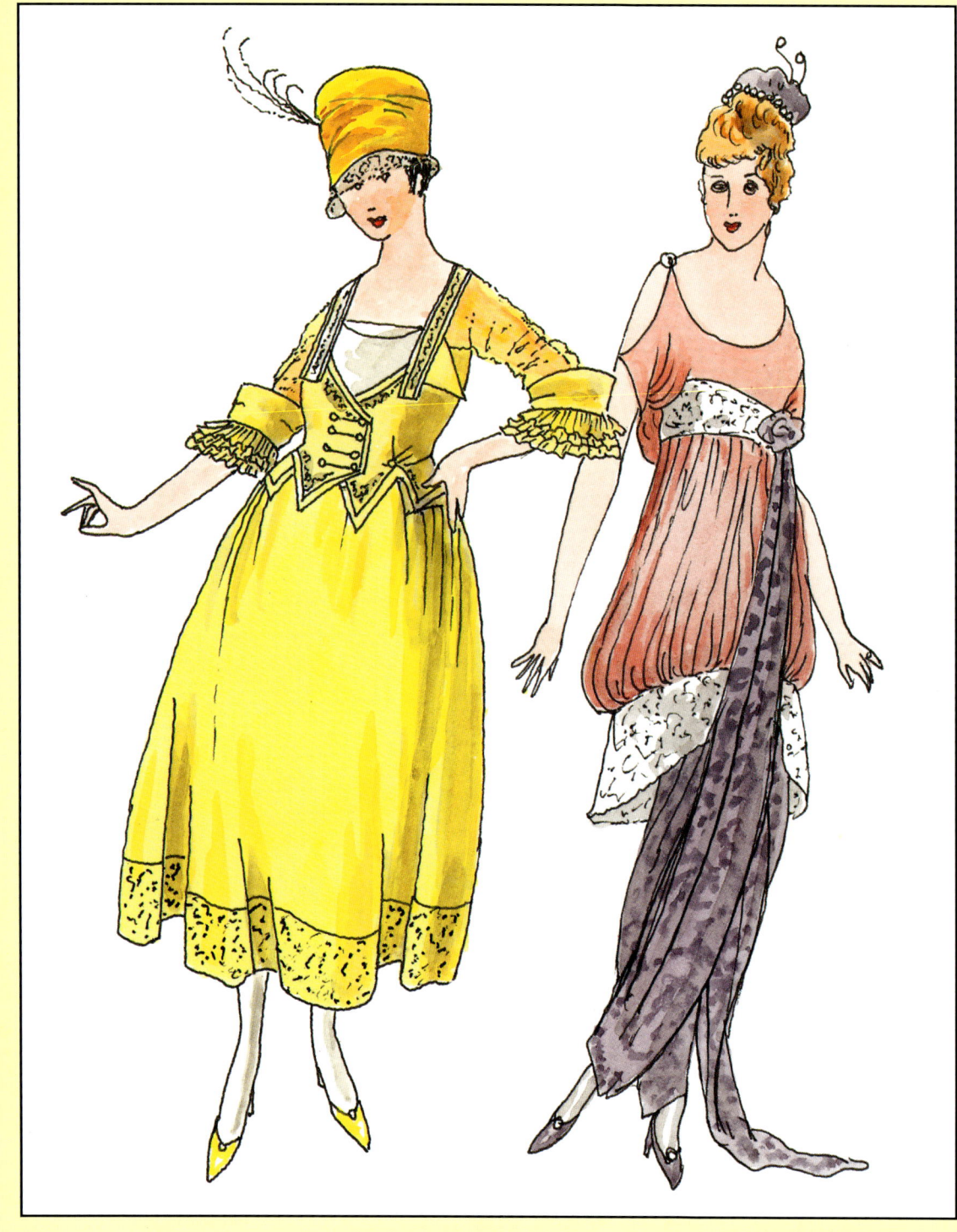

1915-1919 Evening Wear

During the evening, women appear to have ignored the War altogether, except for those who (as during the day) dressed to cheer up the men by looking as pretty as possible. More dining-out went on than ever before, for which a woman (at left) would wear a short, elaborately trimmed, rather bulky dress with a hat. For full evening, the "Turkish" style was still all the rage (at right), with a skimpy, low-necked, high-waisted tunic bulging out at the knees, and an ankle-revealing trained skirt in a different material, often brocade.

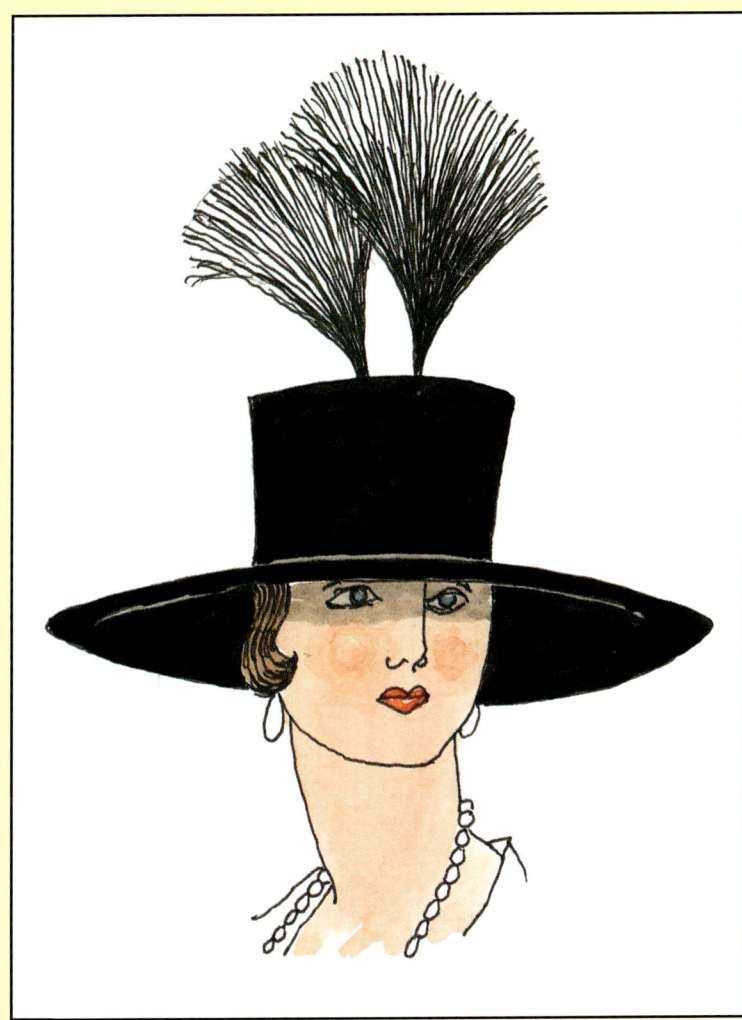

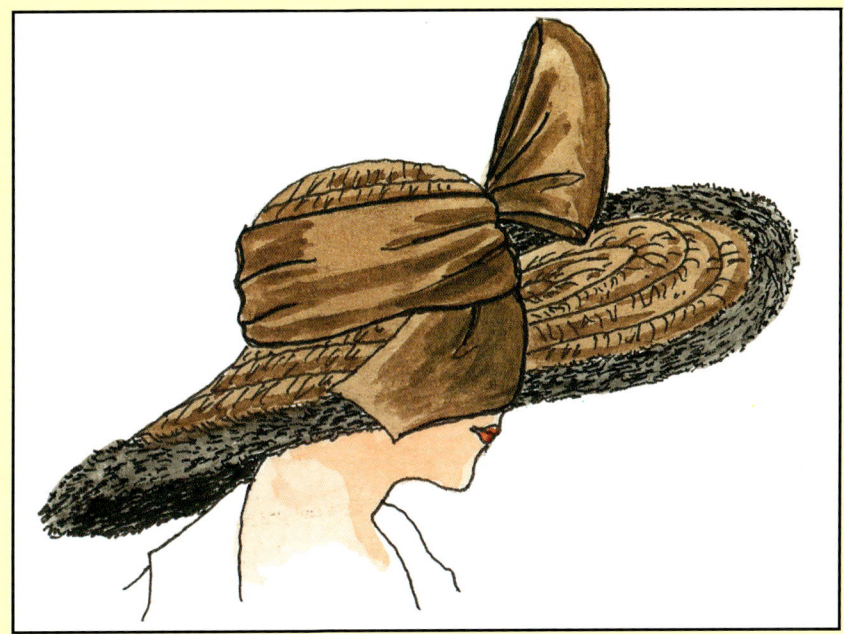

A restaurant hat in ruched grosgrain with a matching bow an edged with skunk fur.

Still in line with Europe, British and American women wore hats in restaurants and theaters. Here, a velvet wide-trimmed "top hat" with "shaving brush" aigrettes is shown.

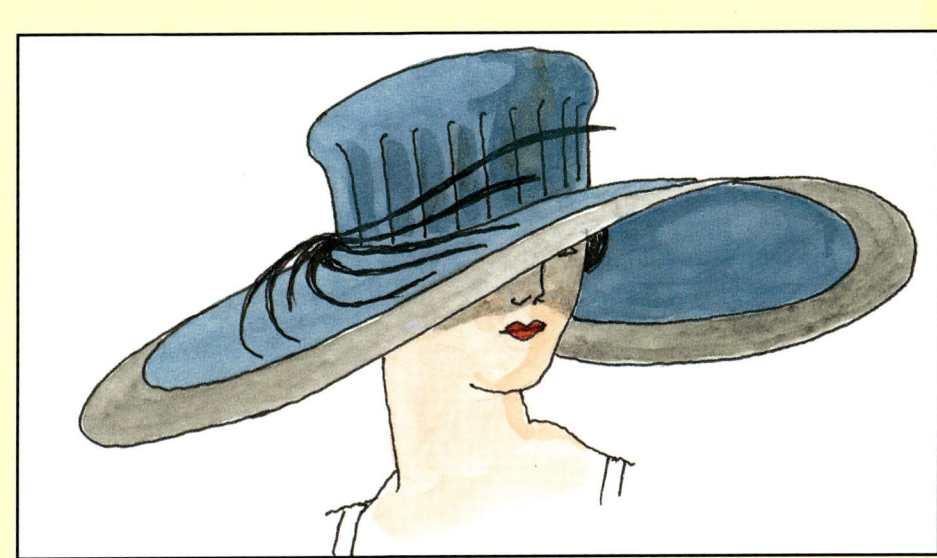

This restaurant hat of swirled velvet is trimmed with silver net.

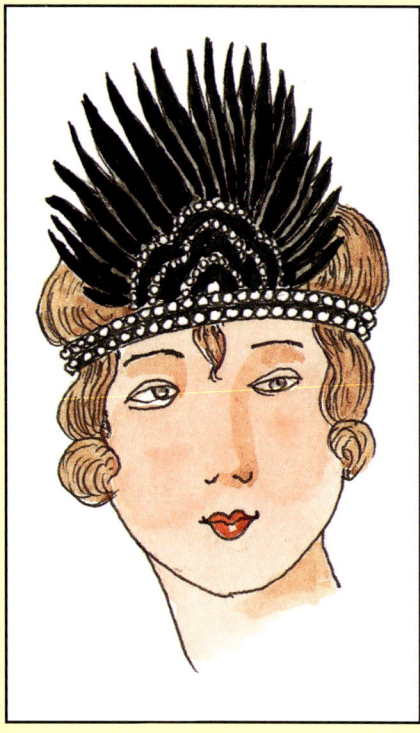

A feathered and jeweled bandeau to wear with full evening dress.

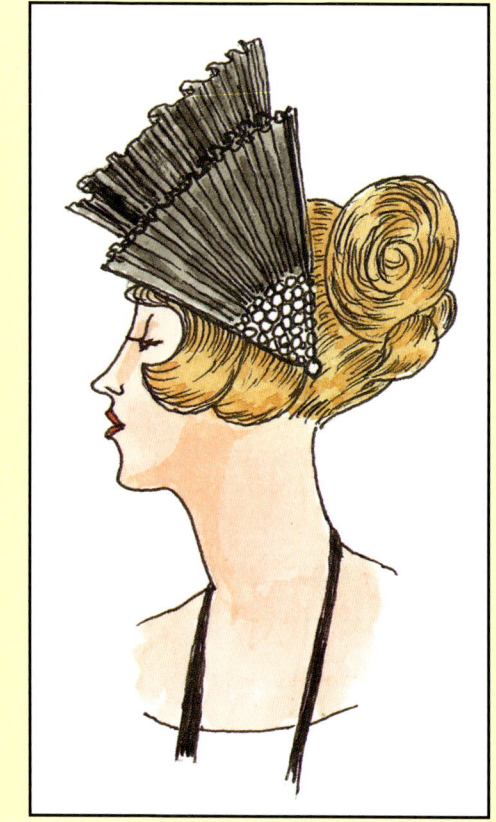

Full evening dress head ornament; pleated tulle fans mounted on a jeweled clasp.

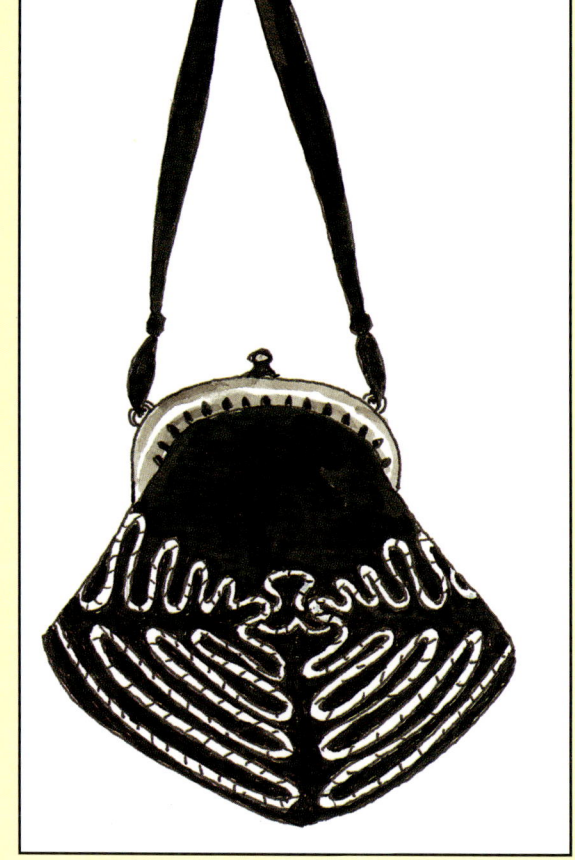

Satin handbag decorated with appliqued cord.

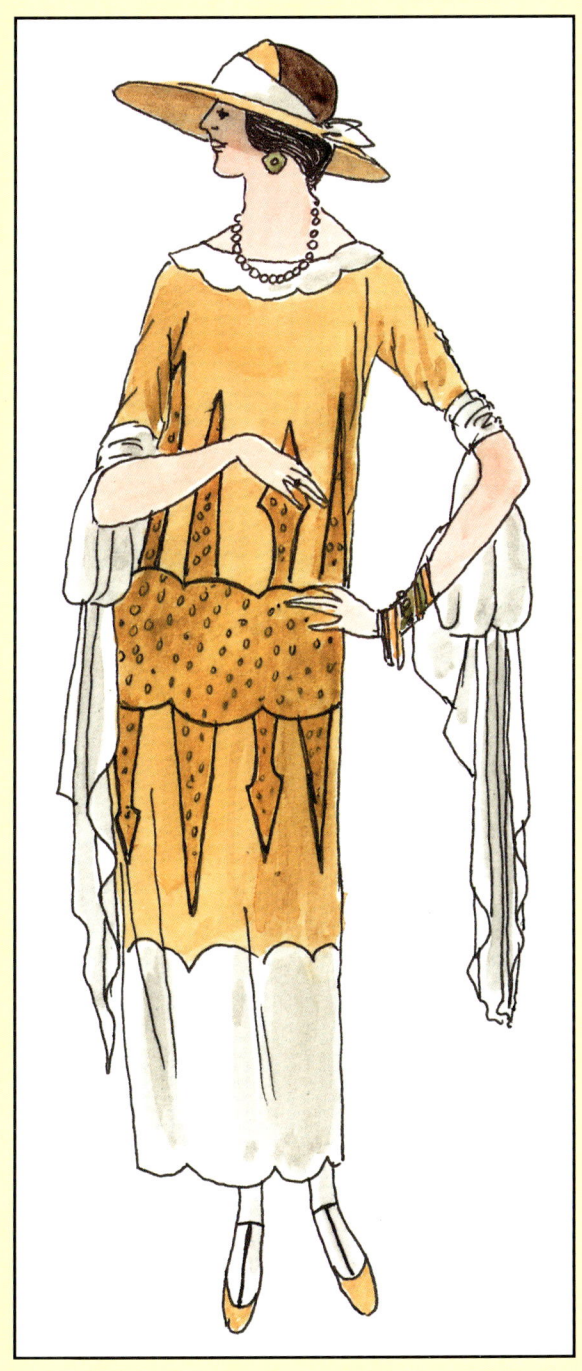

1919-1923 Day Wear

Although the War freed many women from social and sexual repression, this was not immediately evident in post-war fashion. However, dresses were narrower and looser, if somewhat shapeless, with low waists and slightly shorter skirts.

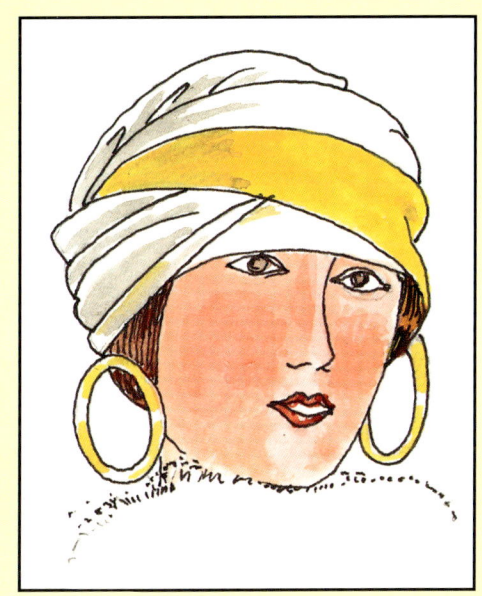

Still influenced by the Russian Ballet, a silk turban worn with "slave" bangle earrings attached to it.

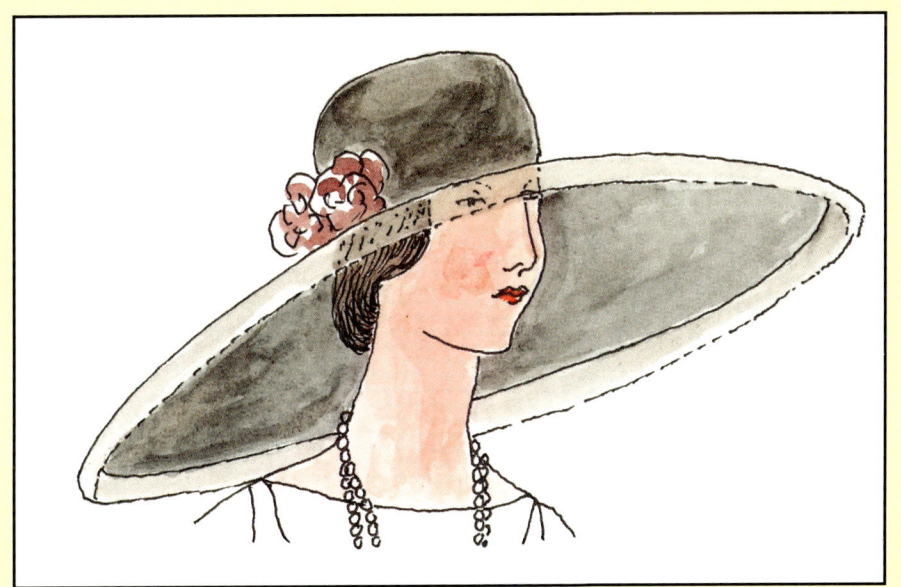

A stiffened chiffon summer hat with silk roses nestling on the brim.

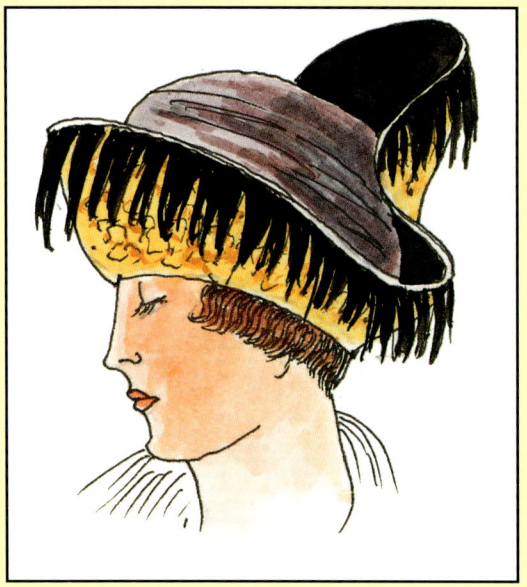

A rather curiously-shaped twirl of a hat: straw and velvet edged with feathers.

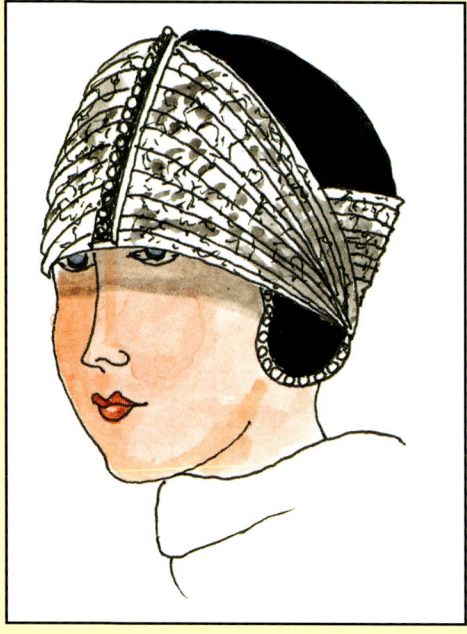

A vaguely Egyptian-inspired hat in velvet, bound with silver lace, fastened by a pearl clip.

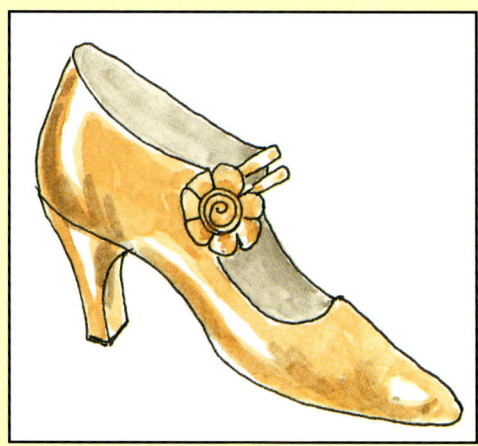

Because beige was the favorite color of this period, this leather shoe went well with a matching ensemble.

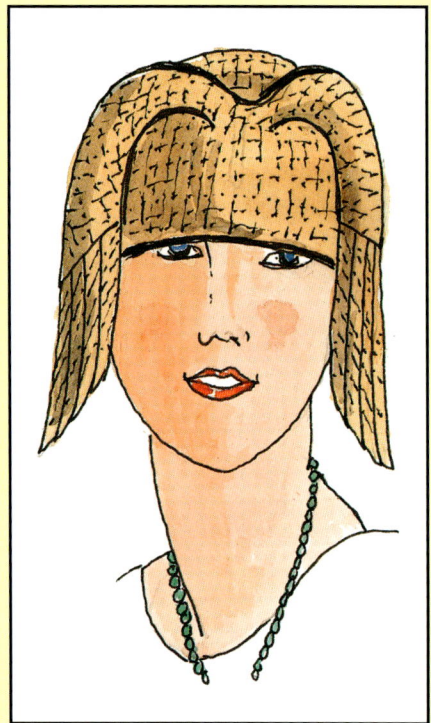

☞ When Tutankhamen's tomb with all its fantastic treasures was opened in late 1922, it spawned a craze for all things Egyptian, such as this molded straw hat with drooping "feathers."

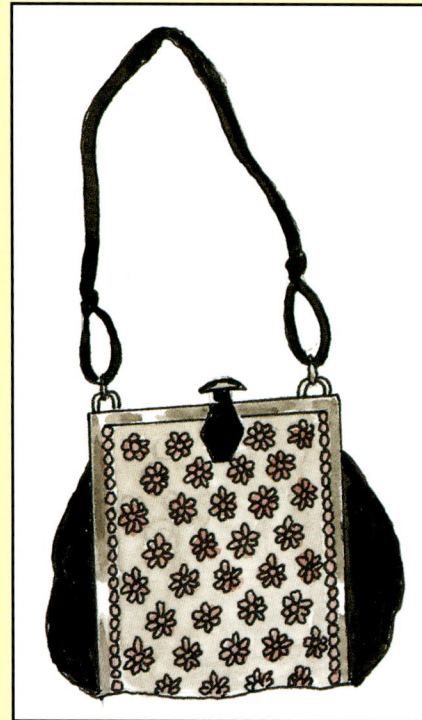

☞ On a metal frame, a velvet handbag sparked up with flower-shaped paillettes.

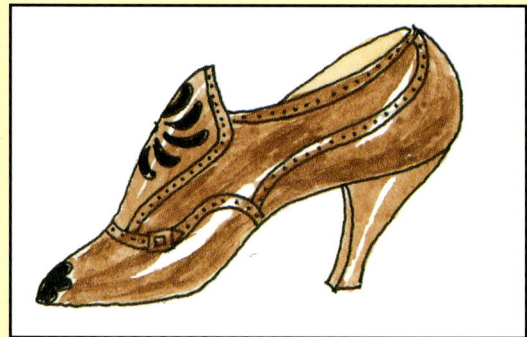

Stitched and punched leather enlivened with black ornamentation.

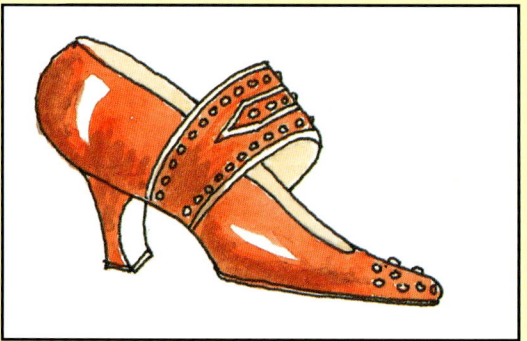

Beaded calf for a dressy occasion.

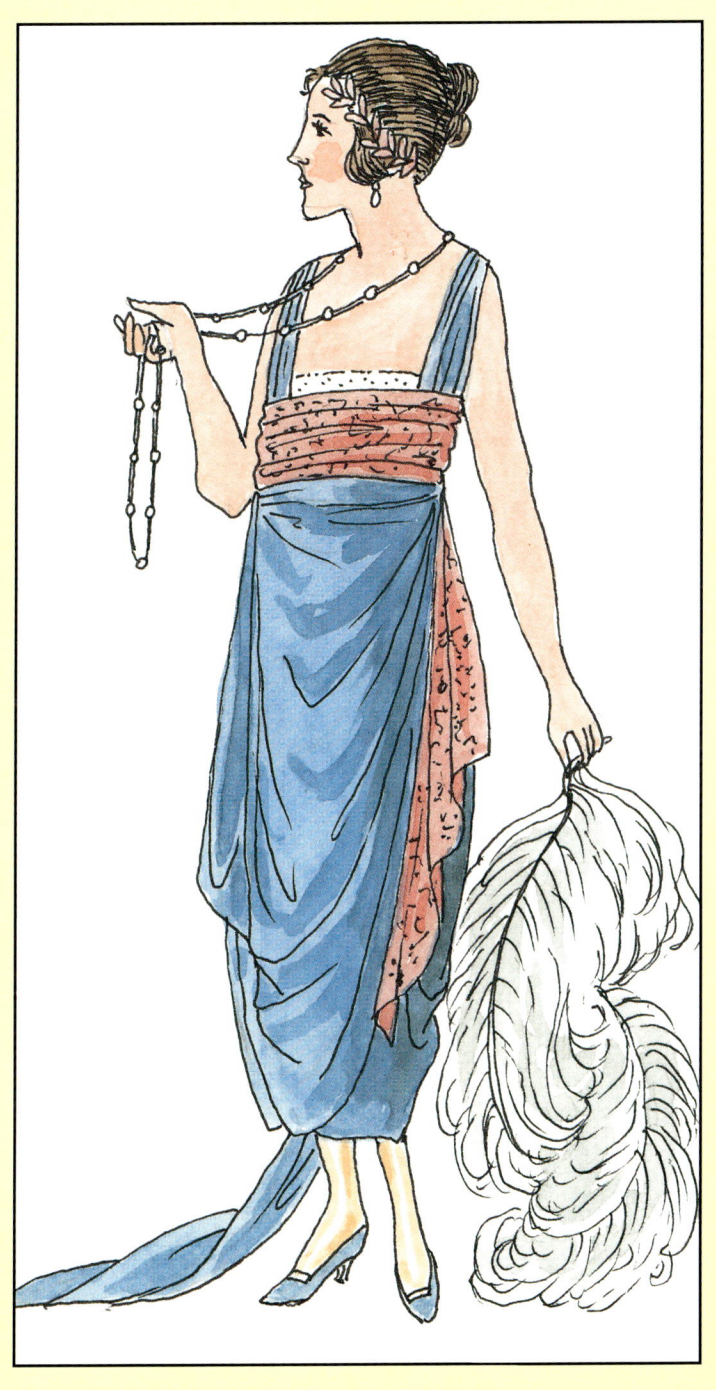

1919-1923 Evening Wear

Dinner and evening dresses of this period consisted of a half-exposed upper body, a flattened bustline, and a loosely-draped, trained skirt—not a particularly flattering look. Long bead necklaces and huge feather fans also were very popular.

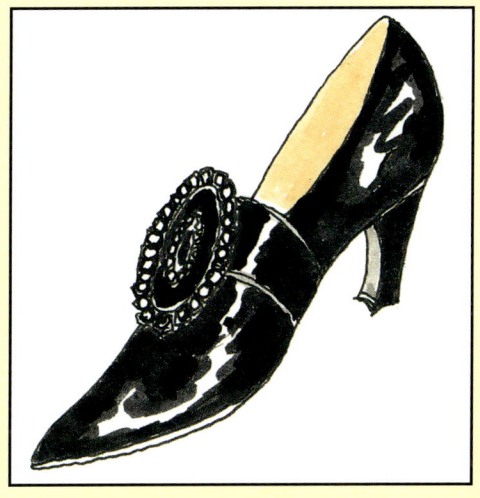

A patent-leather shoe with a huge jet buckle.

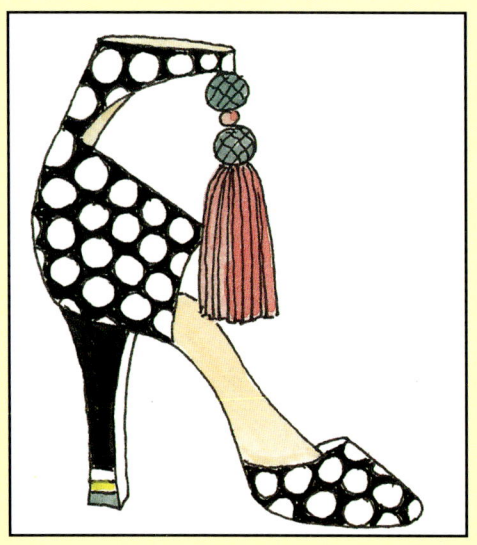

With its very high heel, polka-dot fabric, and large tassel, this kind of shoe would have been worn by only the daring.

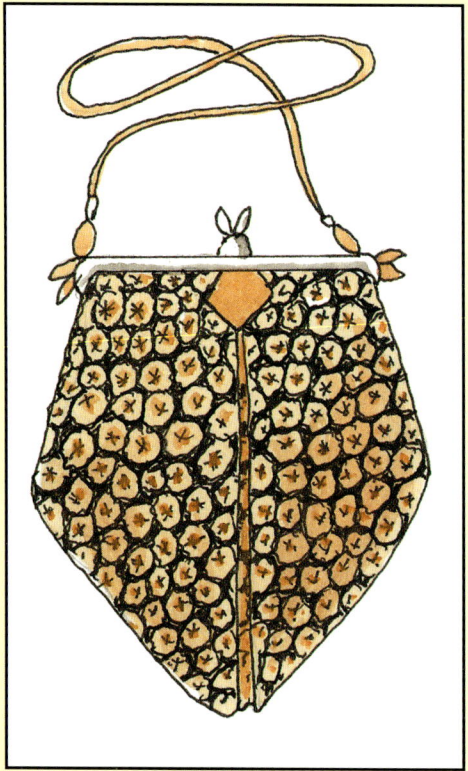

A velvet handbag smothered in gold paillettes.

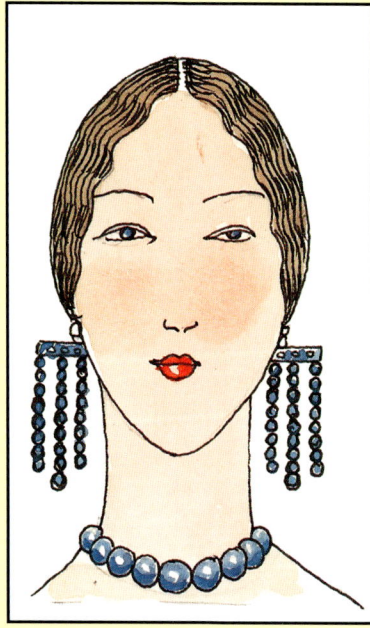

A necklace and earrings in lapis lazuli, which was a semiprecious stone much favored by the ancient Egyptians.

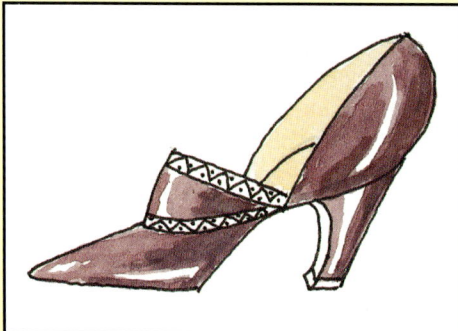

A satin shoe with hands of glittery braid.

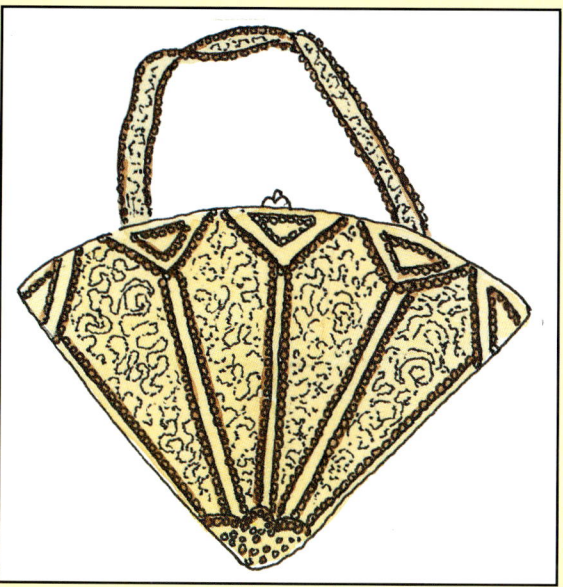

A silk Art Deco bag richly sewn with beads; the reverse is quite plain.

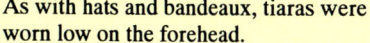

As with hats and bandeaux, tiaras were worn low on the forehead.

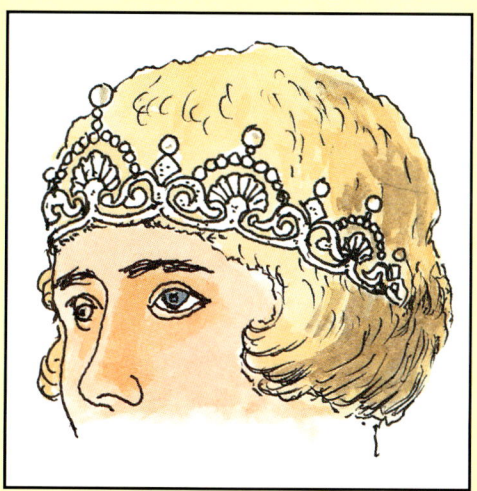

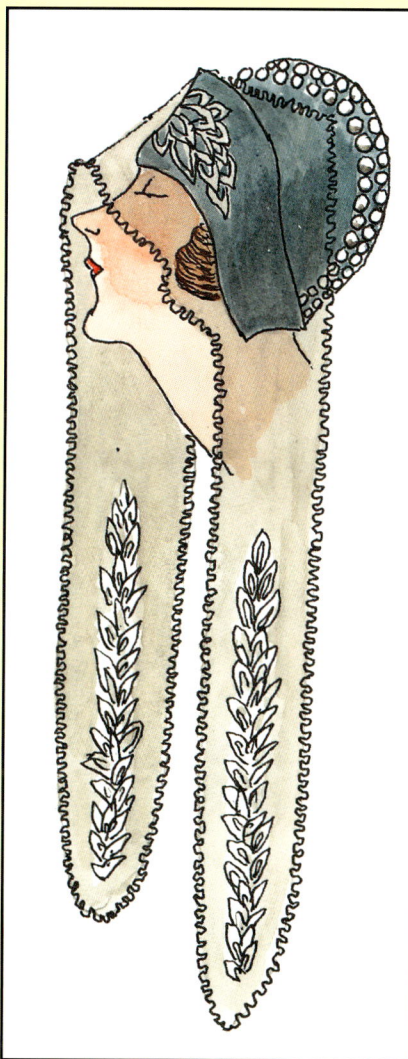

Although this piece of evening nonsense was probably not worn by many, it typifies the extravagance of the 1920s: an embroidered and beaded velvet cap with embroidered chiffon lappets.

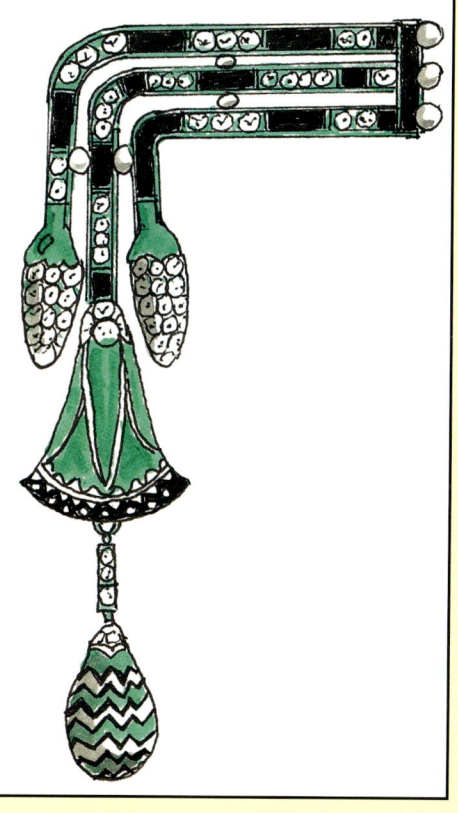

Onyx, emeralds, and diamonds make up this Egyptian-style brooch.

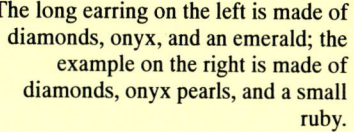

The long earring on the left is made of diamonds, onyx, and an emerald; the example on the right is made of diamonds, onyx pearls, and a small ruby.

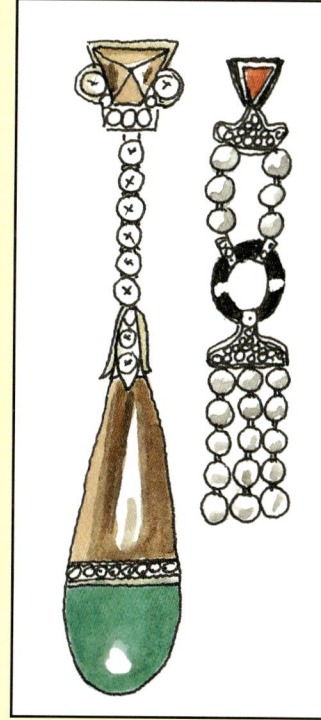

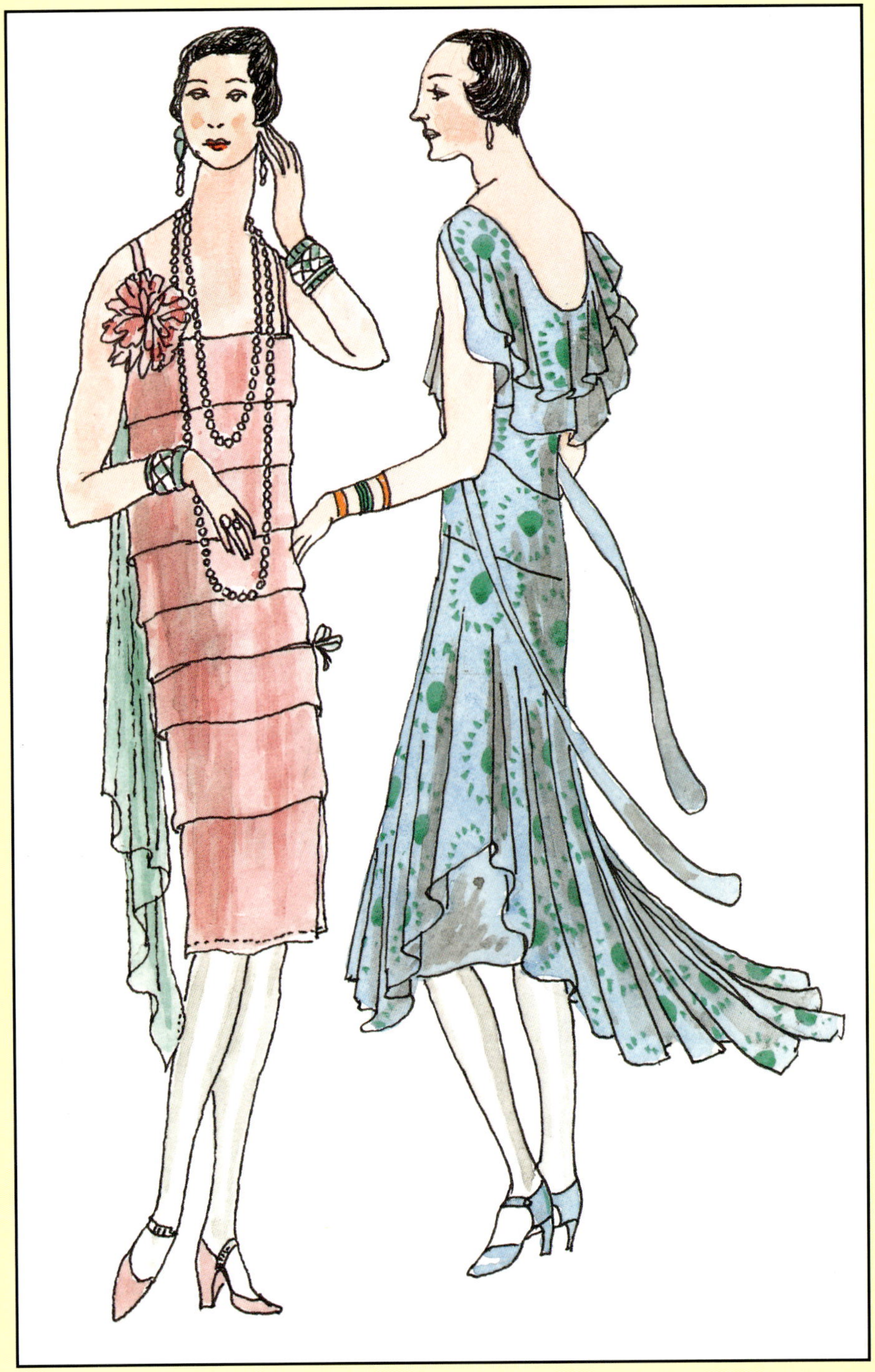

1923-1929 Evening Wear

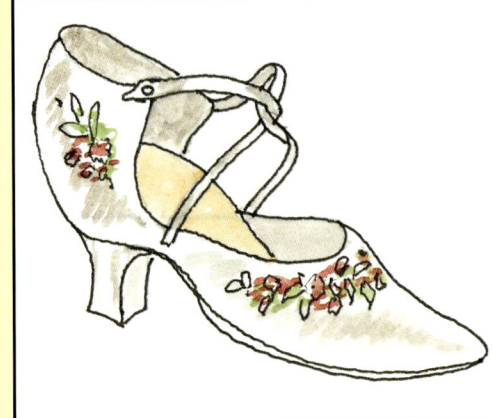

Embroidered silk shoe with a louis heel.

By 1924, evening dresses (at left) were cut on lines similar to day dresses: narrow, flat-busted, and the mere token of a low waist, worn with very long earrings, masses of bracelets and bangles, and a wisp of chiffon. Dresses were made of silk, chiffon, lace, or entirely of beads in black, white, and soft colors. By the late 1920s (at right) there was great uncertainty as to the length and style of the hemline, uneven all around or divided into "handkerchief" points. As for day, short hair, especially the "Eton Crop" was practically universal.

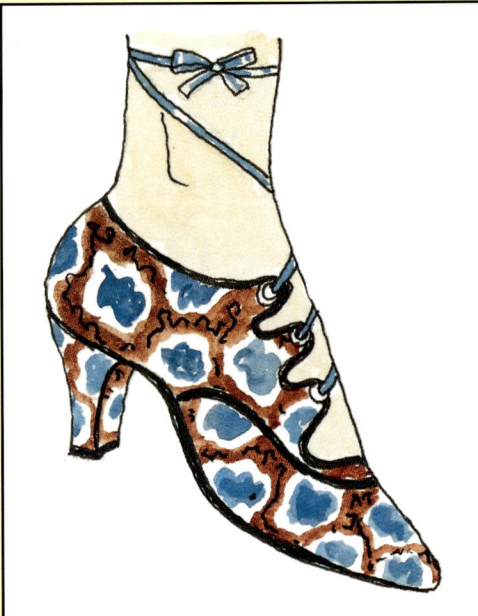

This brocade shoe has a Cuban heel.

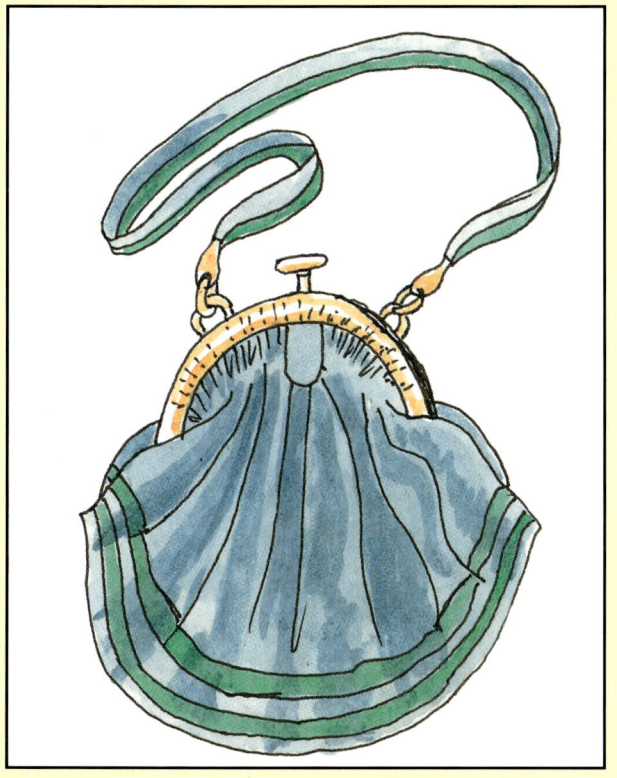

A simple, rather traditional, soft silk bag on a gilt frame.

With the British Empire still flourishing, it was fashionable in Britain to carry an exotic parasol. The check-patterned parasol has a carved "palm" handle; the flower-spotted one has an Eastern-styled handle; flowers and leaves on the third suggest Chinese or Indian influence.

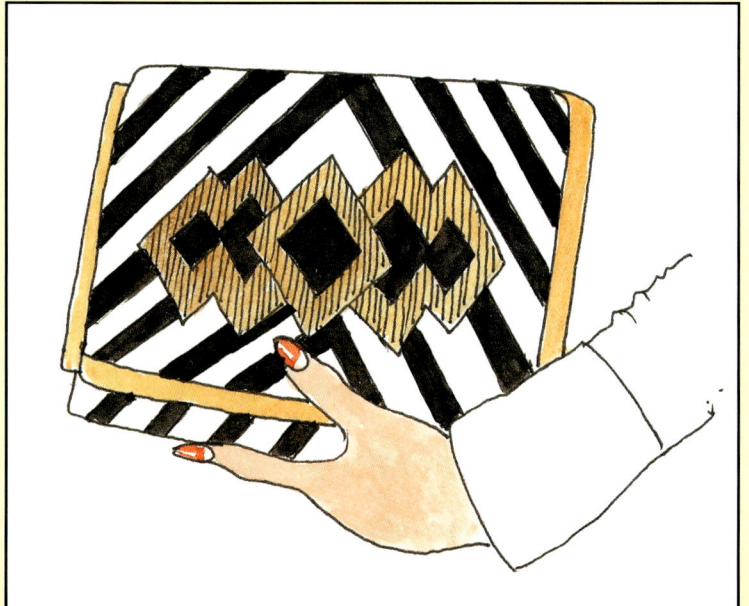

This jazzily patterned pochette is very much of the Art Deco period.

During the era of the "Bright Young Things," emancipation, and Noël Coward, long cigarette holders were much in use, since it was smart for women to smoke in public. *Left to right:* enamel with tiny pearls; onyx; bone and tortoiseshell; silver and onyx.

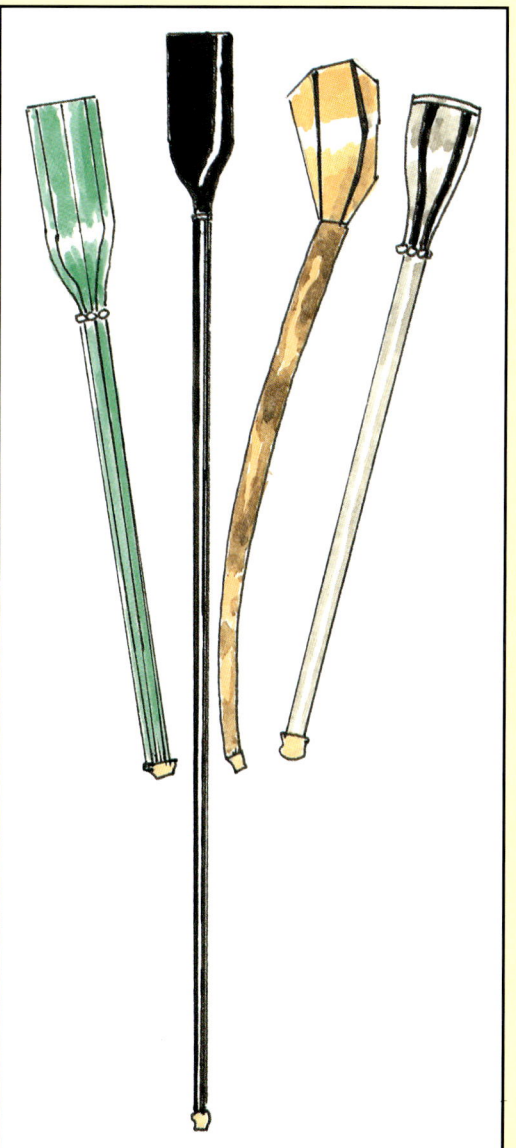

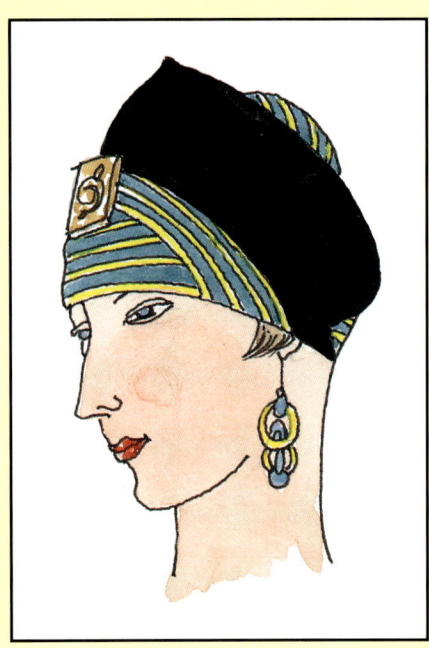

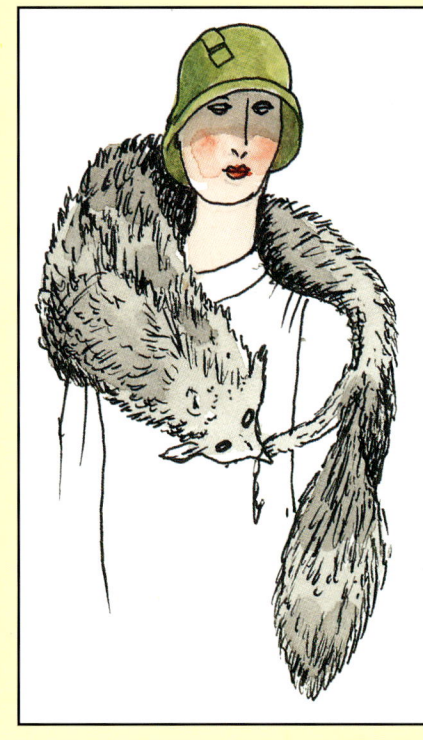

The Egyptian style had by no means died out by the end of the 1920s. Here, a 1928 velvet and gilded ribbon creation is worn with enameled earrings, probably for a cocktail party, a restaurant, or the theater.

What now seems a rather sinister fashion of wearing a whole fox's skin around the shoulders, complete with molded muzzle and glass eyes, was very fashionable from the late 1920s to the late 1930s. Silver fox was the most expensive and most smart.

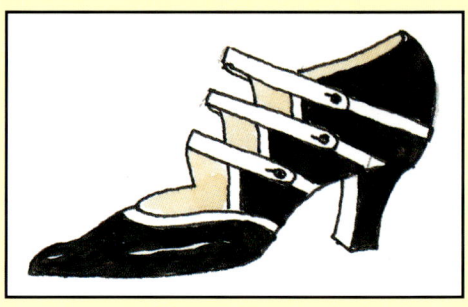

The more straps the better! Two colors of leather.

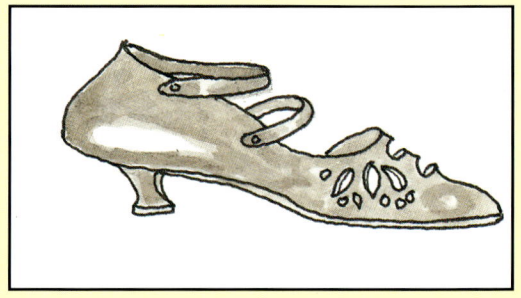

A strapped and pierced silk shoe with a louis heel, also worn for evening.

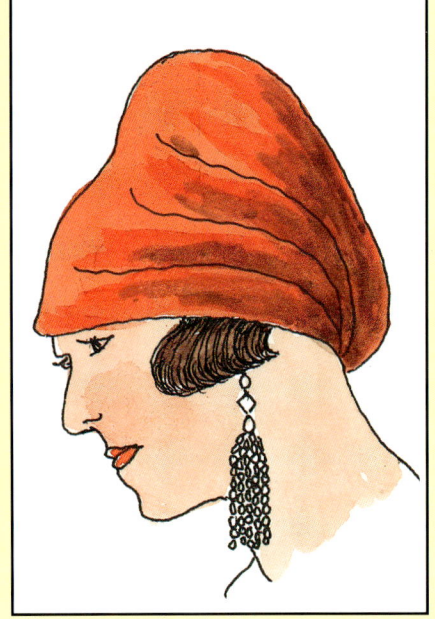

By the late 1920s, a simple velvet "helmet" was almost as popular as the cloche.

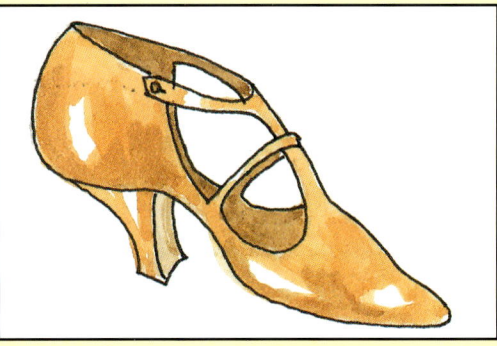

All kinds of strapped shoes with pointed toes were fashionable; here they are shown in leather.

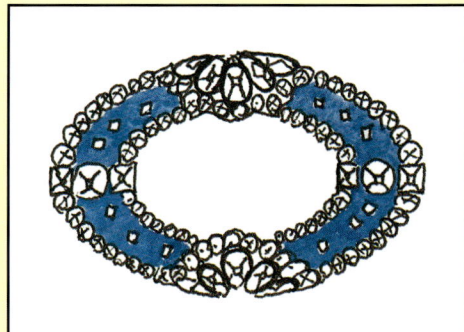

An eighteenth-century style paste and enamel hat buckle.

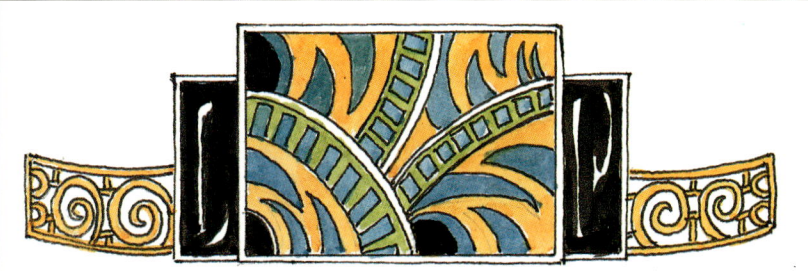

An enameled belt buckle designed in very Art Deco style.

97

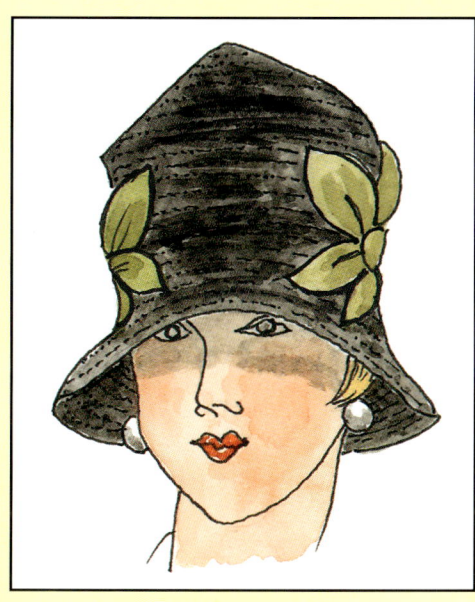

Dyed straw hat with silk "flowers".

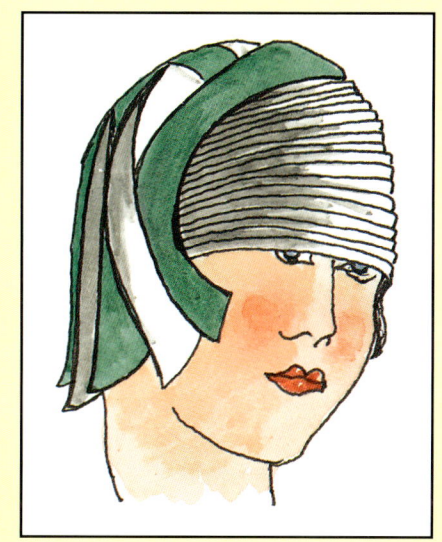

Pleated silk hat with Art Deco flaps covering the ears.

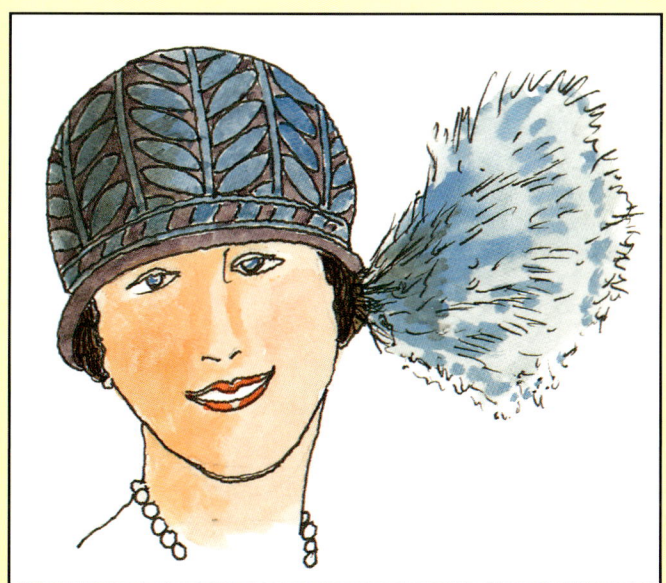

Felt hat twisted with silk ribbon; a bunch of artificial flowers on the shoulder was smart.

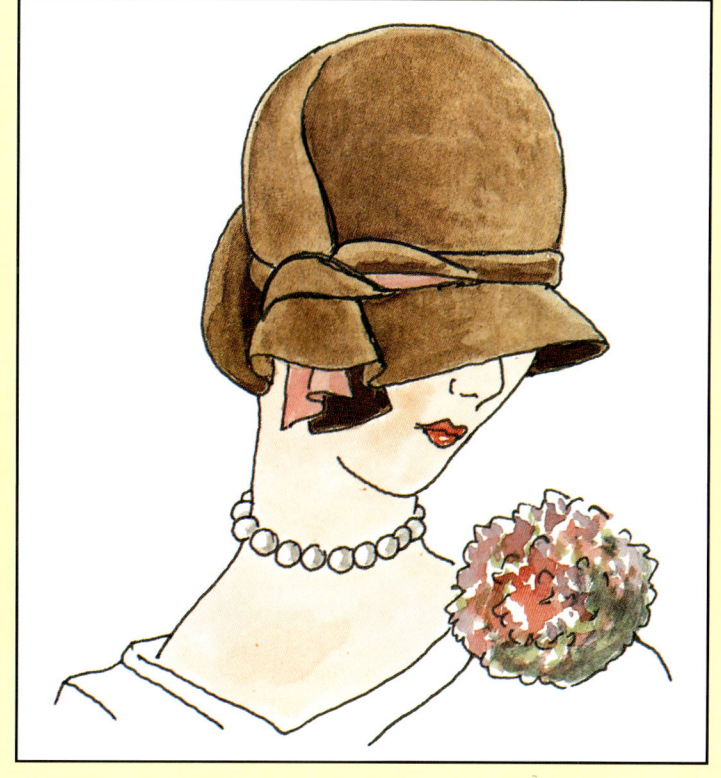

A puff of feathers protrudes at an acute angle from this silk cloche decorated with stylized leaves. Two-colored hats were considered the most chic.

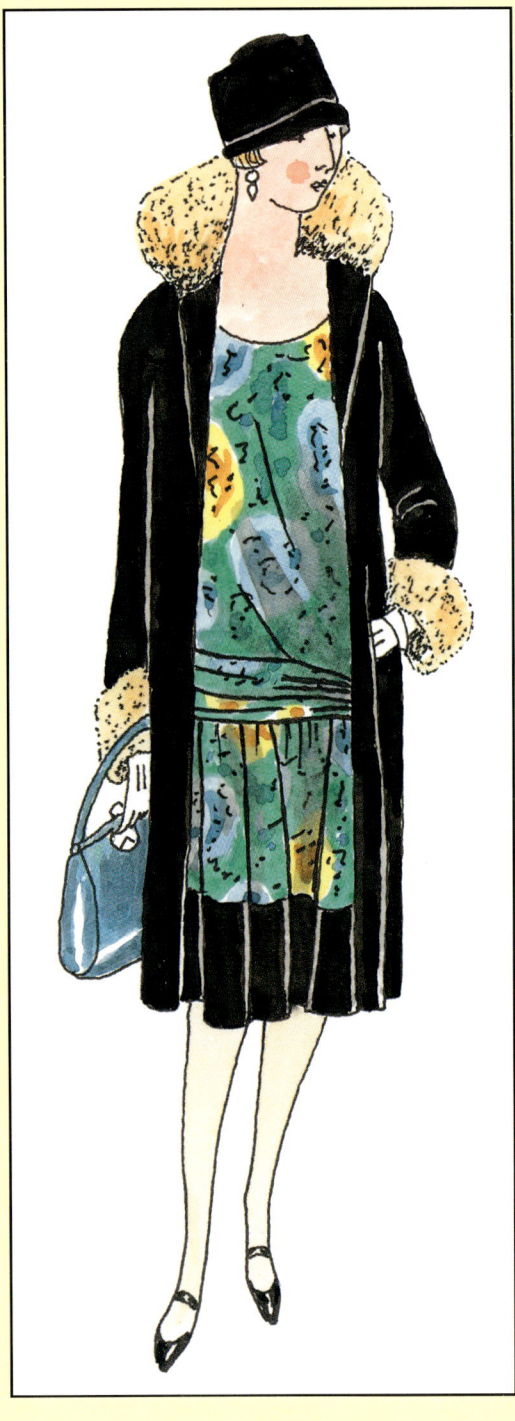

1923-1929 Day Wear

Although the cloche hat, a fashion much associated with the 1920s, appeared in approximately 1922, the popular image of the "Flapper Girl," in her narrow, very low-waisted dress and short hair, did not appear until roughly 1924, with skirts at their shortest in 1926. Equally short coats in velvet, cloth, silk, or fur, with huge fur collars and cuffs, are also a feature of this period. Although older women wore these fashions (sometimes with disastrous results) the emphasis was on youth and women's emancipation, leading young women to adopt a "boyish" look. It was a look promoted by "Coco" Chanel, the French couturier who advocated simple, easy-fitting clothes, long bead necklaces, and a lot of costume jewelry. Women and girls (as well as some men) began to dress like Hollywood film stars. This was also the era of Art Deco, jazzy designs and bright colors.

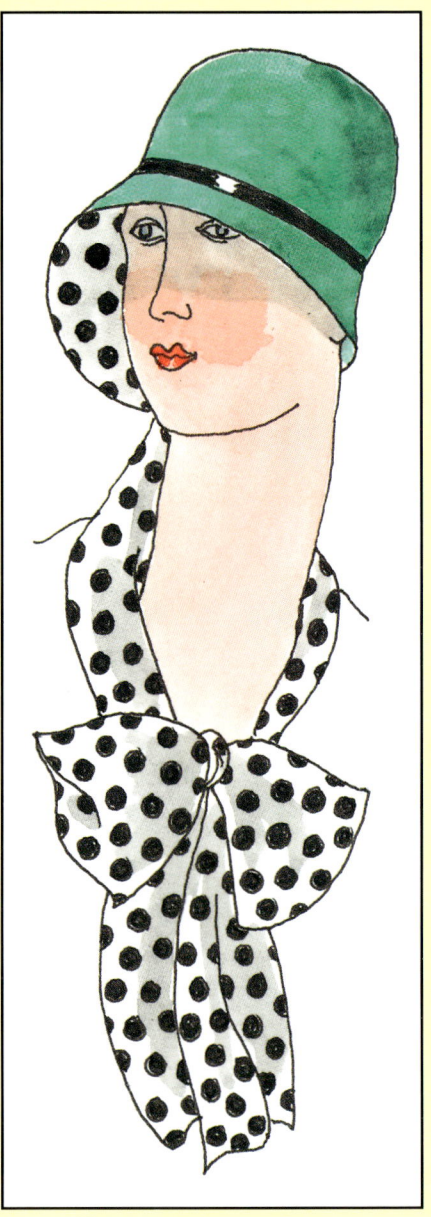

The first cloche hat appeared toward the end of 1922, soon to become the smartest of all hats; here in felt, its crêpe-de-chine lining matching the scarf.

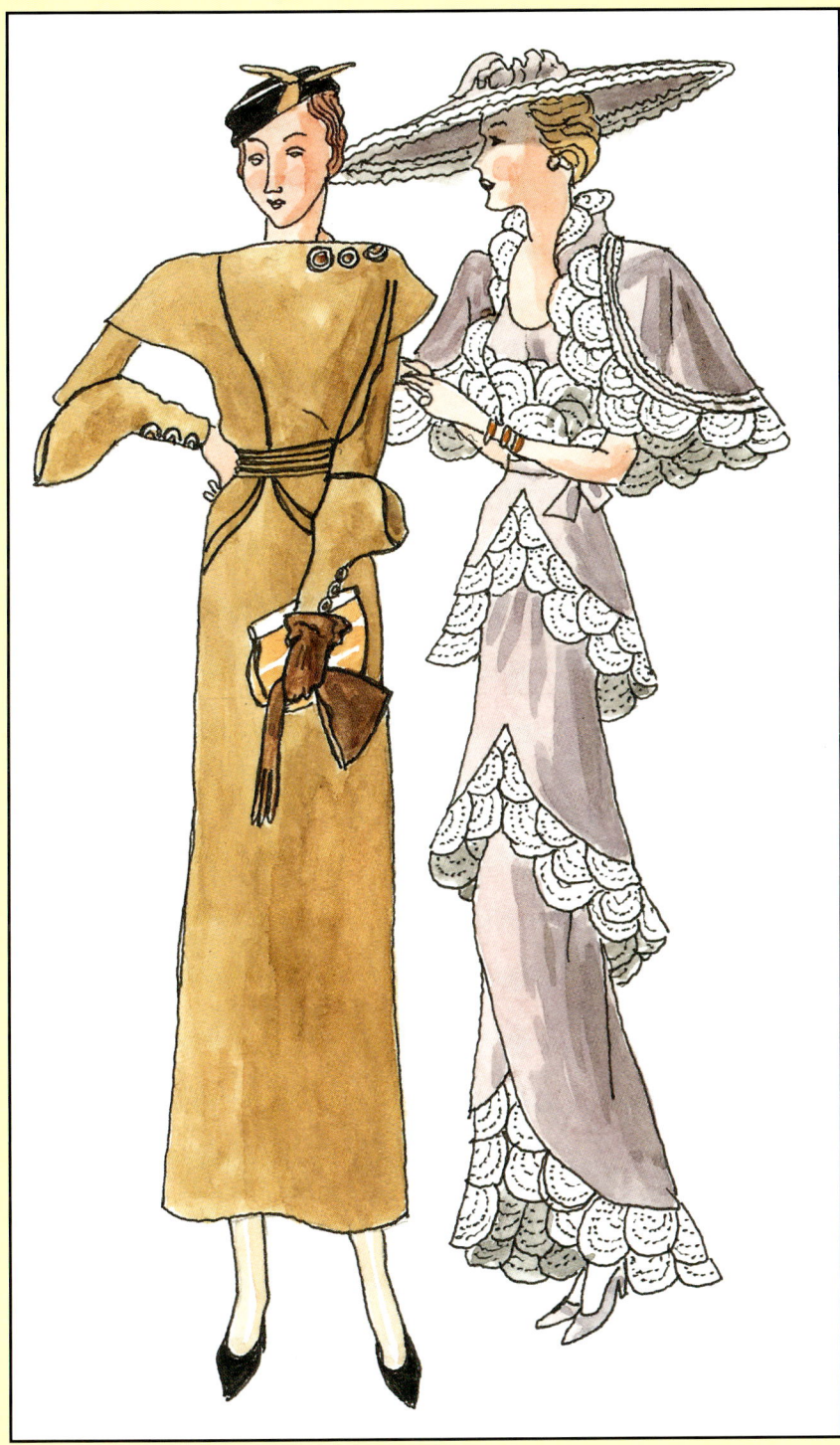

1929-1937 Day Wear

The Wall Street Crash of 1929 coincided with the fall of women's hemlines to below the calf. (The Crash is said to have inflicted a blow to the extravagance of Paris couture, from which it never fully recovered.) The waist returned to its natural level and the ideal style (at left) was to look very tall in narrow, simple, wide-shouldered dresses and coats. Sleeves could be somewhat flamboyant with deep gauntlet-like cuffs echoing gauntlet gloves. The introduction of bias-cutting in 1933, with its many, variously-shaped panels, molded the feminine figure into the fashionable, slim silhouette. Trimming consisted mainly of braid and buttons, although frills could be added to the neck and elbows. Blouses with huge bows also softened the line. Materials included wood, tweed, and rayon in such colors as beige, brown, cream, bright red, dull or shocking pink, green, and gray.

An alternative was the Romantic look (at right), inspired by Hollywood in an attempt to divert attention from the Great Depression with musicals and costume dramas, for example, Jeanette MacDonald in *Summer Time* and Greta Garbo in *Camille*, clothed in frothy, away-from-it-all dresses and hats. Other Hollywood stars (often dressed by the great Adrian) who influenced 1930s fashion included Joan Crawford with her extra-wide shoulders, Jean Harlow in her slinky dresses, and Marlene Dietrich with her insolent elegance. In the later 1930s, the ultra-sophisticated Mrs. Simpson (later the Duchess of Windsor), who patronized French Schiaparelli and American Mainbocher, was also a fashion trend setter.

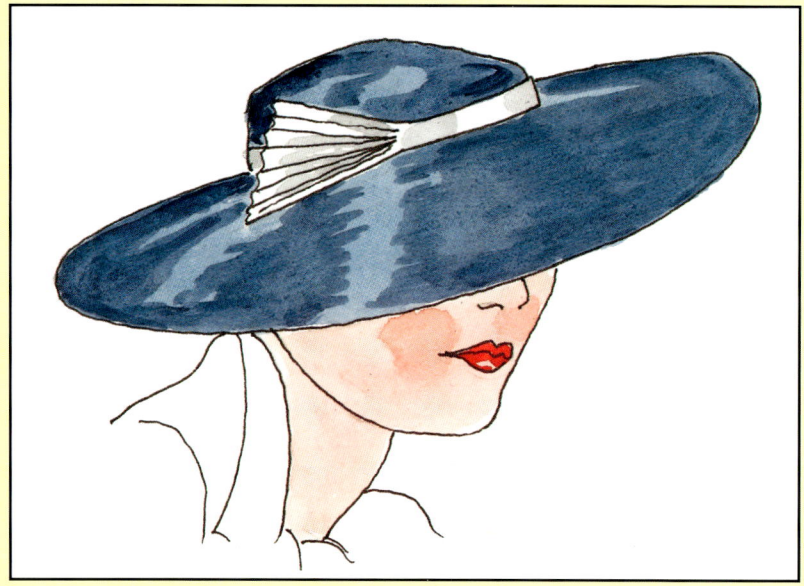

When beautiful, sophisticated, Princess Marina of Greece married the Duke of Kent, King George V's third son in 1934, she immediately became a leader of fashion. She introduced the "Princess Marina" hat, which was wide and shallow. However, she wore it against royal protocol which decreed that royal ladies must not wear hats which concealed their faces from the public.

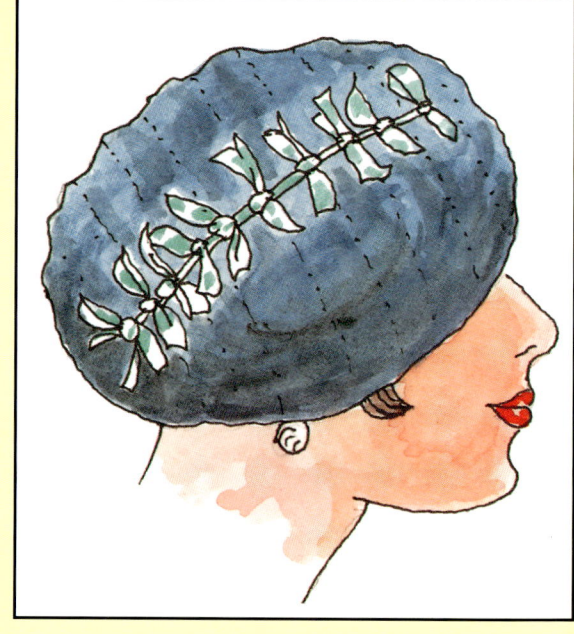

From the early 1930s, a French Basque-style beret was very fashionable, often made of knitted wool, with or without decoration.

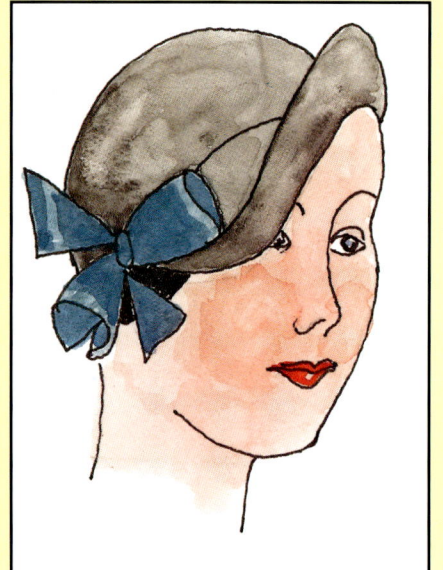

A typical 1930s hat: small, in felt, with a ribbon, and cocked over one eye.

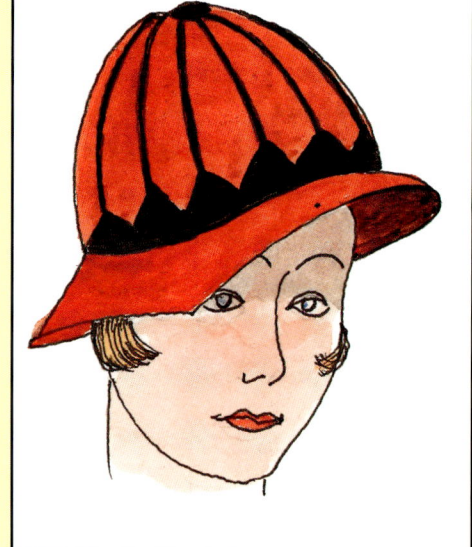

Small but bright felt hat.

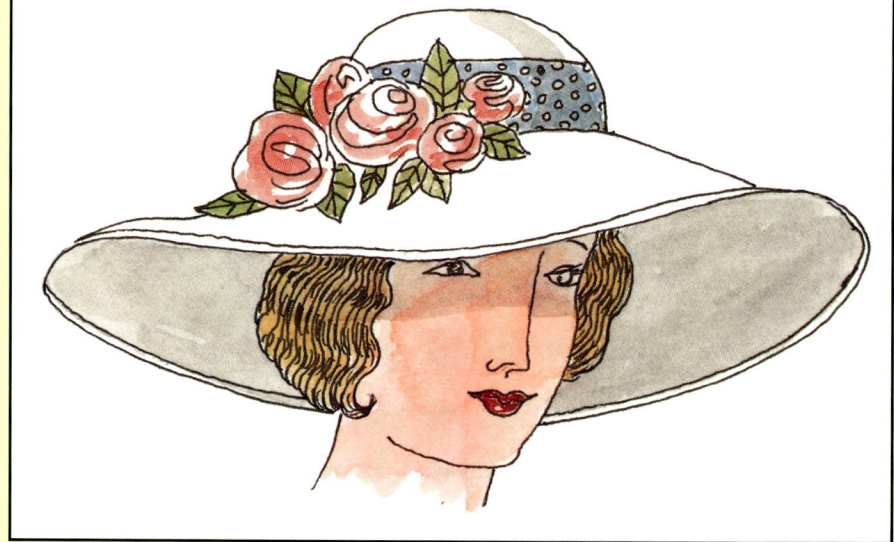

A stiffened organza hat, obviously inspired by Hollywood musicals and costume dramas.

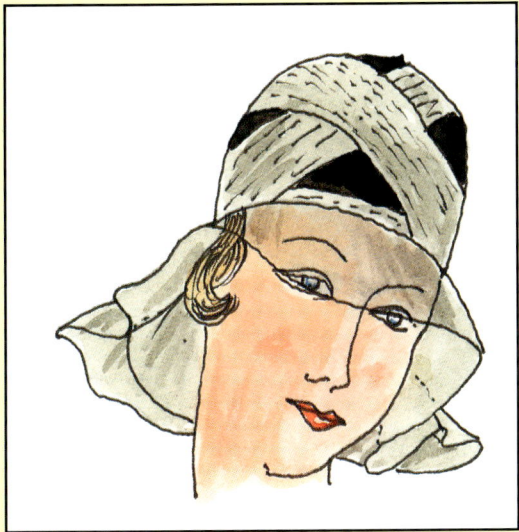

An "escapist" hat worn for dressy occasions: felt, bound and veiled in chiffon.

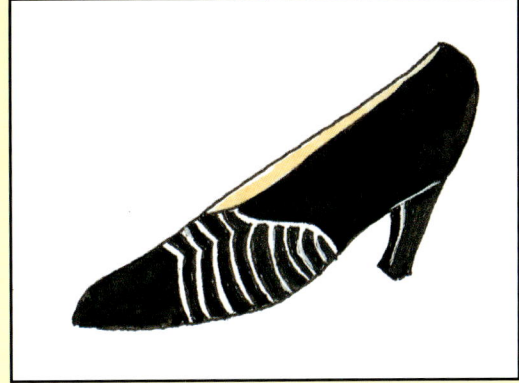

"Court" shoes were all the fashion, plain or, as here, given an Art Deco pattern. These shoes were made in leather or velvet, and navy blue was another favorite color.

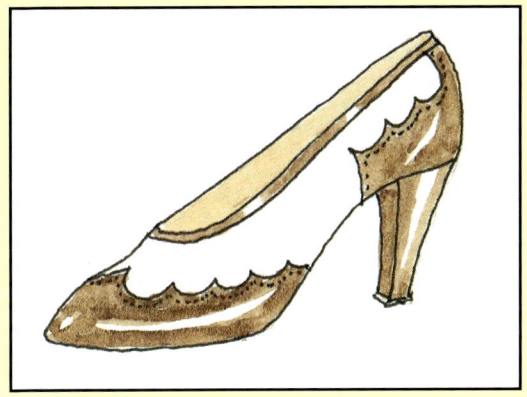

As with men, women also favored two-tone leather shoes.

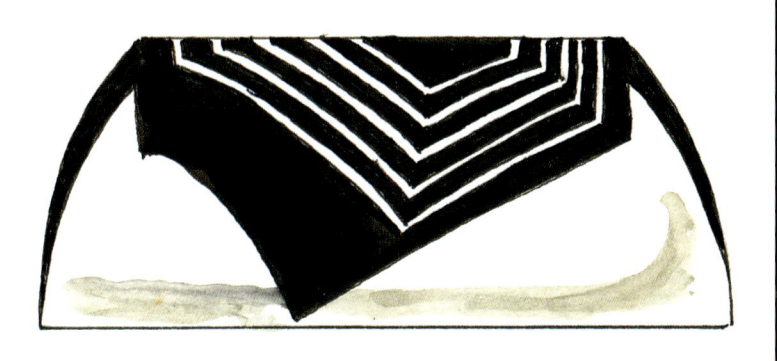

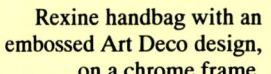 A typical 1930s Art Deco handbag. Navy blue coloring was also smart.

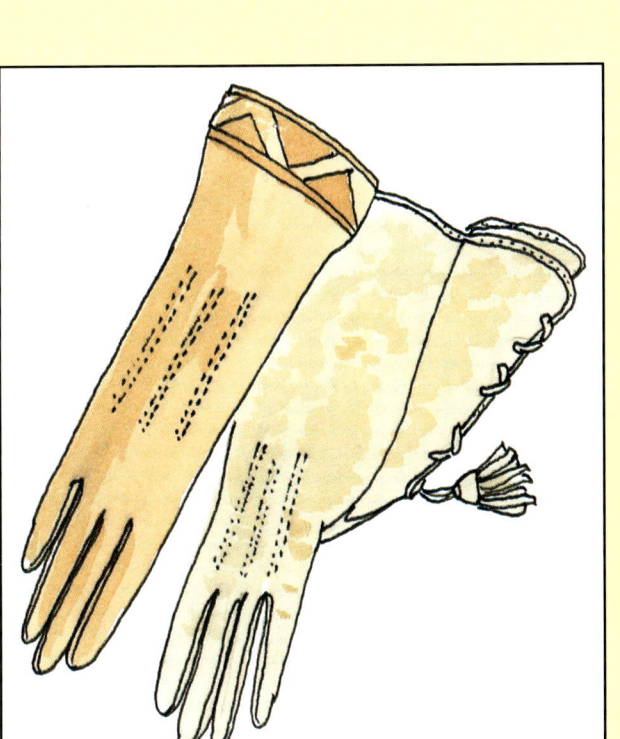

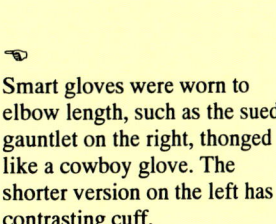 Smart gloves were worn to elbow length, such as the suede gauntlet on the right, thonged like a cowboy glove. The shorter version on the left has a contrasting cuff.

Rexine handbag with an embossed Art Deco design, on a chrome frame.

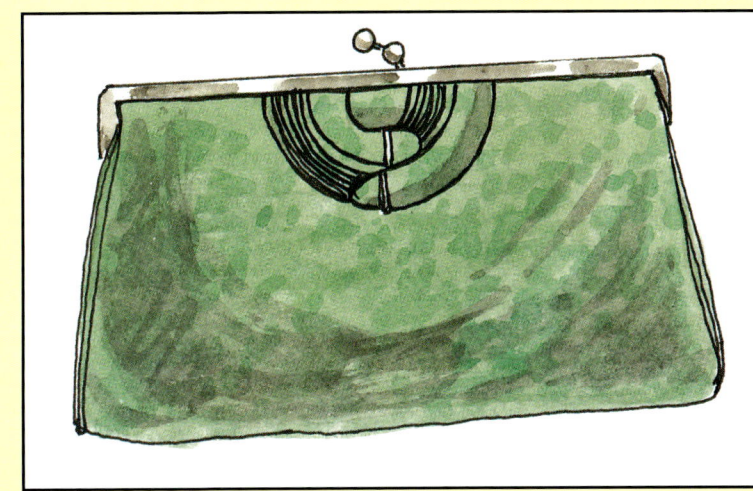

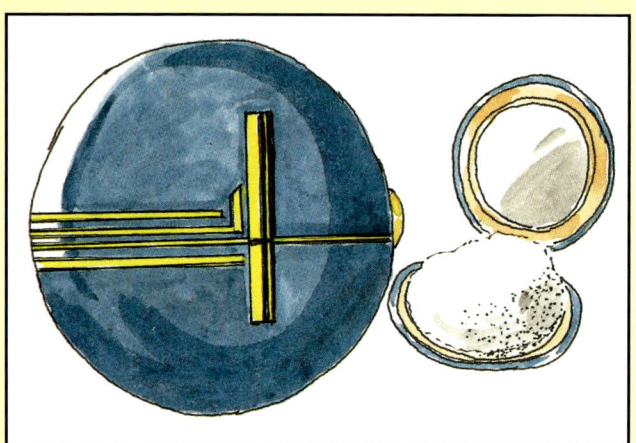

When it became acceptable for women to make-up in public, the powder compact became an important accessory to show off; it was usually made of plastic.

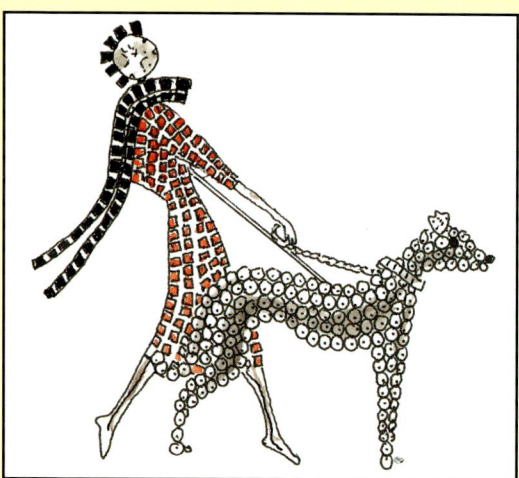

A popular painting called "Diana of the Uplands," a windswept woman with her dog, was reproduced many times and was the inspiration for this silver, diamond, ruby, and onyx brooch.

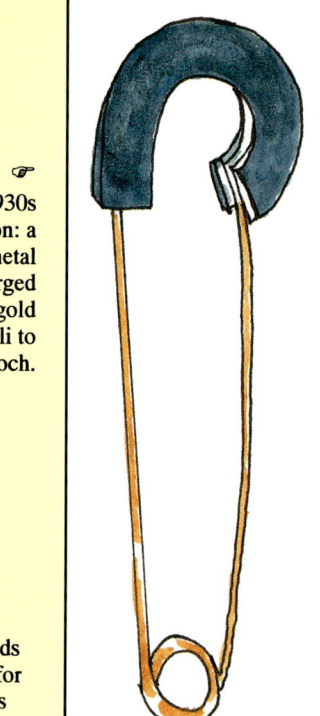

☞ The height of 1930s sophistication: a "common" metal safety pin enlarged and executed in gold and lapis lazuli to form a scarf brooch.

Animals of all kinds were fashionable for jewelry: hence this molded and carved plastic "coral" squirrel brooch.

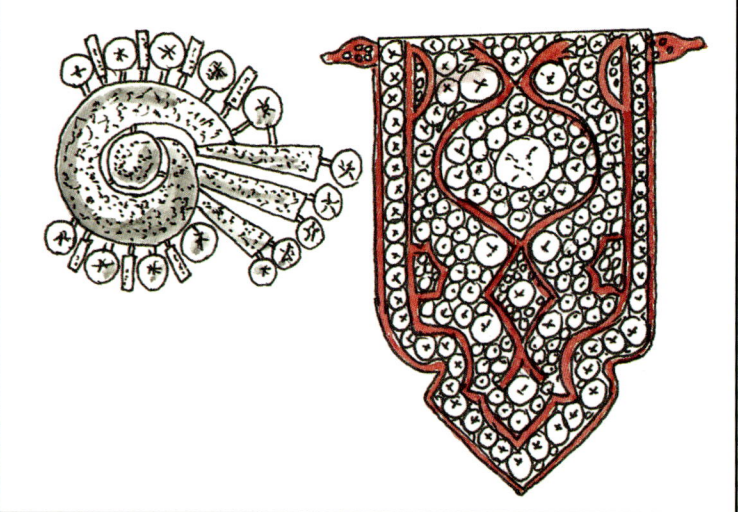

No piece of jewelry, real or imitation, so symbolized the 1930s as the clip. A pair of clips was often worn to the side of the décolletage of a dress. *Left:* in diamonds or paste, in surrealistic style. *Right:* in more traditional mode, a "banner" clip in real or imitation diamonds and rubies.

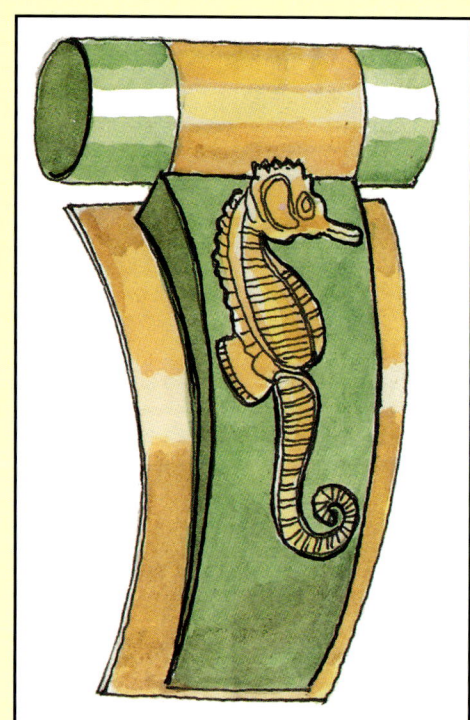

Costume jewelry (i.e., not real) was becoming more and more popular and acceptable, as in this Art Deco molded plastic brooch.

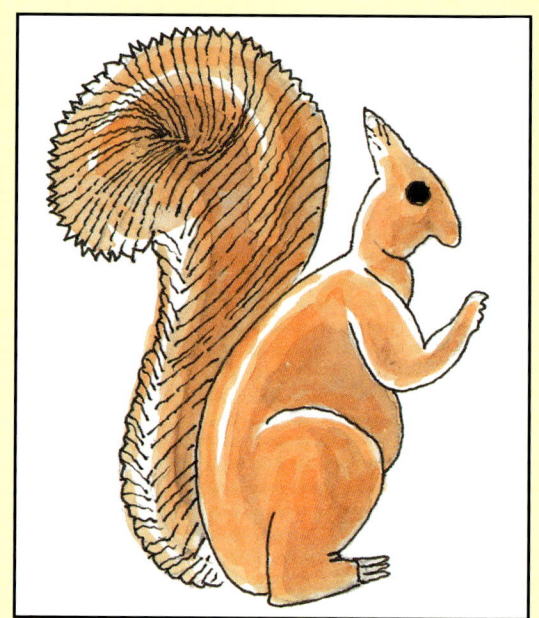

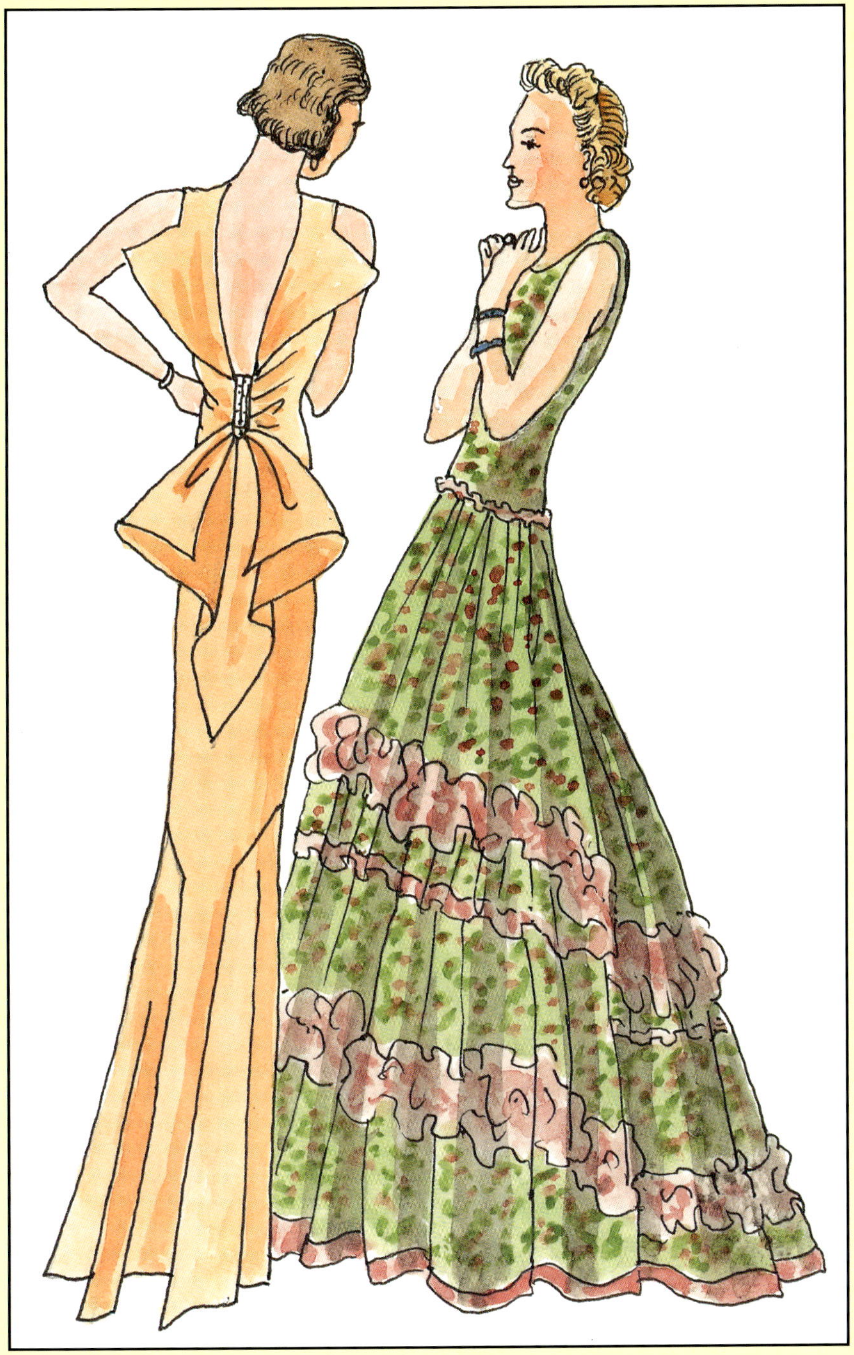

1929-1939 Evening Wear

Up to the late 1930s, bias-cutting was nowhere more evident than on the dance floor (at left) with dresses either halter-necked or so open down the back as to nearly reach the waist, with skirts that flared out at the hem. Silk, chiffon, georgette, and rayon were used in plain, muted colors or multi-colored prints.

I have extended the period here, because accessories were much the same up to 1939 and also because the Romantic look was also evident in the evening, often more covered up, and with almost crinoline-like skirts. After their coronation in 1937, when King George VI and Queen Elizabeth (later the Queen Mother) paid a state visit to Paris, the Queen stunned Parisians by wearing a magnificent white crinoline dress.

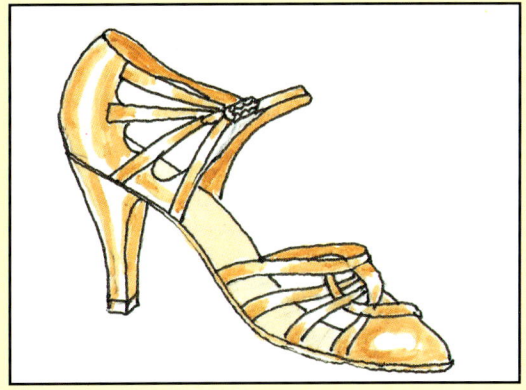

A gilt kid sandal such as those Ginger Rogers might have worn when dancing with Fred Astaire.

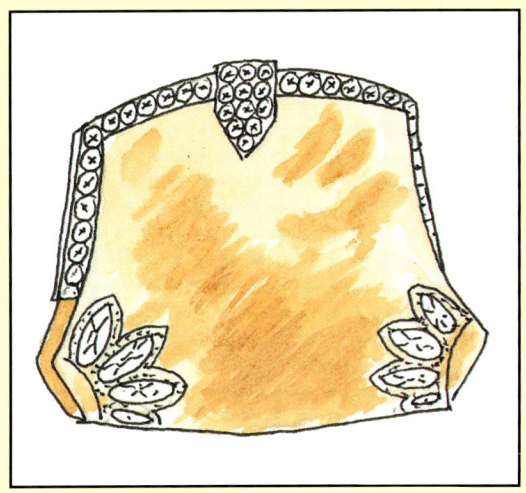

Gold lamé sewn with brilliants and more brilliants on the metal frame and clasp.

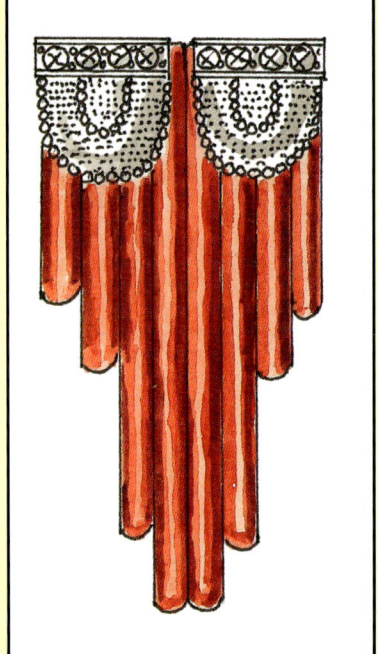

The kind of clip (this one in plastic), which would have been fastened to the back of an evening dress, as seen in the full-length figure.

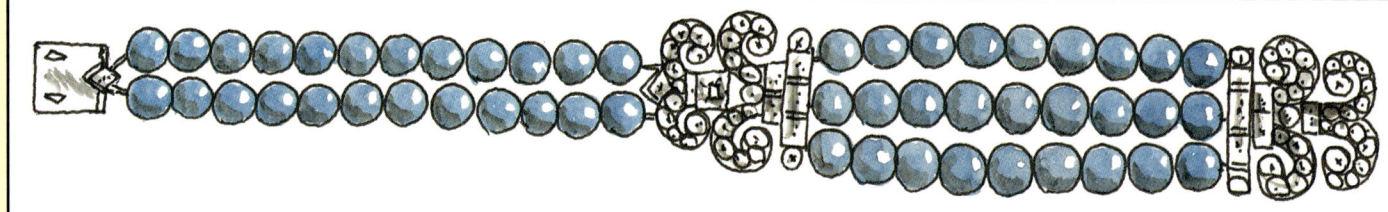

A magnificent diamond and chalcedony bead bracelet.

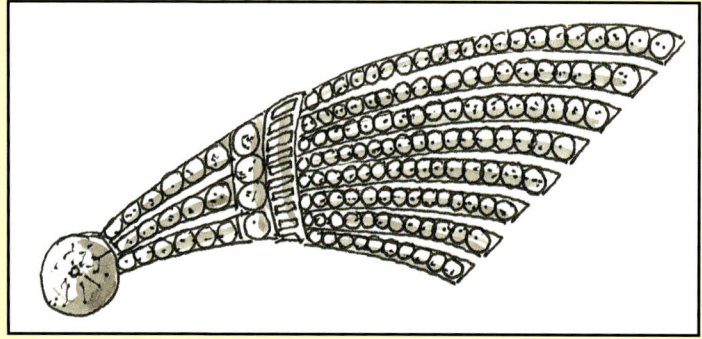

A grand, comet-shaped or shooting star-shaped evening clip.

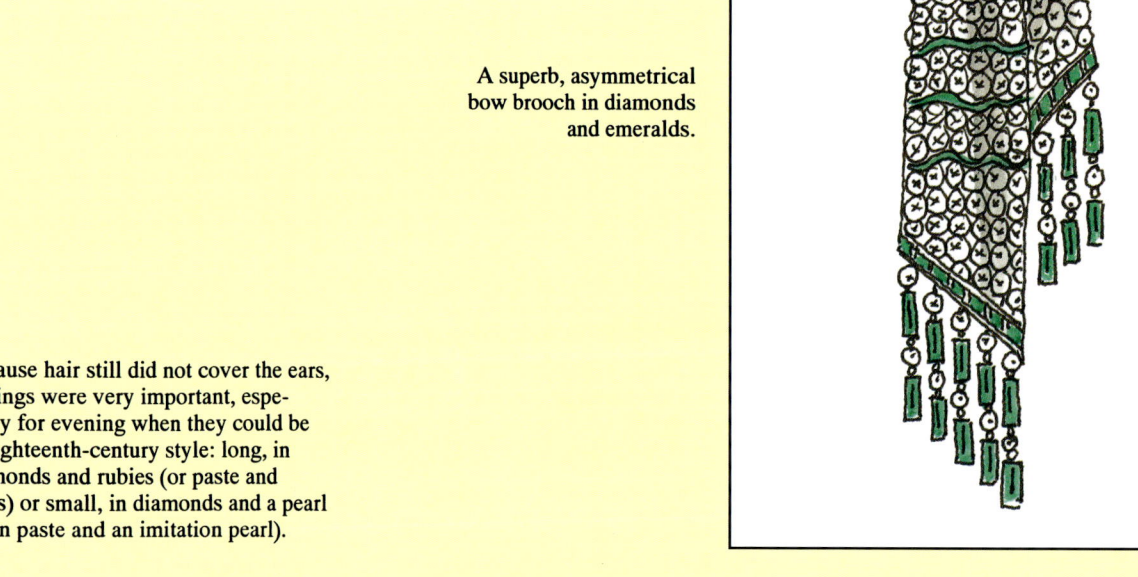

A superb, asymmetrical bow brooch in diamonds and emeralds.

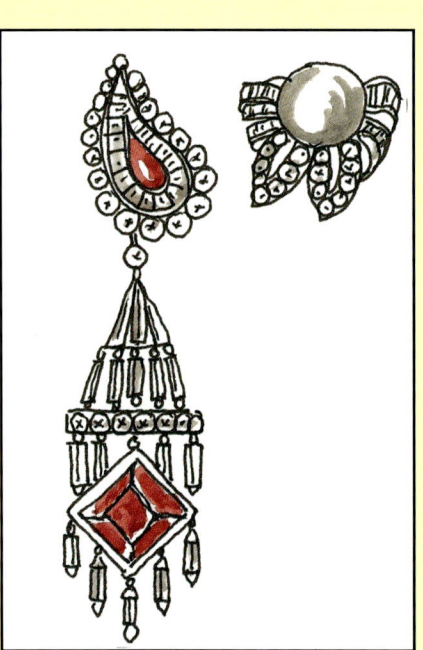

Because hair still did not cover the ears, earrings were very important, especially for evening when they could be in eighteenth-century style: long, in diamonds and rubies (or paste and glass) or small, in diamonds and a pearl (or in paste and an imitation pearl).

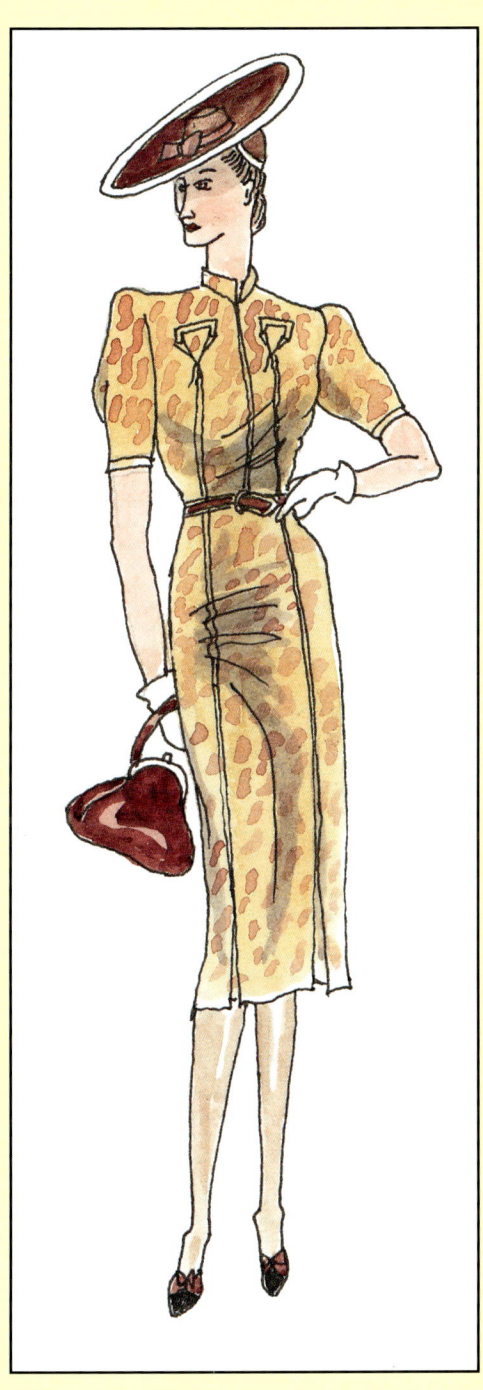

1937-1939 Day Wear

By the late 1930s, skirt hemlines had risen to just below the knee. Short sleeves had puffed shoulders but the whole look was rather skimpy. This style was likely a reflection of the anxiety people felt, knowing another big war was on the horizon, an anxiety relieved by some crazy hats.

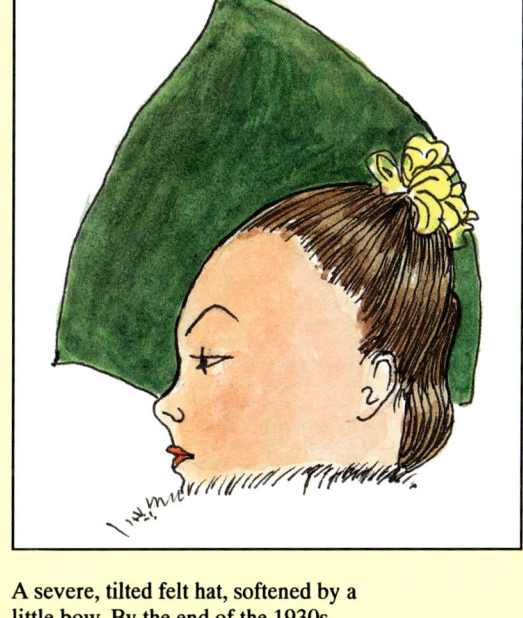

A severe, tilted felt hat, softened by a little bow. By the end of the 1930s, many women wore their hair swept up, with coils at the nape of the neck.

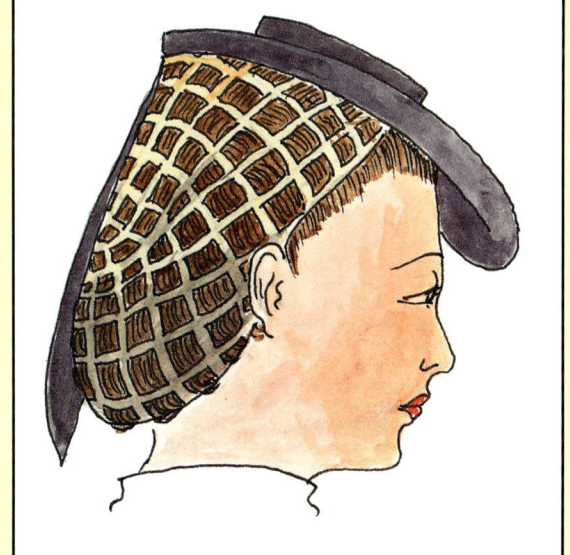

Once popular in the 1860s, a coarse net snood was revived in the late 1930s and continued to be worn in the early 1940s. Here the net is shown with a minute hat.

By the close of the 1930s, hats were more varied in shape but often rather absurd, such as this huge "dinner plate" in velvet. Displaying that women had not lost their fascination with the reptile, the woman here also wears a thin gold, snake necklace.

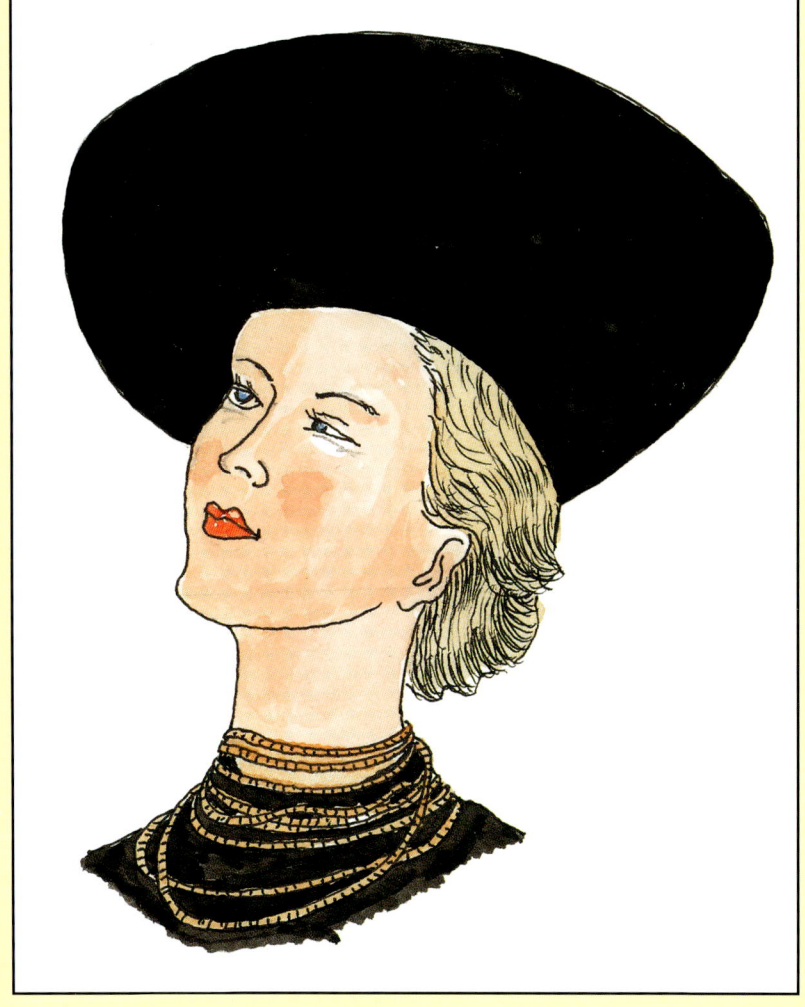

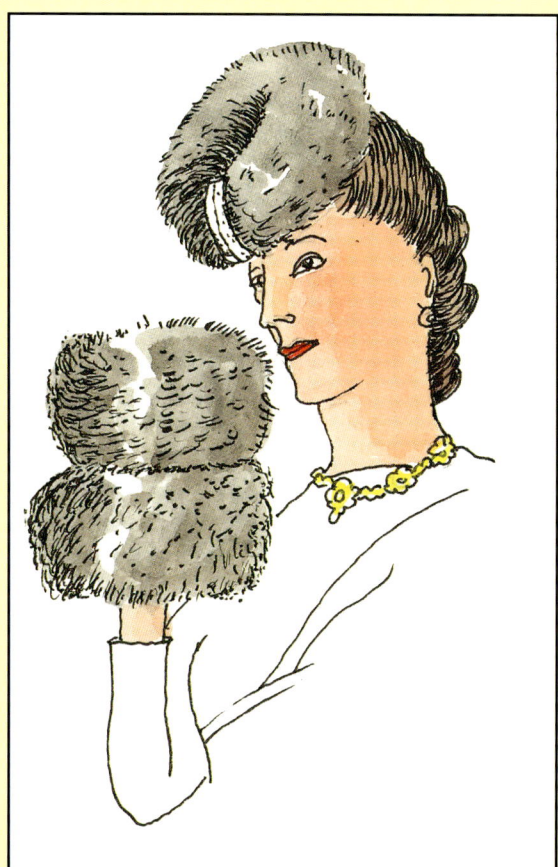

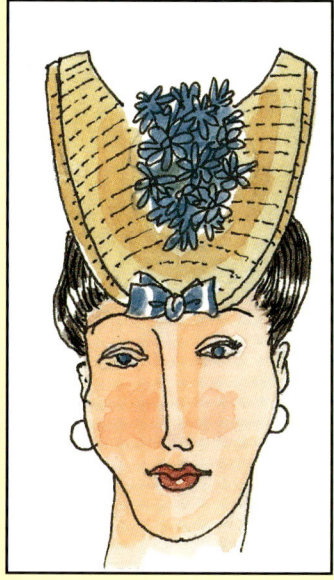

A saucy little straw hat, intended to provoke and amuse.

As a whole coat, a stole, or as trimming, silver fox was still the smartest fur. Here, it is used to make a brooch-clasped hat and muff.

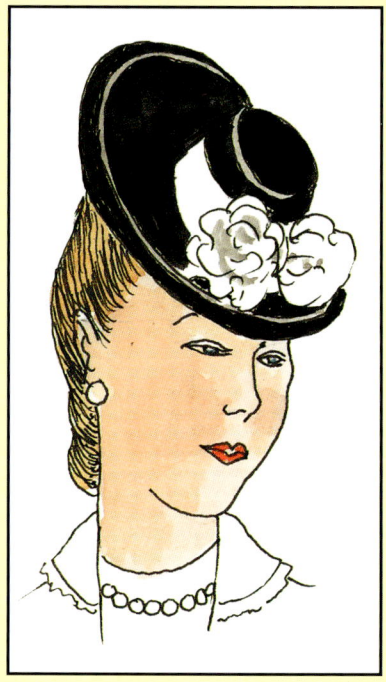

This mannish little hat is made feminine by ribbon and flowers.

Very high-heeled, much strapped, and thick-soled, such sandals were worn for informal occasions and holidays.

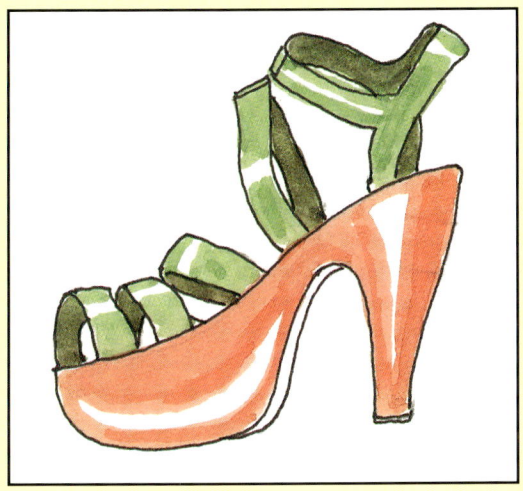

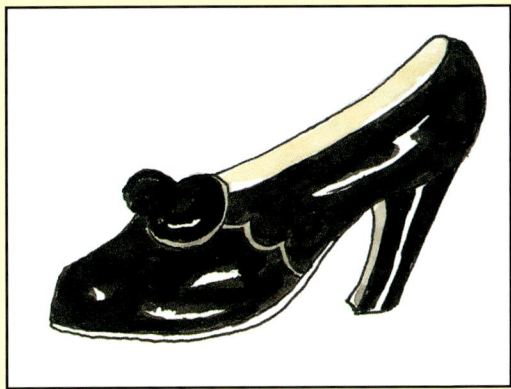

A rather clumpy version of the leather court shoe.

Mrs. Simpson, then Duchess of Windsor and one of the smartest of late-1930s ladies, did much to promote bold if somewhat vulgar jewelry. Much of hers was in the form of animals and birds, made for her by jewelers in le Place Vendome in Paris when she was in exile there. Her favorite and most famous piece is this flamingo brooch, encrusted in diamonds, rubies and sapphires; lesser mortals made do with plastic. This piece was much copied in all sizes well into the 1960s.

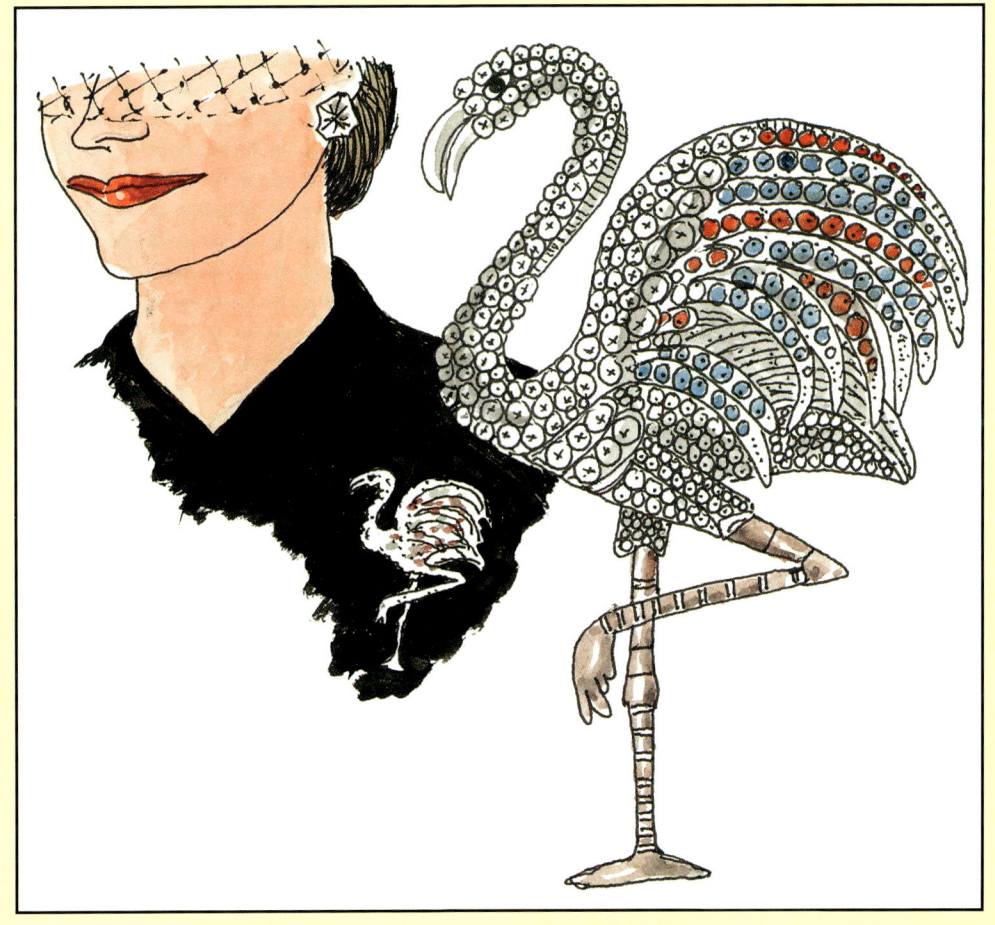

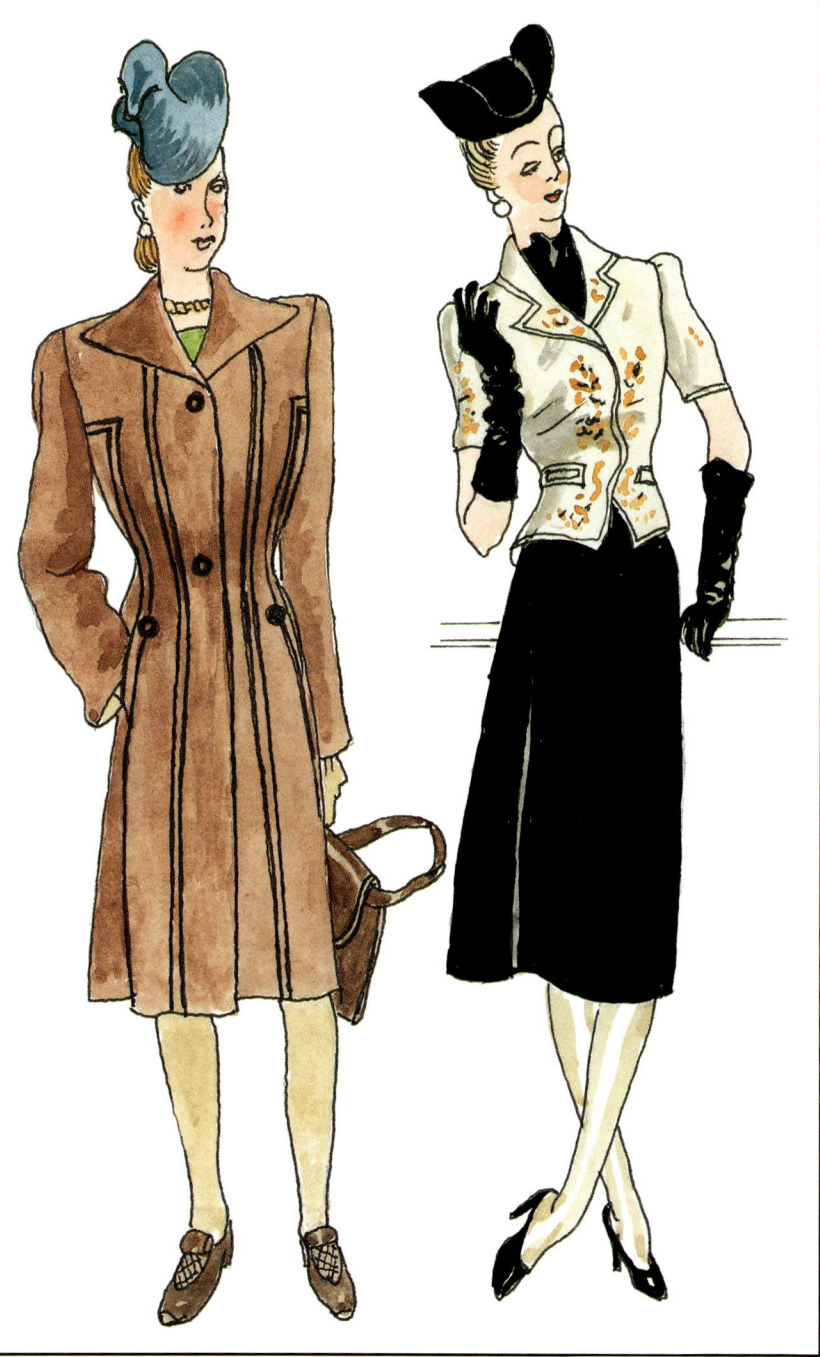

1940-1945 Day Wear

The Second World War (1939 to 1944) had a far greater effect on fashion, particularly in Britain and in Europe, than the First World War. Although Britain declared war on Germany in September 1939, it was not until May 1941 that the government, in an attempt to cut down on materials, introduced Utility Clothes, pared-down versions of pre-war styles. Despite the introduction of this clothing, coats (at left) were bulkier. After America entered the war in 1941, there were some restrictions as to the amount of material and trimming used in American fashions, but nothing as extensive as in Britain. Cut off from Paris, American designers had to create their own styles (at right), with a number of elegant hats.

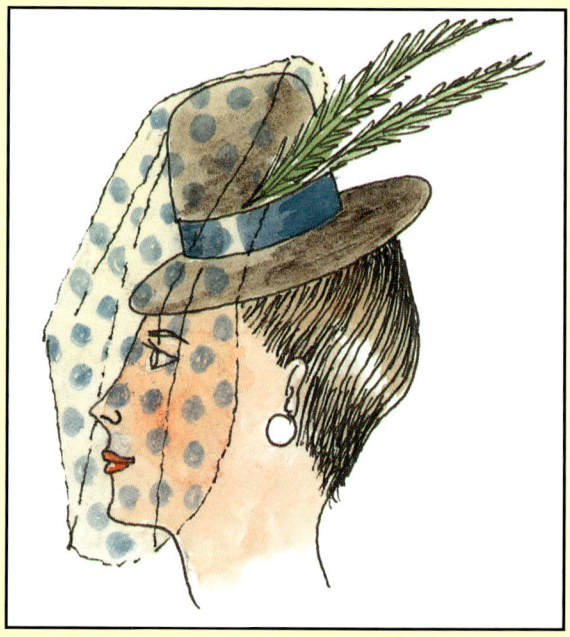

A perky little British nonsense hat with a velvet-spotted veil. As one fashion writer stated in 1940, "A spring hat is a tonic. It's good for the spirits. It's fun for your friends."

Even after the German occupation of Paris in June 1940, a number of French couturiers carried on, some as an act of defiance or, some in collaboration with the enemy. Soon after Paris was liberated in August of 1944, its fashion influence was once more in full force on both sides of the Atlantic.

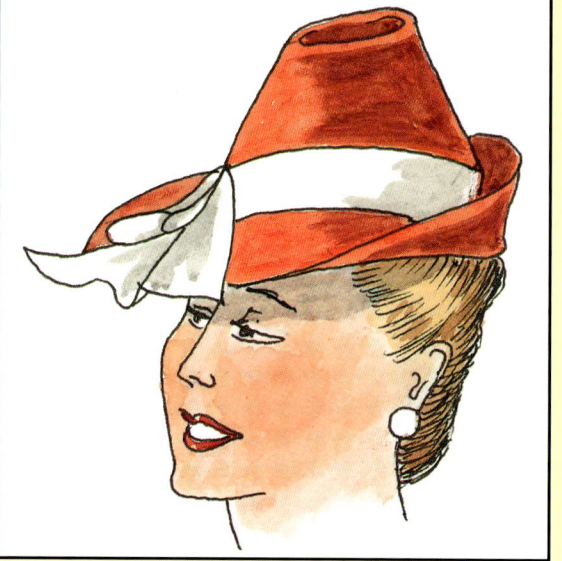

A felt and ribbon "Robin Hood" hat, probably inspired by a similar one worn by Errol Flynn in the title role of the 1938 movie.

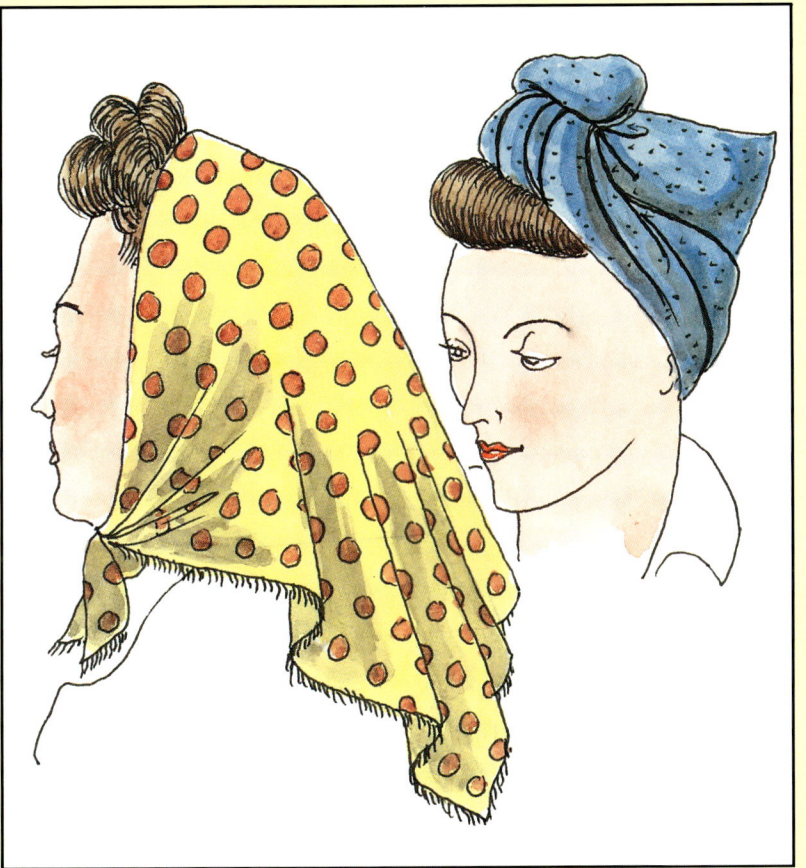

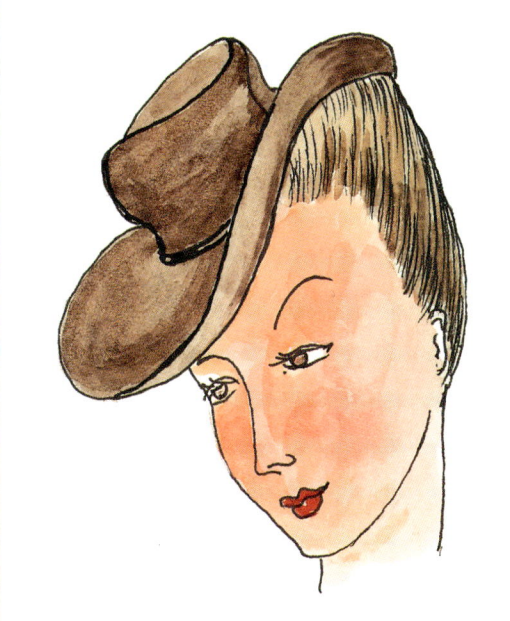

A French felt hat.

Despite the War, many British women did not cease to be stylish, especially when it came to hats which were unrationed. This woman looks particularly smart in a velvet pillbox-cum-turban with matching handbag. Note the heavy gilt and enamelled Art Deco bracelet.

The head scarf (still worn today by all classes in Britain) was very popular during the War, worn loose and in many tied-up variations. The most usual and most symbolic of Britain in war-time, was the form seen at right: tied as a safety measure by the many women who worked in factories and on the land.

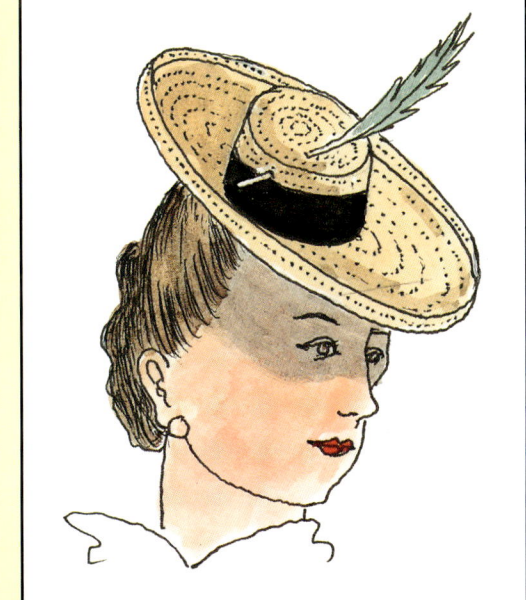

A French creation: a straw hat with an impudent feather.

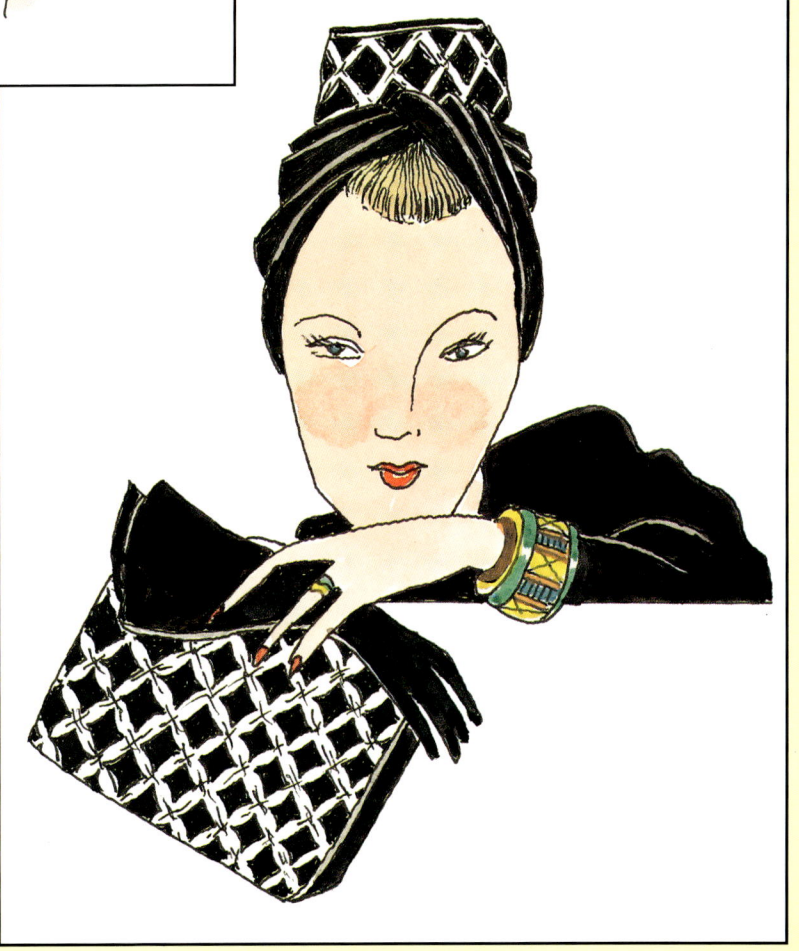

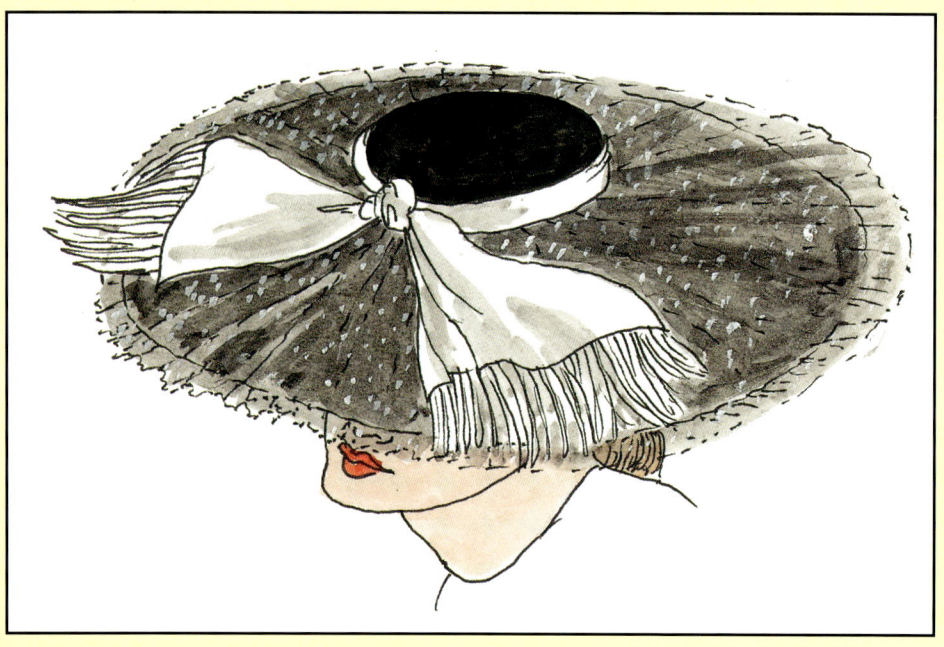

An example of American sophistication: a hat of a low-crowned circle of velvet covered in spotted net, completed with a flamboyant silk bow.

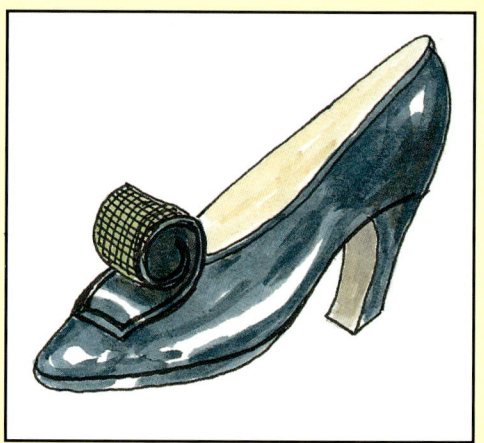

Stylish leather shoe, the swirled ornament lined with tweed.

With severe clothes rationing in Britain, "to eke out the nation's leather" a number of leather shoes were given wooden soles and heels. Critics referred to them as "clogs". The arrows indicate the necessary hinges.

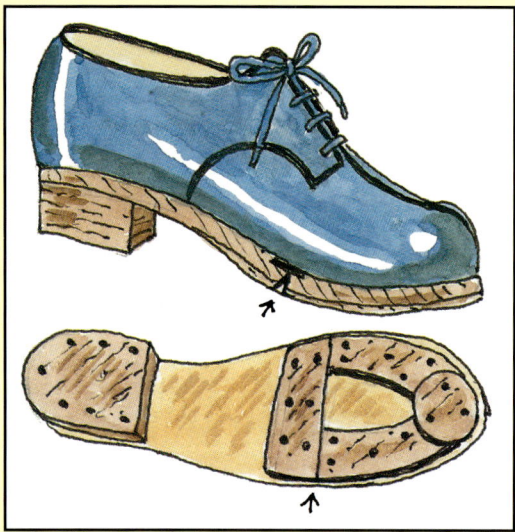

Shoes were still clumpy and blunt-toed. However, this shoe in suede is made elegant with trimmings.

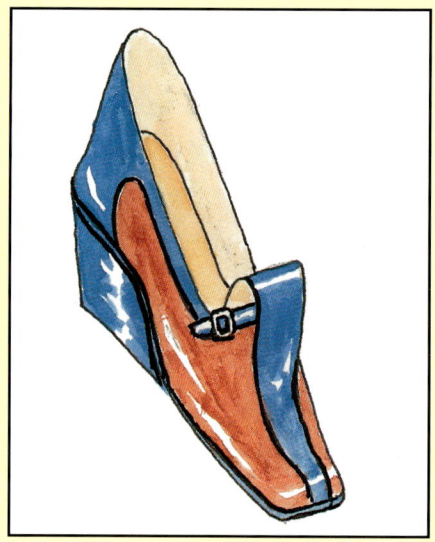

By the end of the War, British shoes began to loose their heavy look; as in this narrow, squared-toed leather example with wedge heel.

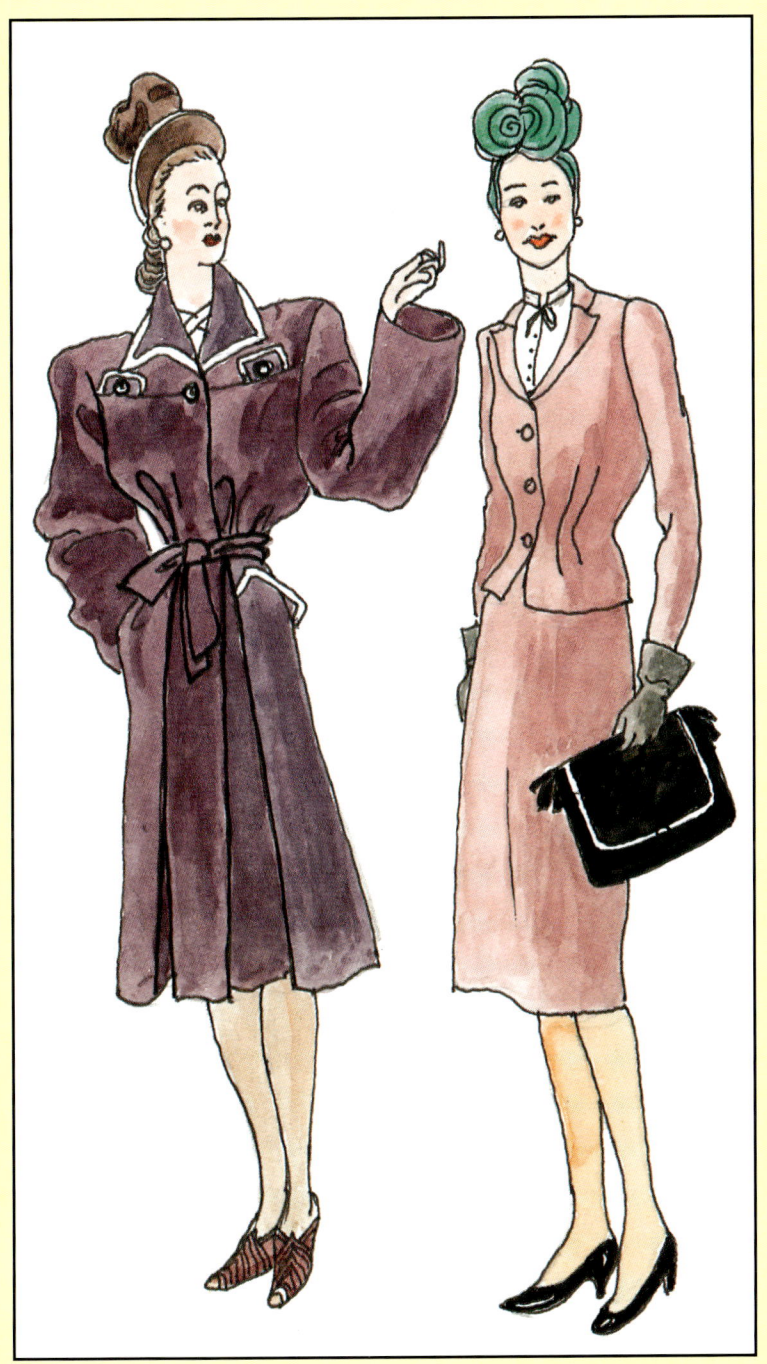

1945-1947 Day Wear

In Britain, where severe post-war austerity affected all aspects of life, fashion remained much as it had been, with bulky coats (at left) and little suits (at right) which did manage to look quite elegant, especially in popular "strawberry" pink. Despite equal deprivations, French couturiers produced extravagant but stylish clothes with gusto. America was particularly noted for its creation of fashions for the teenager (girls in full skirts, tight pants, blouses, or sweaters), a consumer who was to become an important fashion and economic factor in the years to come.

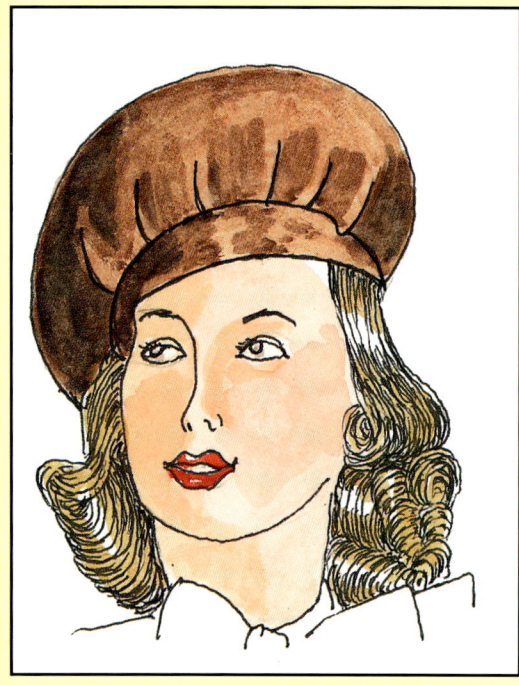

In Britain, symbolic of post-war austerity, even hats, such as this felt "sailor" style, were sober.

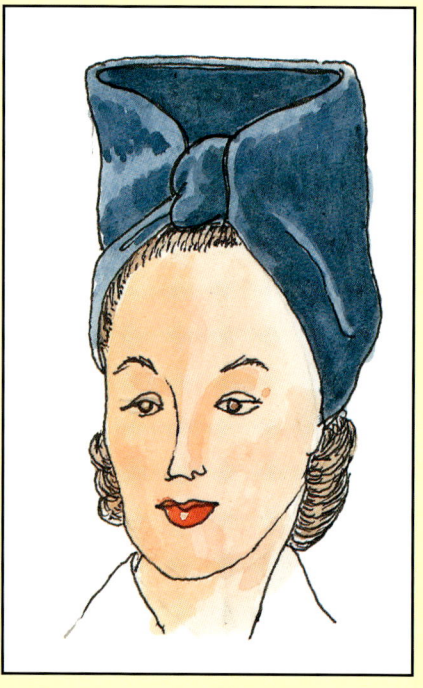

The war-time tied-up scarf, given elegance in the form of a velour creation.

Although still rationed, shoes began to take on a more elegant, even flippant air, as in this "peep-toe" leather example.

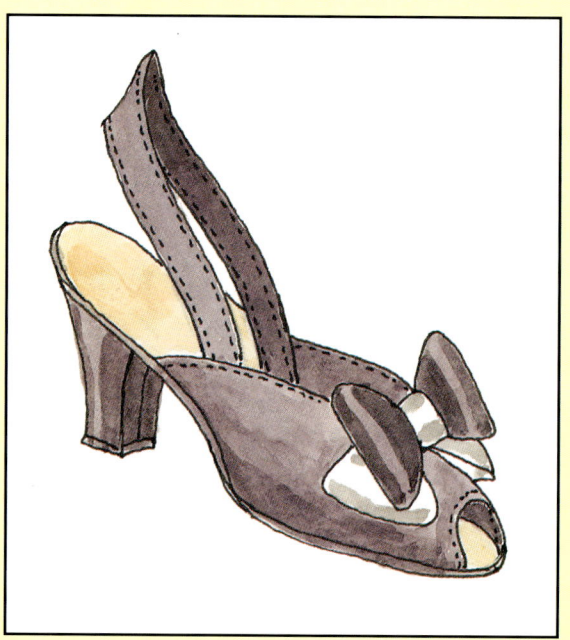

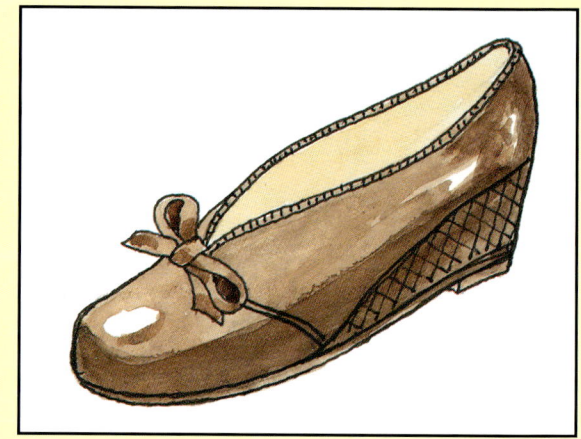

However, austerity is still evident in this simple leather shoe with its blunt toe and wedge heel.

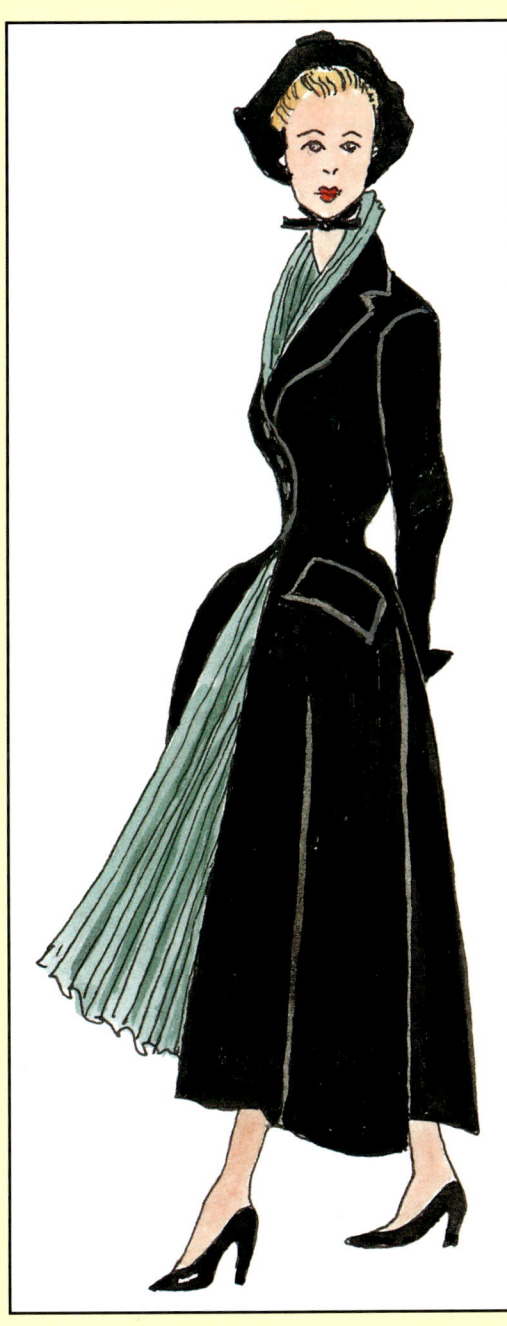

1947-1948 Day Wear

This was a short but important fashion period. Although the 1946 Paris Collections were reported to be "fabulous" and feminine, femininity still had a post-war restrictiveness about it. It was not until February 1947, when Christian Dior launched his famous "New Look," that "real" femininity was in the air again. Dior filled out and lengthened the skirt 7 to 8 inches above the ground, tightened the bodice, pinched in the waist, sloped the shoulders, and narrowed the sleeves; one garment could use 50 yards of material. Although much criticized for its waste, the style was quickly taken up (or adapted) by glamour-starved women, especially in America where shortage of material was not much of a problem. Ironically, the look was not really "new"; it was more of a nostalgic look back to the 1880s. However, this style did set the pace for the greater femininity of the 1950s. In Britain, it was difficult to wear the whole look, because clothes rationing did not end until March 1949.

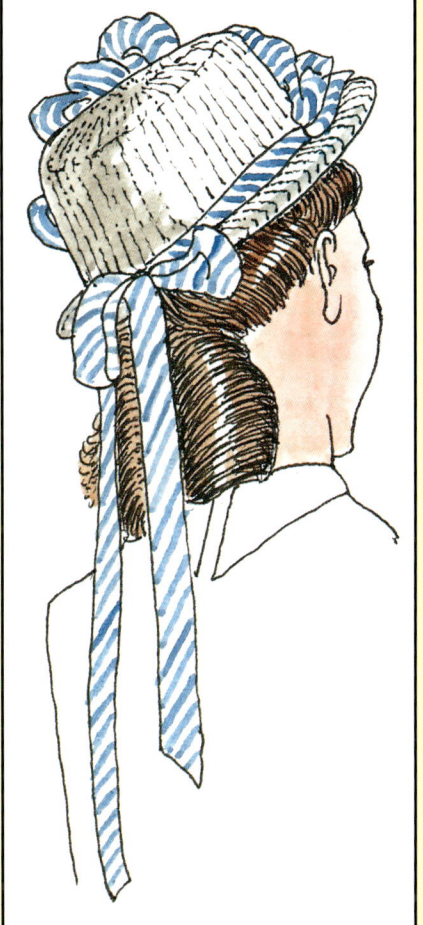

As explained in the text, Dior's 1947 "New Look" was also a nostalgic glance to the past. This stitched silk hat with its ribbons would not have looked out of place in the early 1880s.

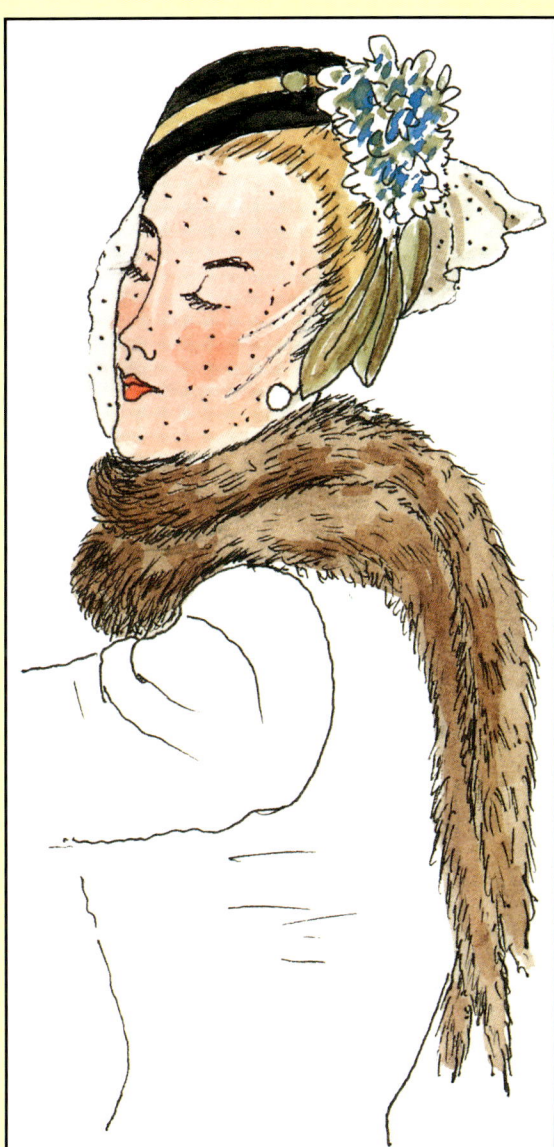

"New Look" chic. A tiny velvet pillbox and a spotted veil, worn with a fur stole.

A very "New Look" sandal, also made in black and dark colors. It was, ironically, favored by both Royal Family members and streetwalker prostitutes!

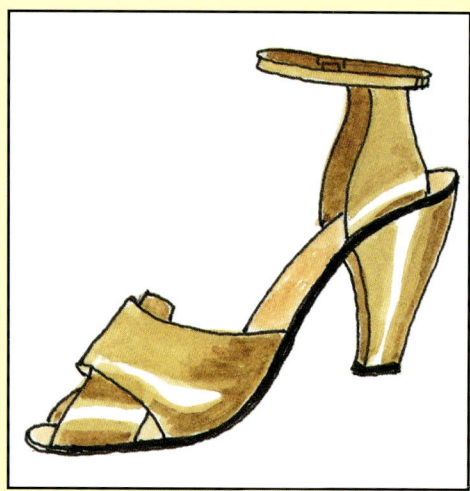

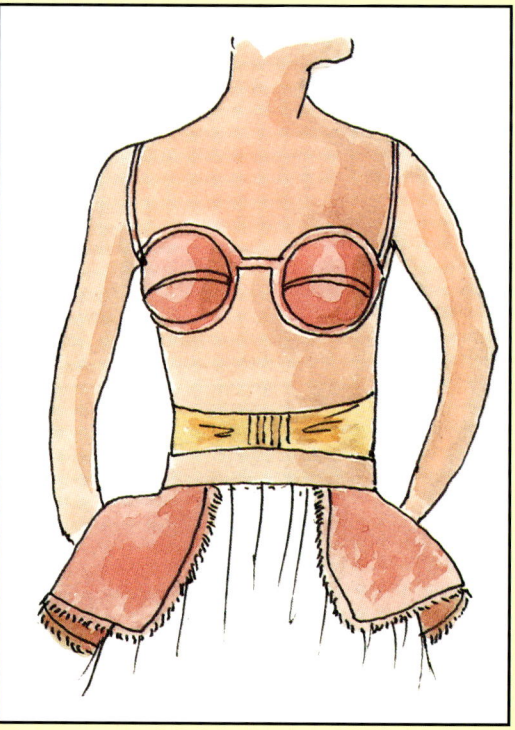

Not since the "S"-bend corset had women needed so much underpropping as the "New Look" demanded: padded brassiere; constricting waist-band, and padding for the hips.

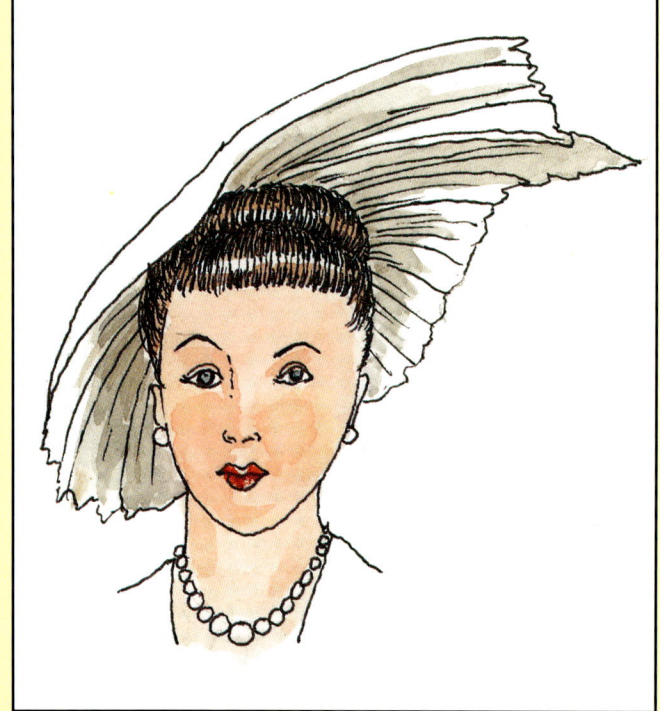

The "New Look" produced some strange hats, such as this swirl of stiffened, pleated silk.

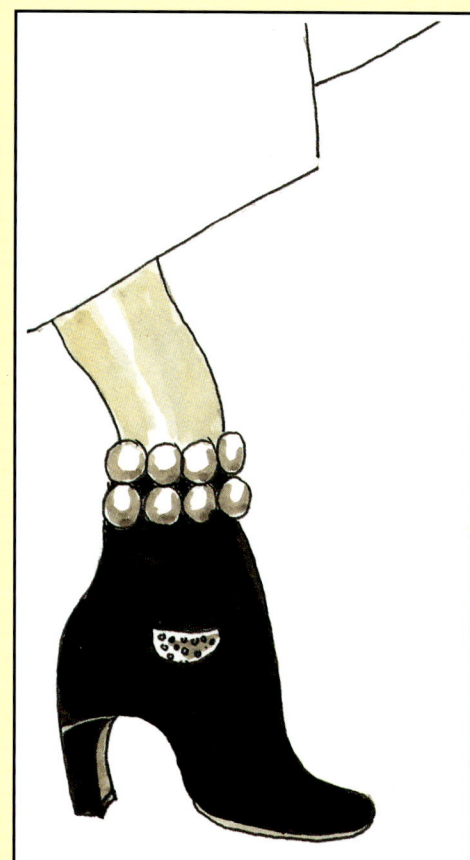

America took to the "New Look" with avidity, as in this 1880s style velvet boot, embellished with huge beads and a diamond clip.

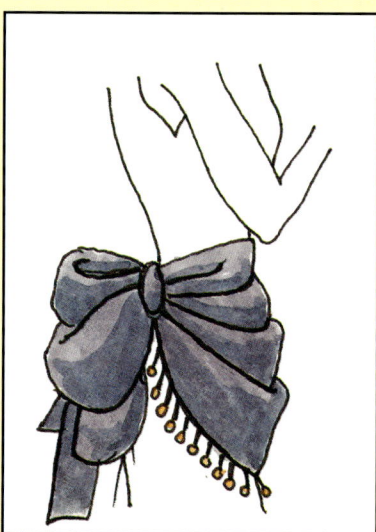

☞ For those who could not afford the "New Look," a number of tricks were employed to achieve it, such as this bustle-and-peplum effect made out of fringed velvet.

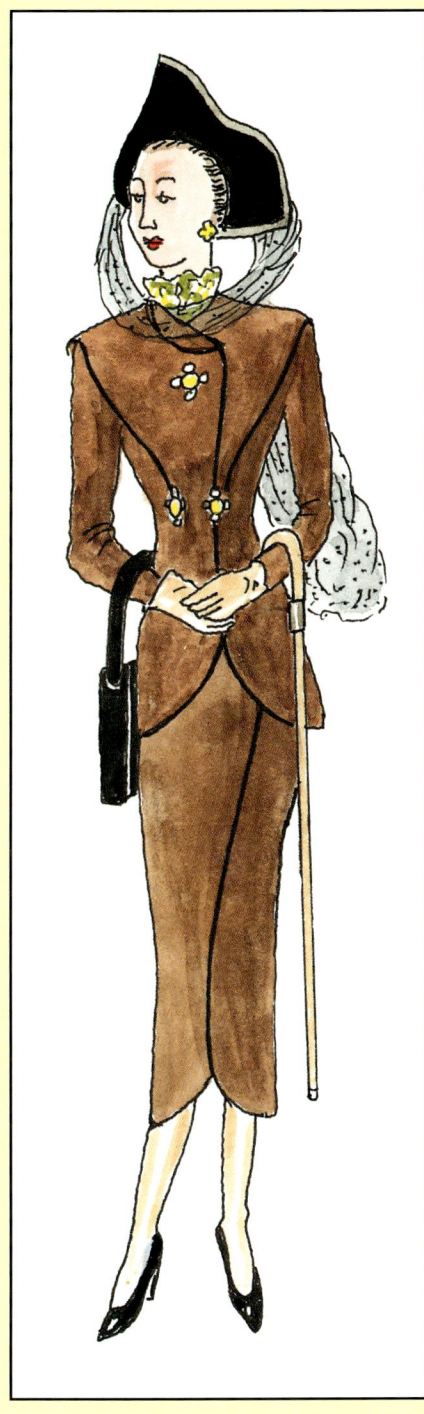

1947-1950 Day Wear

Despite restrictions in Britain, suits and dresses were becoming more elegant, with nipped-in waists, narrow hips, wide shoulders, and often wrap-over, calf-length skirts.

An important factor governing fashion after the War was the adoption of technological and scientific lessons learned during the War, introducing such new materials as melamine, polythene, PVC (vinyl), and molded plastic for jewelry.

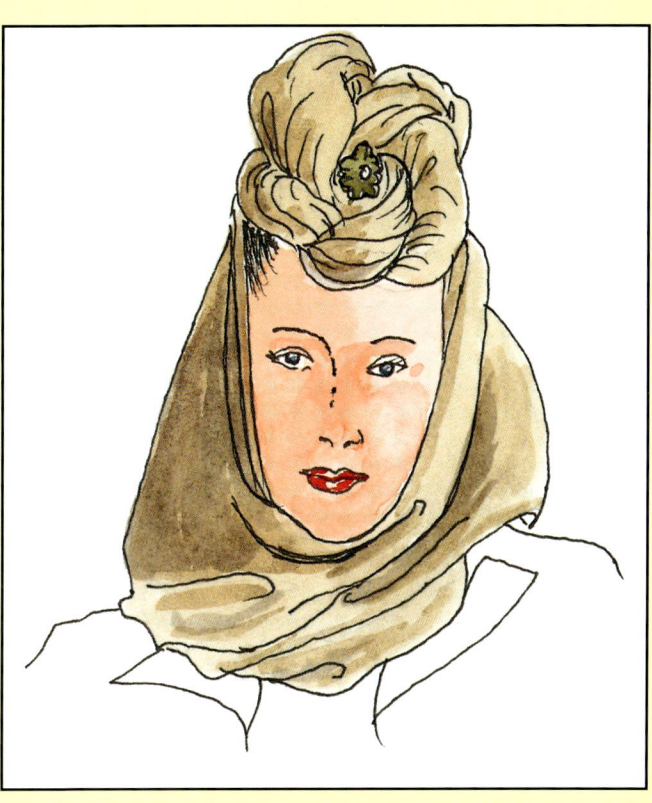

The "New Look" was for the relatively few, so that post-war styles, especially in Britain, were still very much around, as in this heavily swathed jersey turban and scarf.

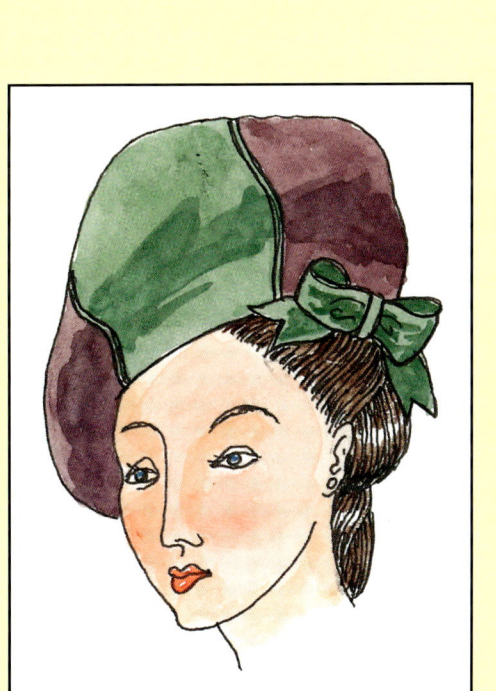

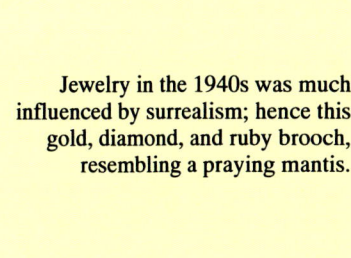

Jewelry in the 1940s was much influenced by surrealism; hence this gold, diamond, and ruby brooch, resembling a praying mantis.

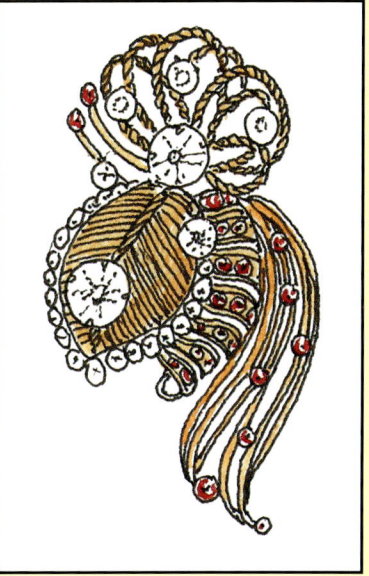

A plain, high, felt beret was also popular.

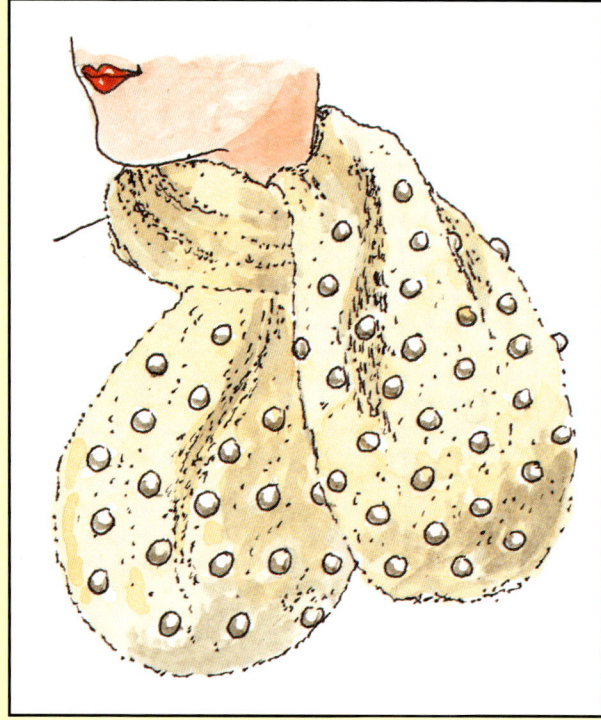

A piece of cocktail-time extravaganza: a lamb's wood muffler studded with imitation pearls.

This style of jeweled basket brooch, with gem fruit or flowers, known as a *Giardinette* (a little flower garden) and dating from the eighteenth century, was revived in the Art Deco period. Made popular when King George VI gave such a basket brooch to his daughter, Princess Elizabeth, in 1941 and another in November 1947 to celebrate the birth of Prince Charles. This particular diamond basket is filled with ruby and sapphire "fruit" and enameled "leaves."

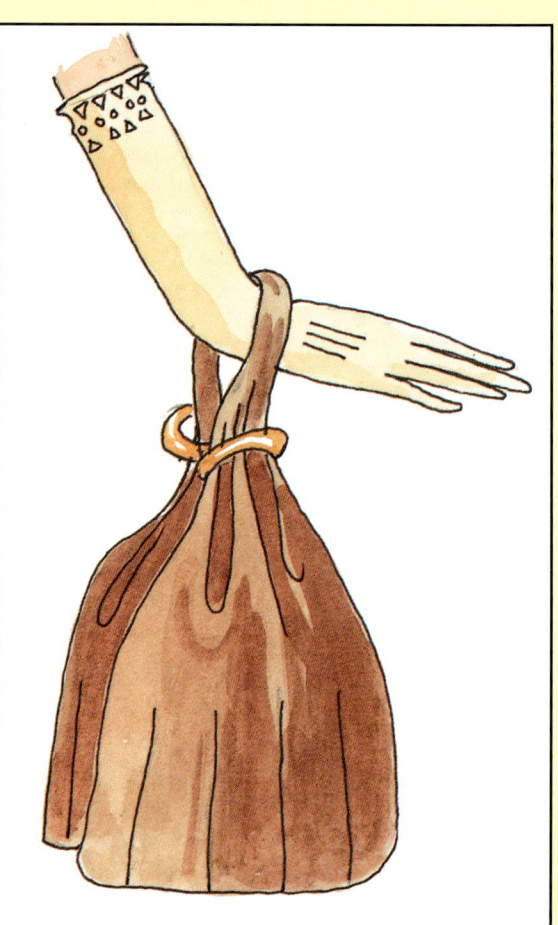

A cloth beach bag with wooden ring fasteners. Significant to the period is the fact that gloves were worn even on the beach.

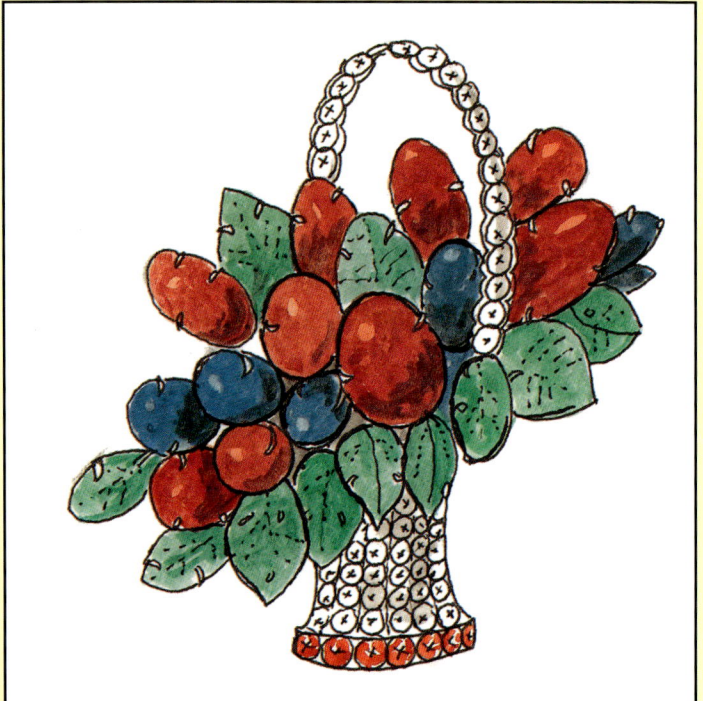

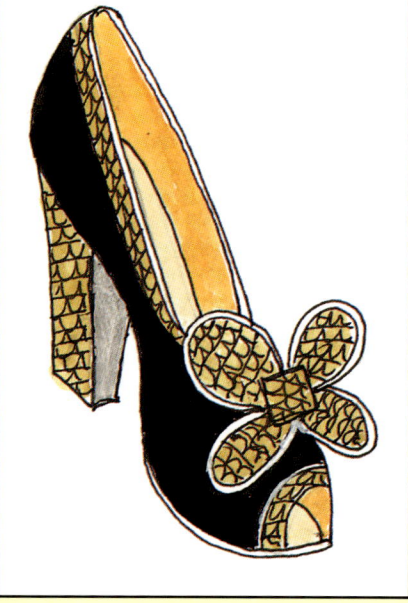

This fanciful "peep-toed" leather shoe is adorned with snakeskin.

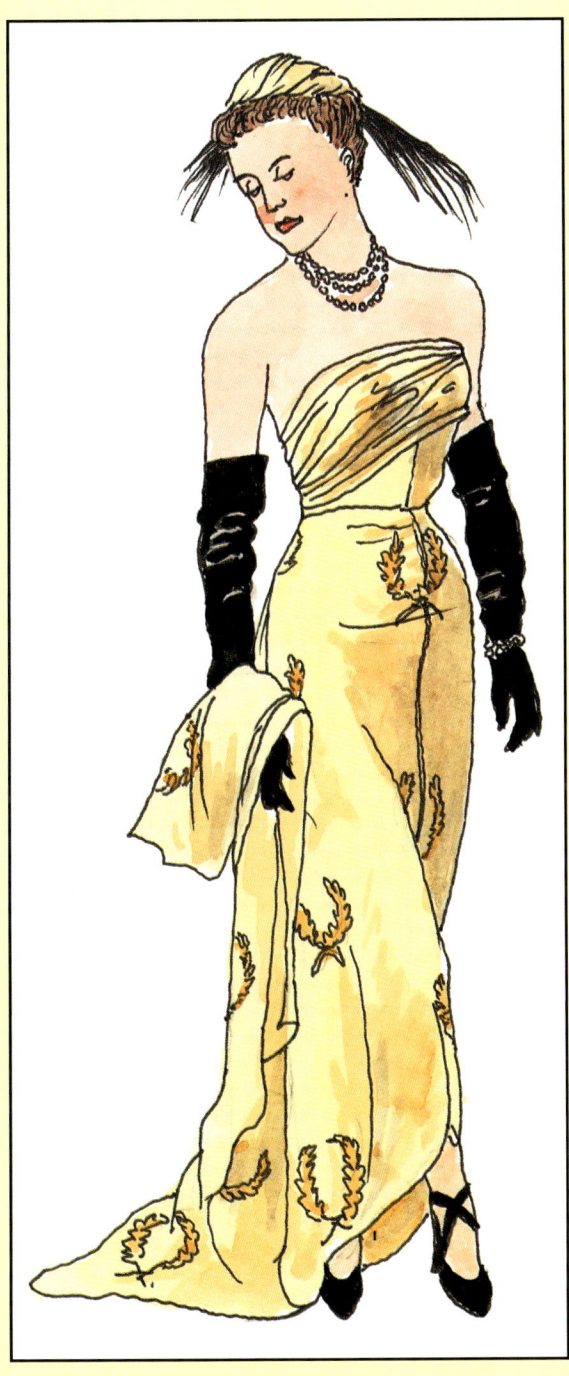

1945-1950 Evening Wear

During the Second World War, evening dresses retained much of their pre-war opulence, but after the War, some new styles were coming in, such as the strapless, boned bodice; tight, long skirts, often with trains, and much beaded embroidery.

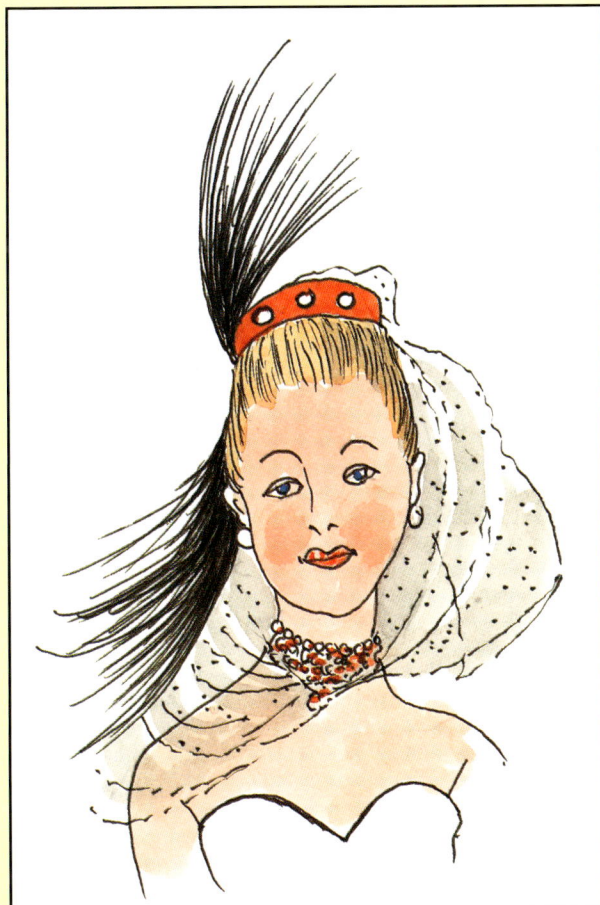

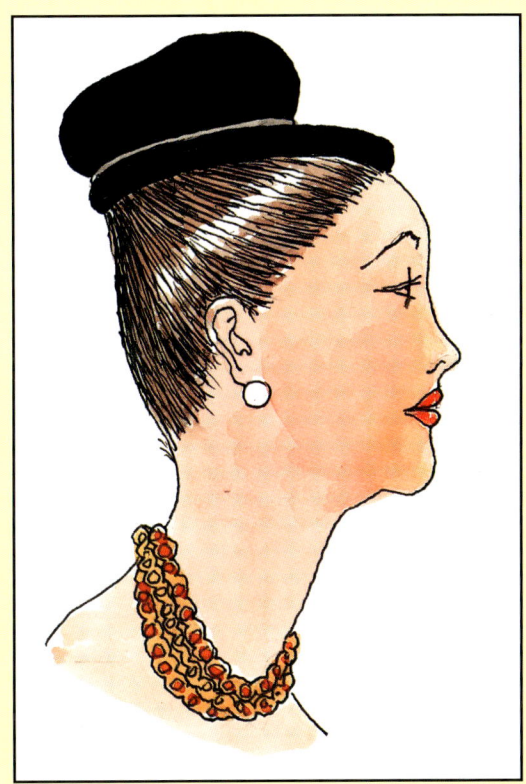

A tiny velvet hat worn with a simple pearl earring and an elaborate three-string real or costume jewelry necklace.

Because evening fashions did not change greatly between 1945 and 1950, accessories also remained much the same over this period. Little velvet "pearl"-decorated hats were popular as were little turbans, veils, and sweeping feathers.

Colored long gloves were fashionable. It was also smart (and continued to be so for day as well, into the 1950s) to wind a necklace around the wrist; shown here, diamonds and gold.

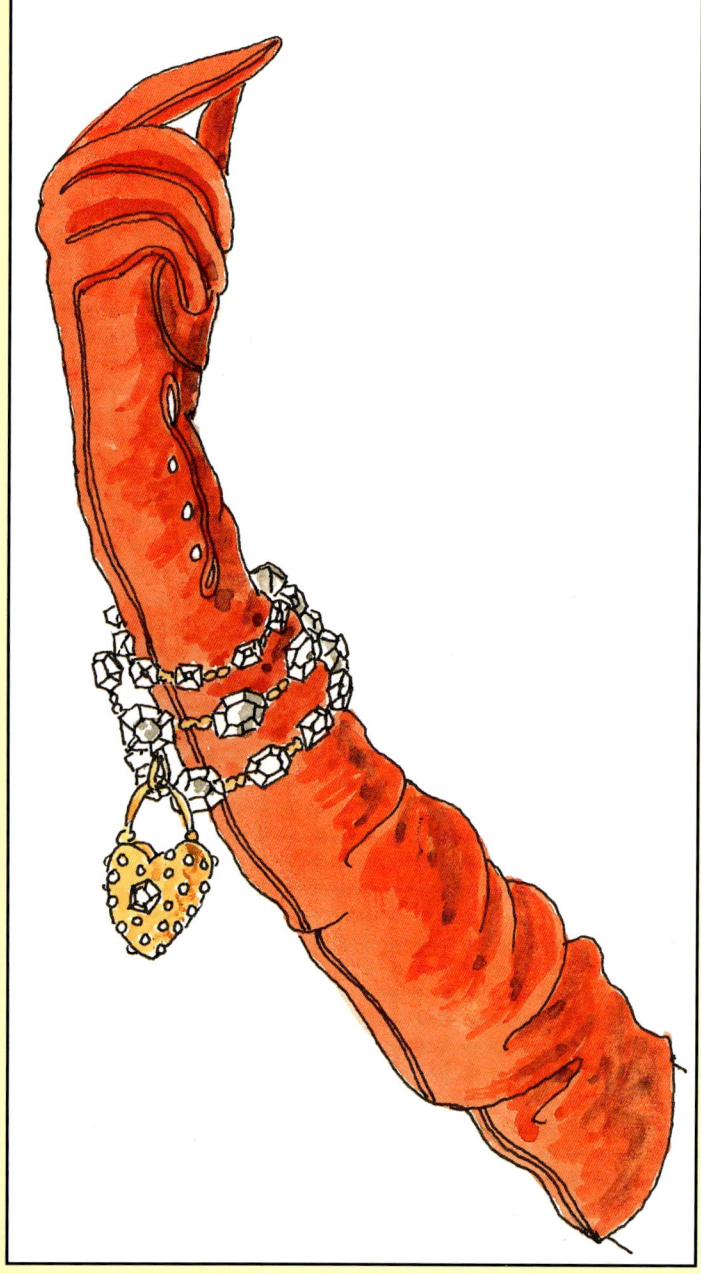

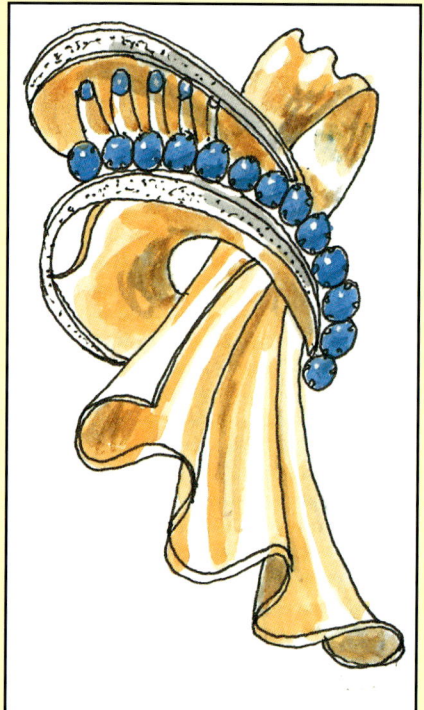

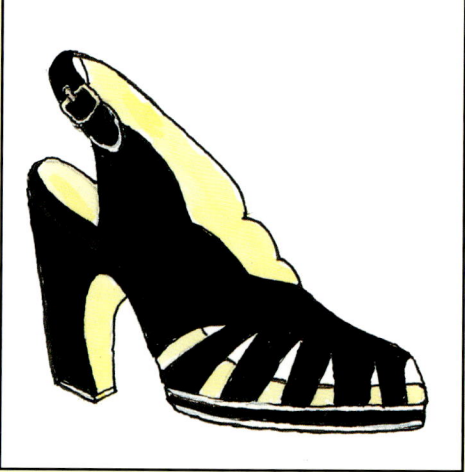

As for day, evening shoes tended to be clumpy, as in this suede "peep-toed" example.

This gold and sapphire brooch was worn during the day, but for evening could be tucked into a coiled-up hairstyle.

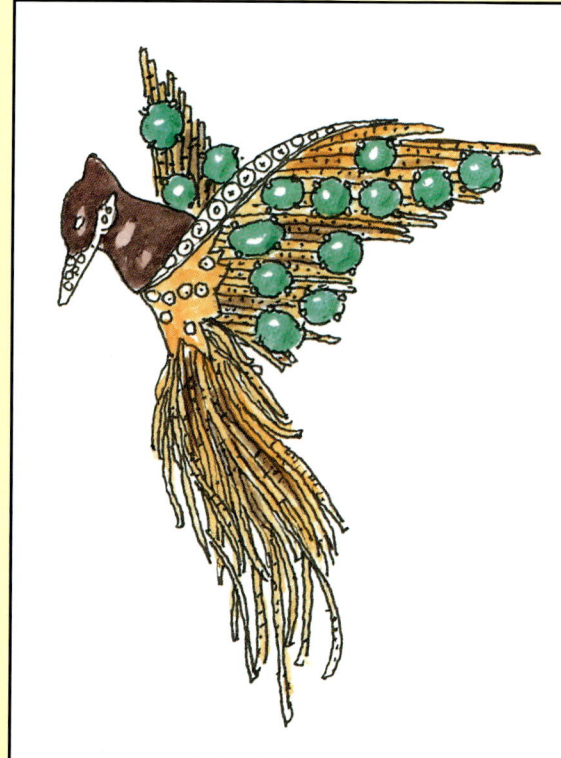

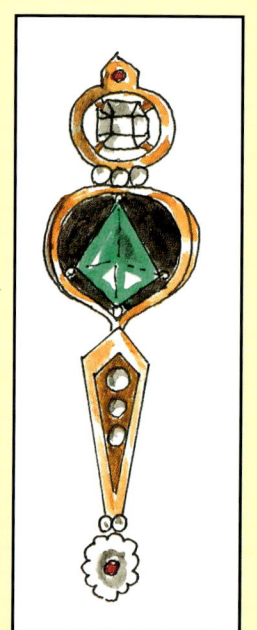

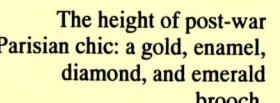

Part classic, part Art Deco, a gold and many-gemmed long earring.

The height of post-war Parisian chic: a gold, enamel, diamond, and emerald brooch.

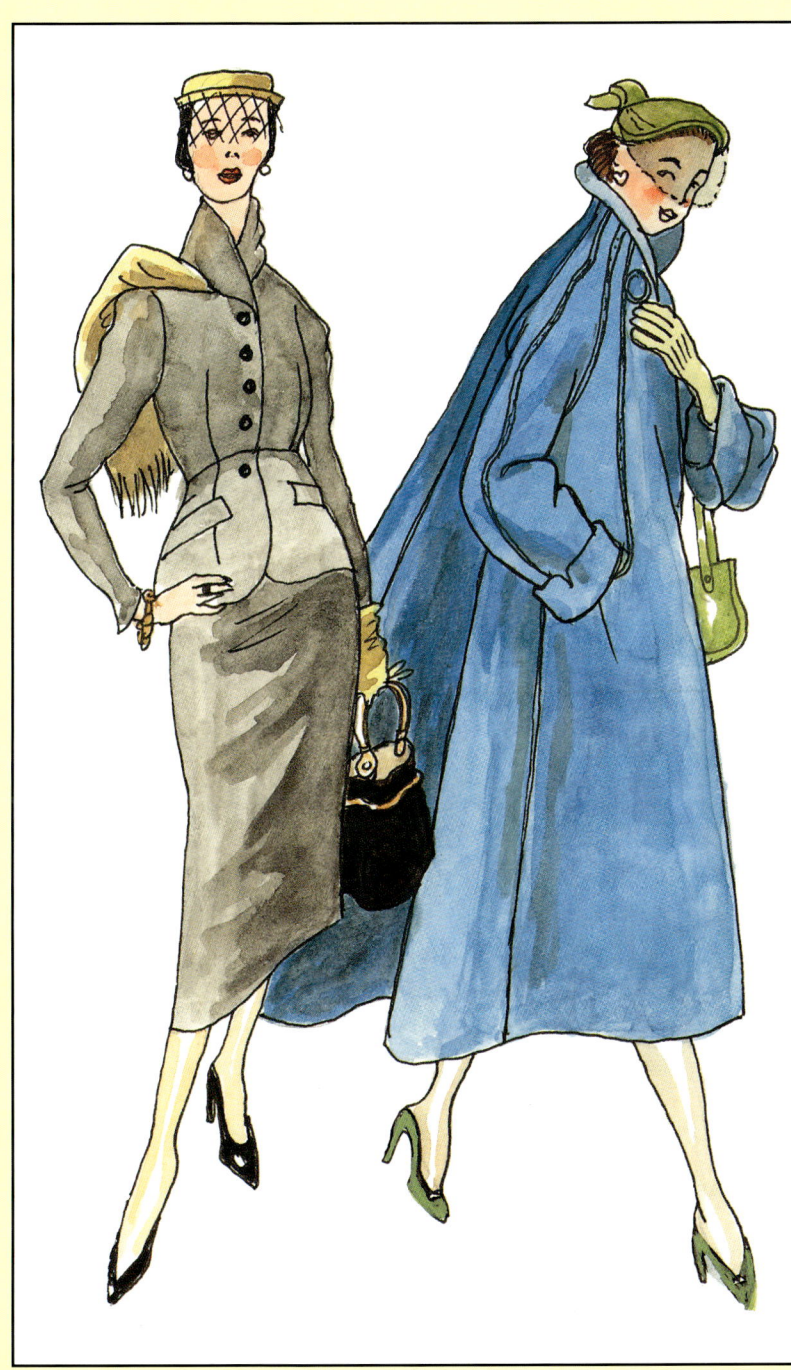

1950-1955 Day Wear

The 1950s in Britain have been dubbed the "drab" decade, but there was a new air of confidence about this period. The 1951 Festival of Britain gave public morale and all the decorative arts, including fashion, a boost. The economy was thriving with nearly full employment and more women were going out to work, although the ideal woman in Britain and America was still the housewife.

Despite having to wear the last figure-constricting corset, an early 1950s woman (at left) stepped out proudly and confidently in her impeccably tailored, tight-waisted, wide-hipped, pencil-slim, just-below-the-knee skirt. Grooming was described by British *Vogue* in 1951 as "our look depends so much on fastidiousness, upon spotless hands and nails, clean, well-brushed hair, and a smooth, soignee look." Wearing the correctly colored accessories was believed to be so important that, during this period, British *Vogue* ran a series of "What to Wear with What" charts. With flannel or wool, clerical gray was the most fashionable color, followed by dark blue and black. In contrast to narrow suits and dresses, coats were voluminous and tent-like and were actually called "tent" coats. Paris couture was probably at its most sophisticated and wearable best, reigned over by such masters as Dior, Balenciaga, and Fath.

America promoted and exported wide and full dirndl skirts, the shirt-waisted dress, and the "sweater-girl." For the first time in centuries, Italian fashion designers entered the international field, with their clever casual clothes and accessories, especially the stiletto heeled shoe, which did more damage to floors than any shoe before or since that time.

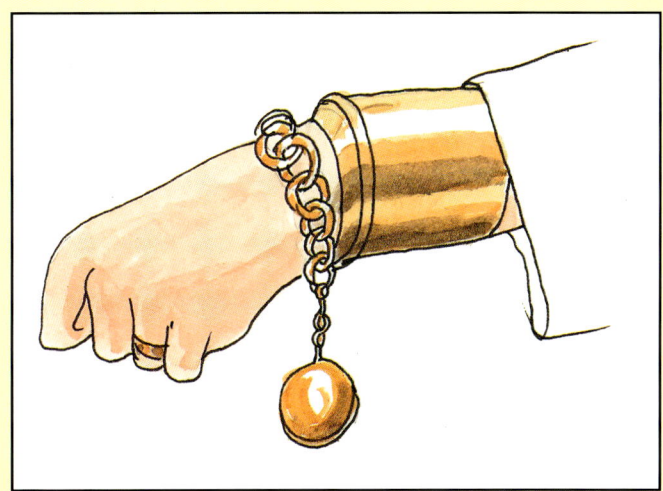

A heavily "armored" wrist weighed down with wide gilt and chain bracelets.

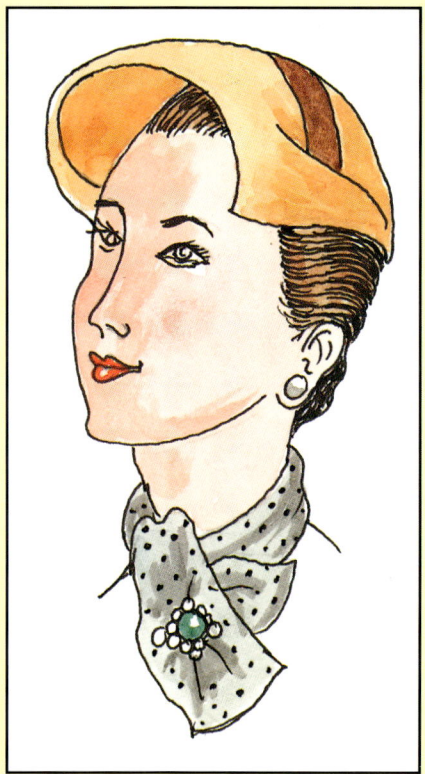

This little shell-like felt hat is archetypical of early 1950s headwear.

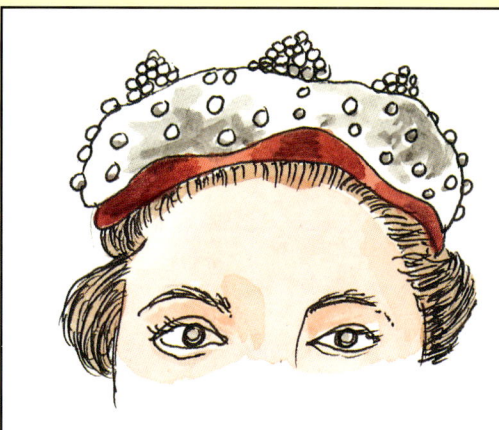

In 1953, Queen Elizabeth II's coronation year, British designers competed in manufacturing suitable items. This "pearl" decorated padded silk hat is in red to suggest velvet and white to simulate ermine, in imitation of a peeress's coronet.

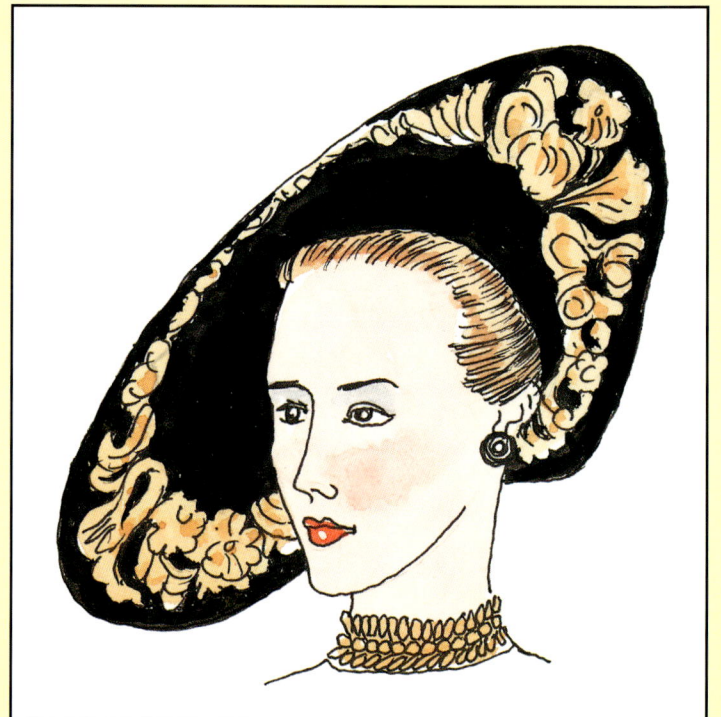

A velvet "halo" hat, richly decorated with embroidered braid.

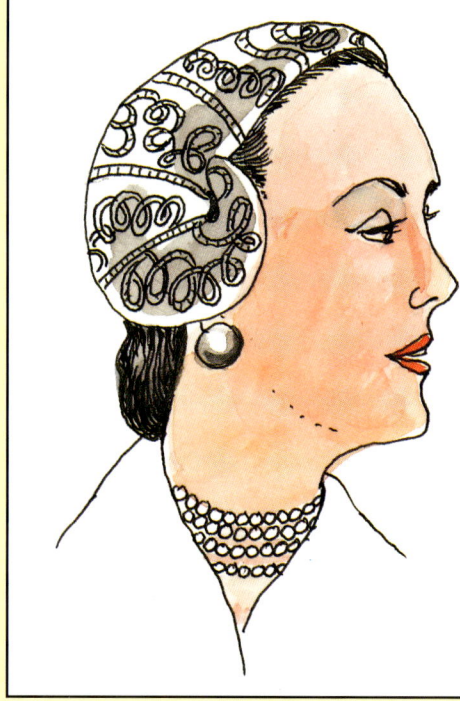

Cord and braid ornament this padded silk "ram's horn" version of the little hat.

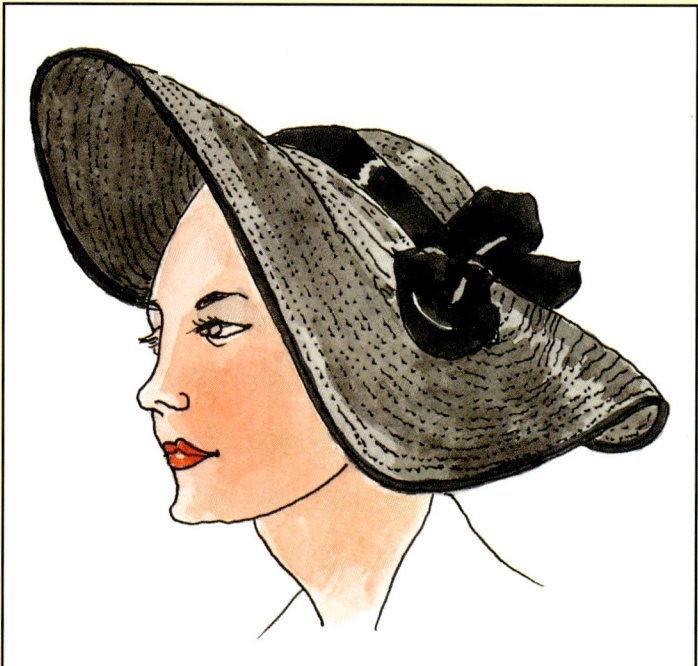

Hats could also be wide, such as this leghorn straw hat for summer.

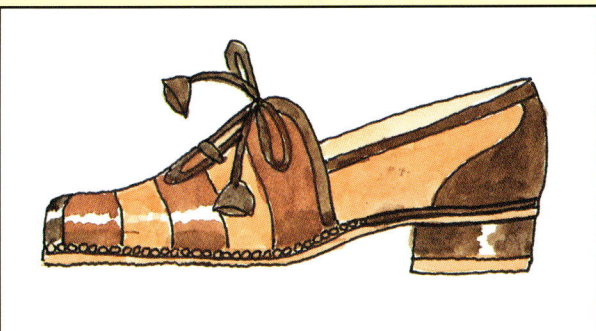

A country shoe in shades of leather.

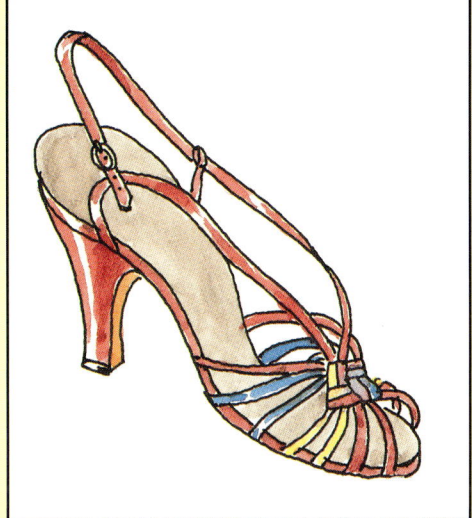

This kind of sandal was much worn for such British occasions as garden parties, weddings, and at Ascot.

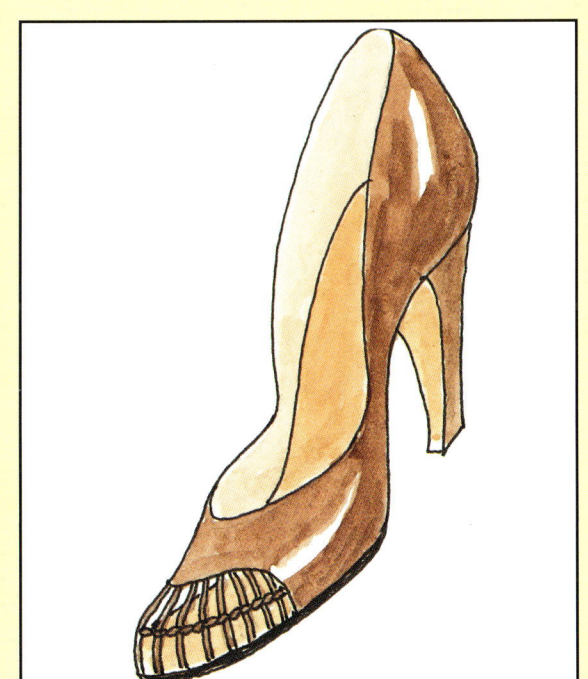

The ever-popular court shoe: in leather with an unusual open-work "birdcage" toe.

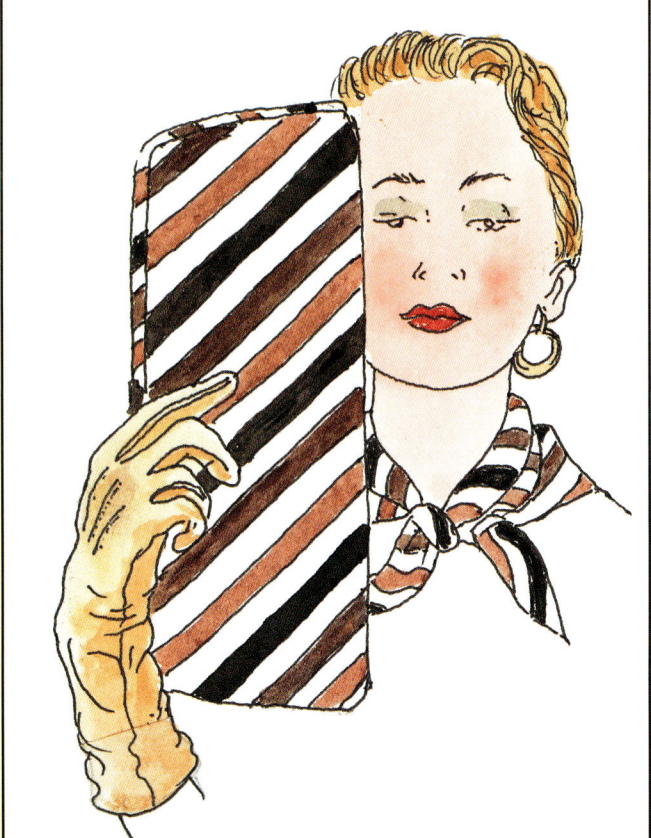

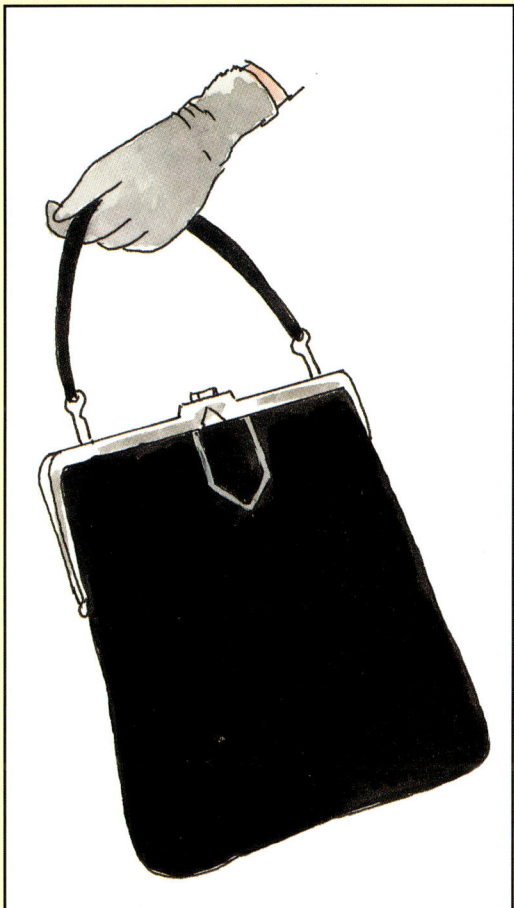

An instance of fashion repeating itself: this huge, thin, flat, and metal-framed reversed calf handbag is reminiscent of those carried during the First World War.

Pochette handbag with matching scarf. Note that long suede gloves were worn during the day as well as in the evening.

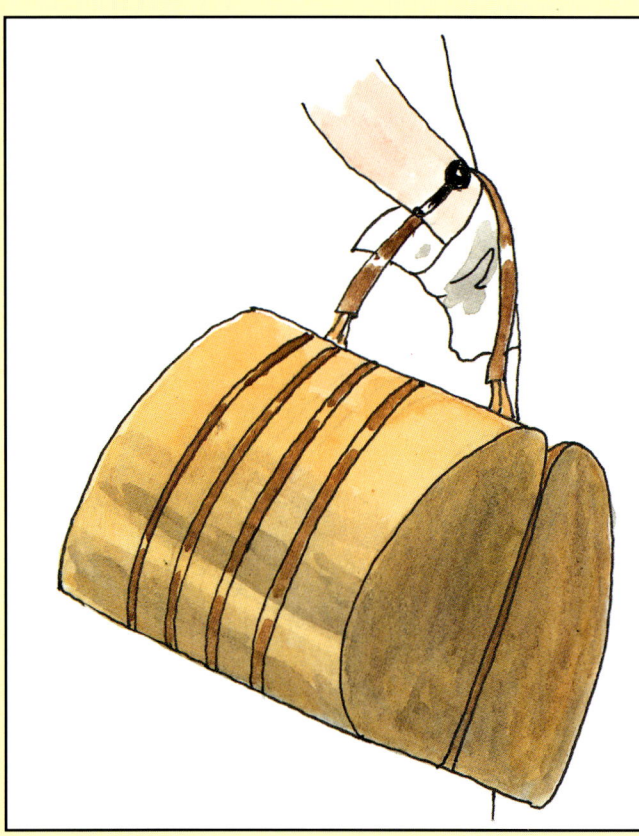

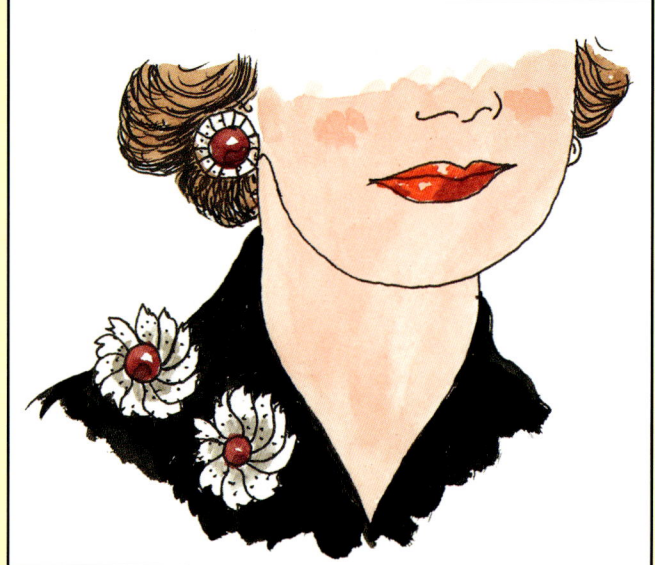

During the first half of the 1950s, it was fashionable to wear brooches, usually in pairs, in unusual places, such as here, in paste and imitation rubies on the shoulder of a cocktail dress. Other places to wear pairs were pockets of suits or anywhere where they would stand out.

☞ A bulky, calf bag for the country.

In the 1950s, costume jewelry is said to have come of age, acceptable everywhere and very much worn. Here, a paste brooch fastens a neck scarf with paste earrings to match.

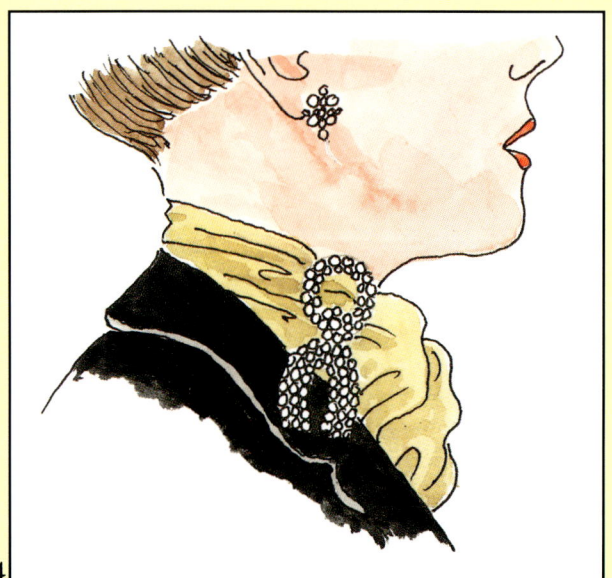

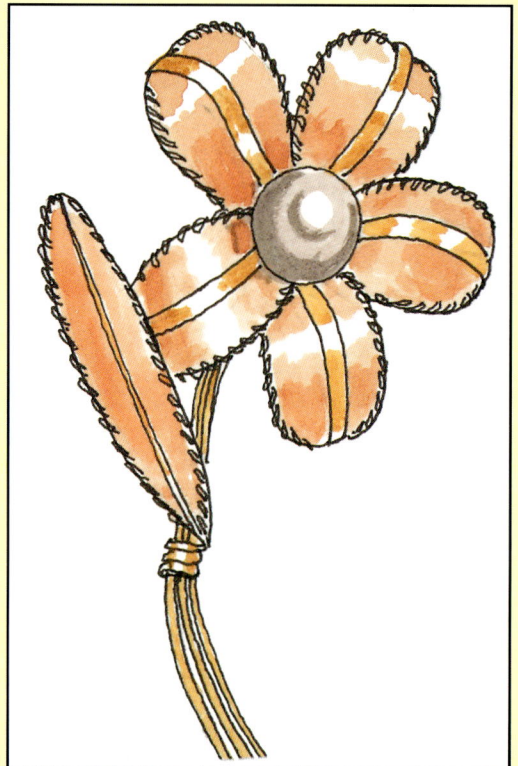

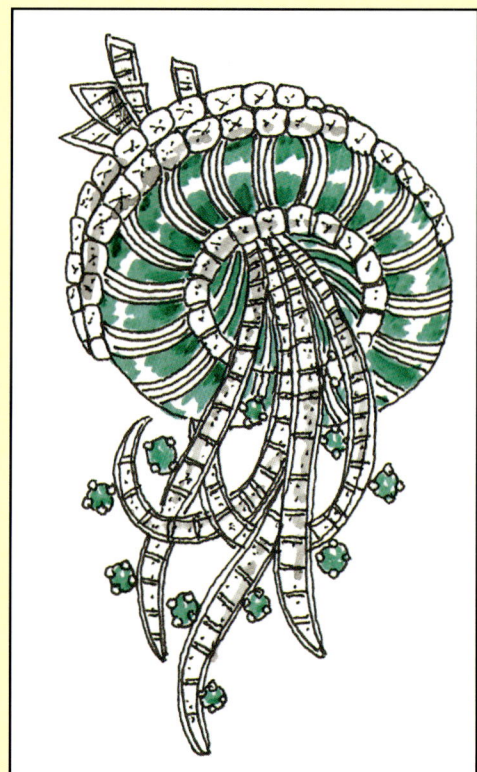

A sea-anemone of a brooch in diamonds and emeralds.

This simulated flower brooch is made of plastic to imitate coral and a pearl and bound about with and given a stem of gilt.

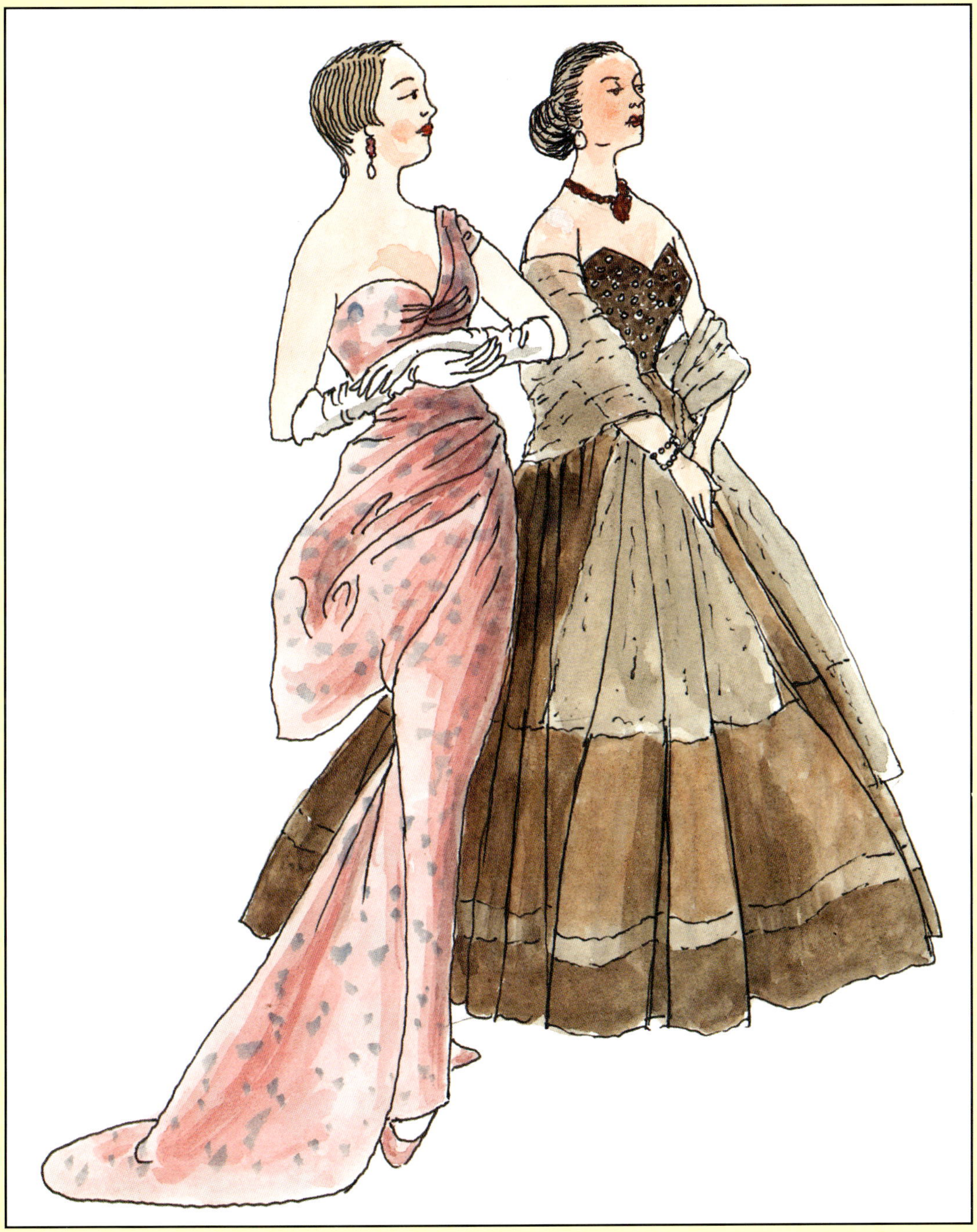

1950-1955 Evening Wear

Glamour reigned supreme in the evening during this period. At left is shown a bare-shouldered, strapless, half-swathed boned bodice, a swathed long skirt and a train in patterned (or plain) silk. At right is the crinoline dress (much favored by the British Royal Family) in tulle or organdie with a beaded or sequined bodice or sequined all over and worn with a long chiffon stole.

Satin gloves with gilt ball-fringe for cocktail wear.

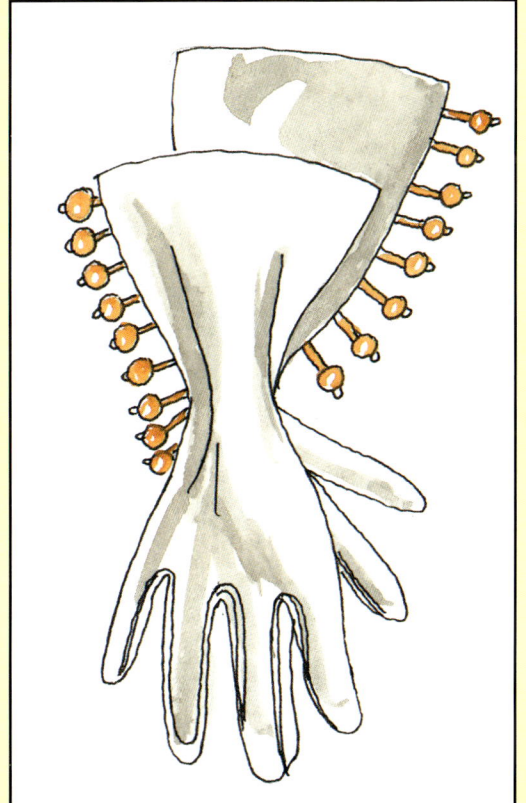

In costume jewelry, gray "pearls" were fashionable. Shown here is a necklace with huge simulated ruby, gilt, and pearl drops.

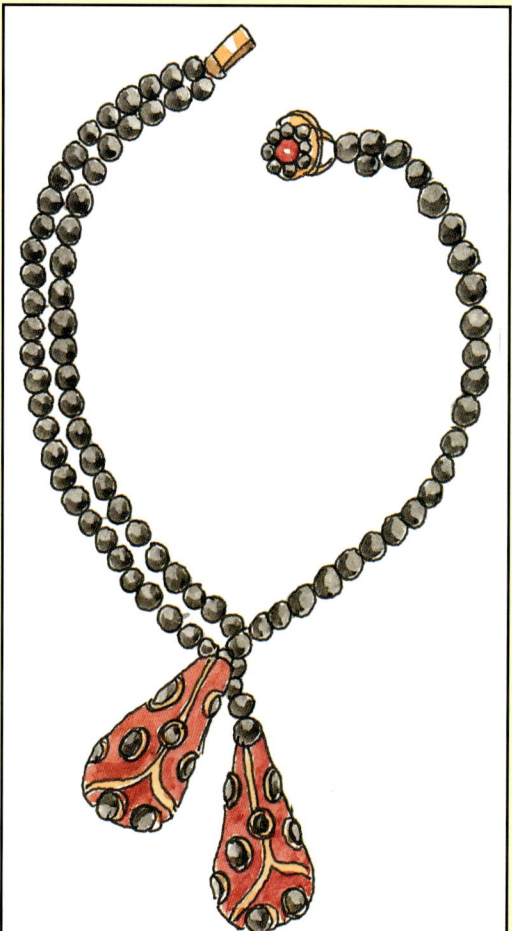

Asymmetric jewelry was still very fashionable, as shown here in gold, pearls, and diamonds with matching earrings.

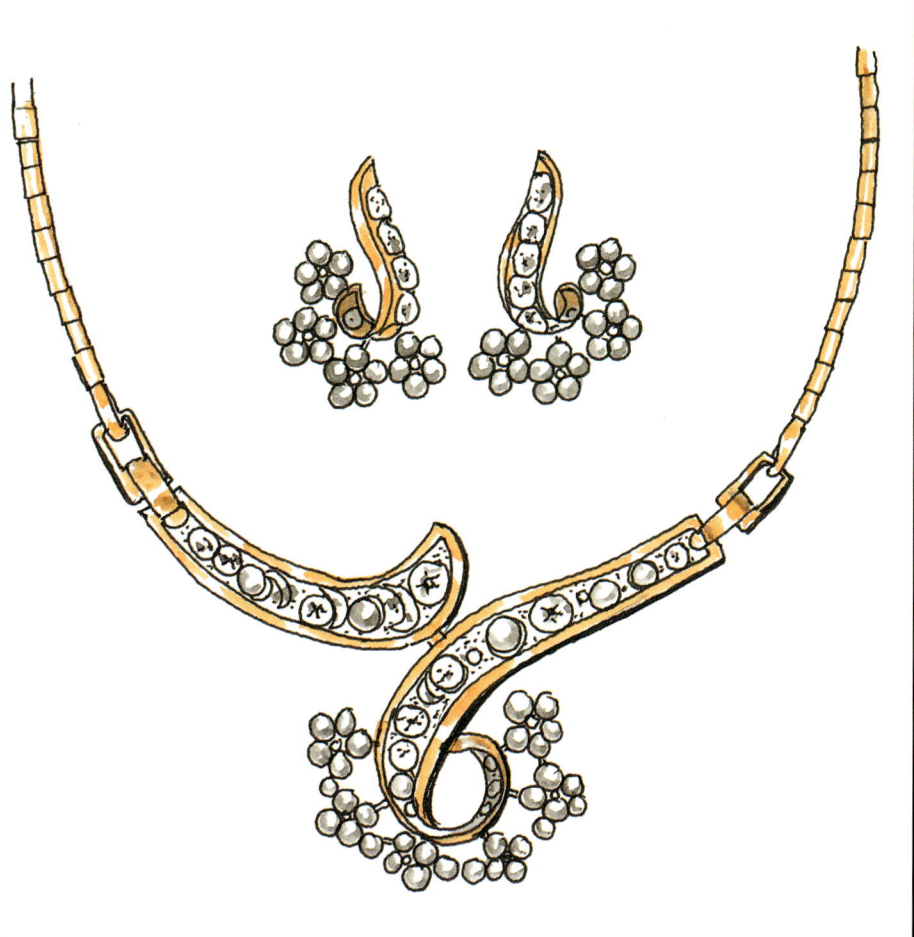

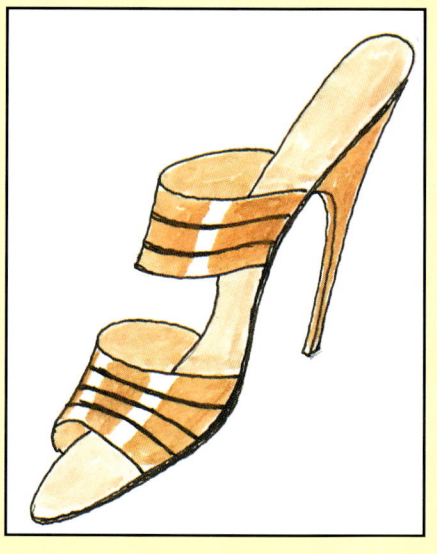

A gilded leather sandal with a very high heel.

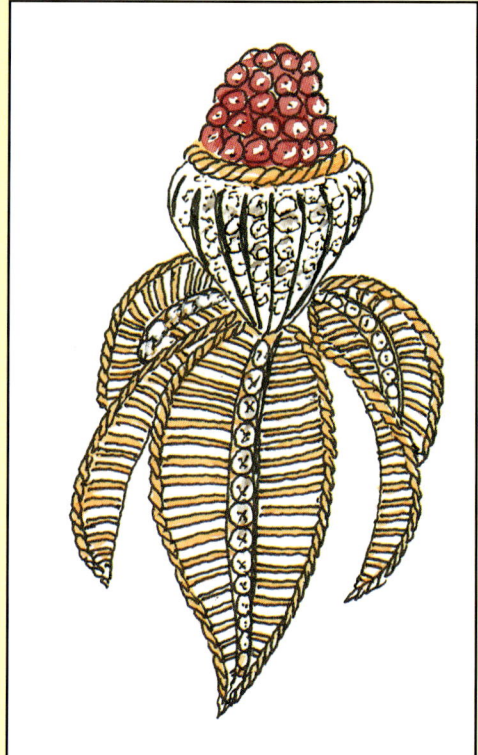

Like something by Dali: an acorn-shaped brooch with ruby "fruit" diamond core, gold, diamond, gold, and platinum "leaves."

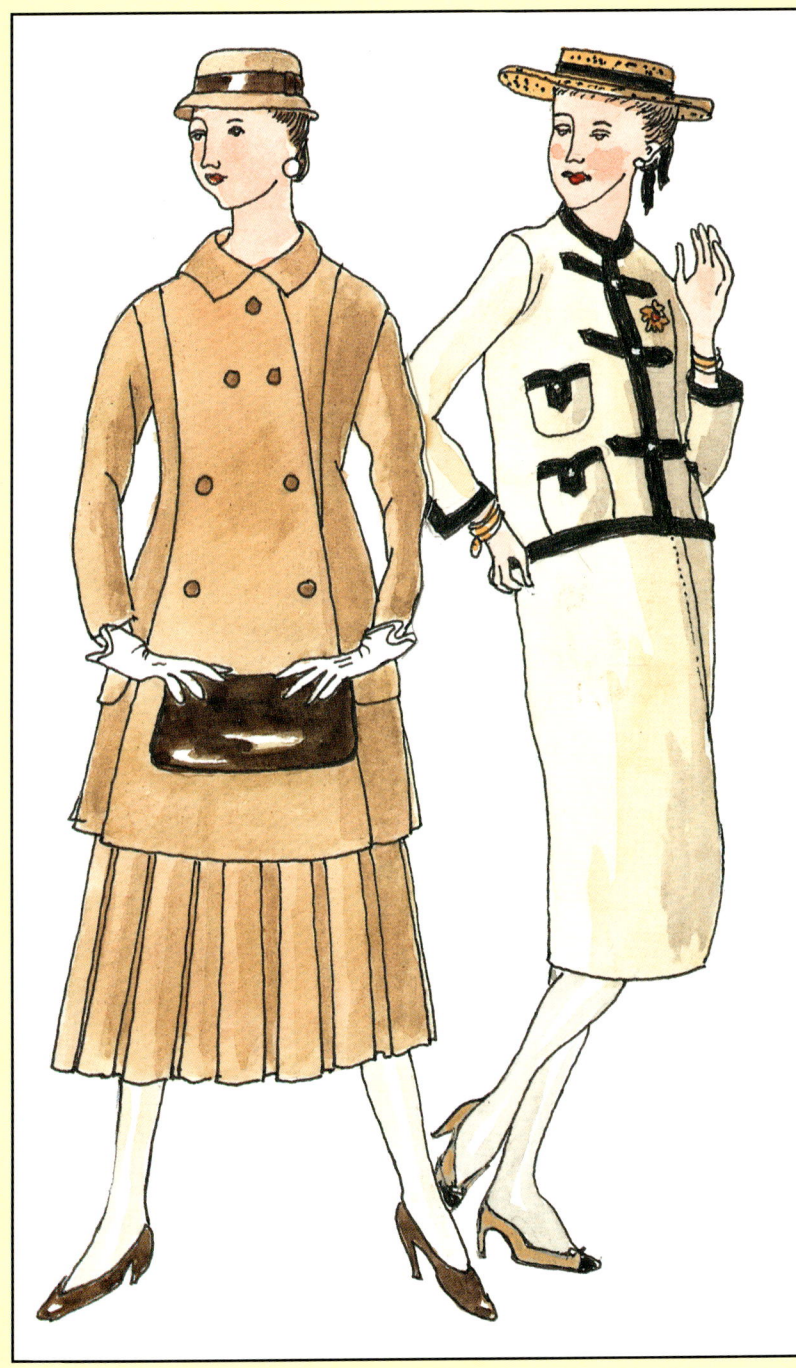

1955-1960 Day Wear

Formality and grooming were still the order of the day, but other silhouettes were coming in from Paris, such as Dior's "A" line (at left) and the rather unattractive "sack dress." The great surprise of 1954 occurred when Chanel came out of retirement and showed her first Paris collection since 1939. One of her sensations has now become a fashion classic: the Chanel suit (at right), in soft jersey trimmed with braid and accessorized with a "sailor" hat, costume jewelry, and always with beige and black shoes. It was immediately adopted in America and made especially famous in the 1960s by America's First Lady, the beautiful and stylish Jacqueline Kennedy.

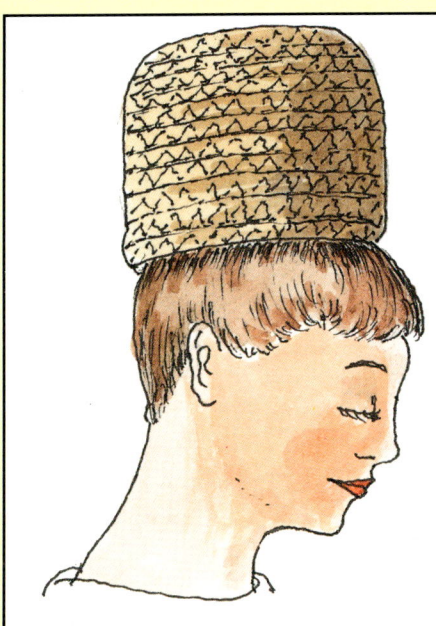

An upturned straw "basket" sits atop fashionably short hair.

Twisted tweed bands make up this head-hugger.

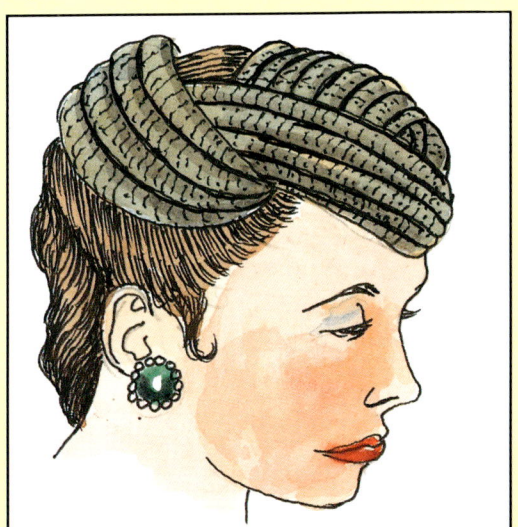

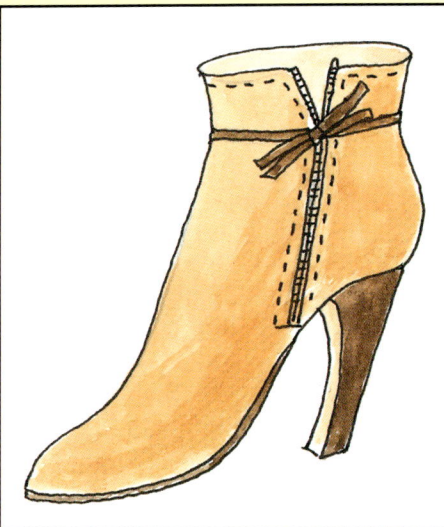

For the country, a suede boot with a zipper fastener and very high heel.

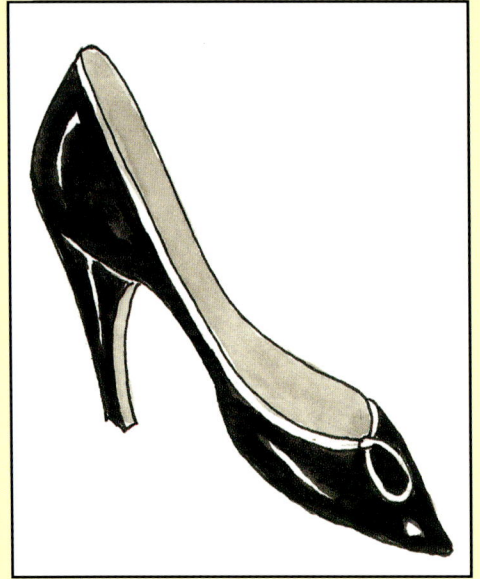

Patent leather and cord with a stiletto heel.

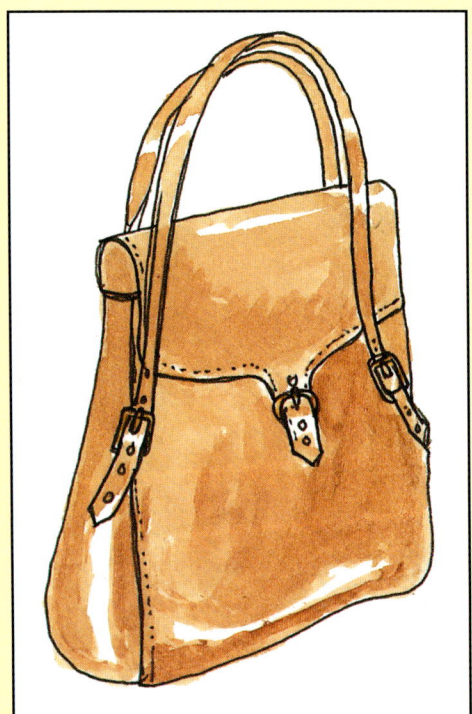

A sturdy leather traveling or country bag.

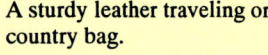

From a pheasant: a circle of small feathers tipped with tail feathers; worn with a fur muffler.

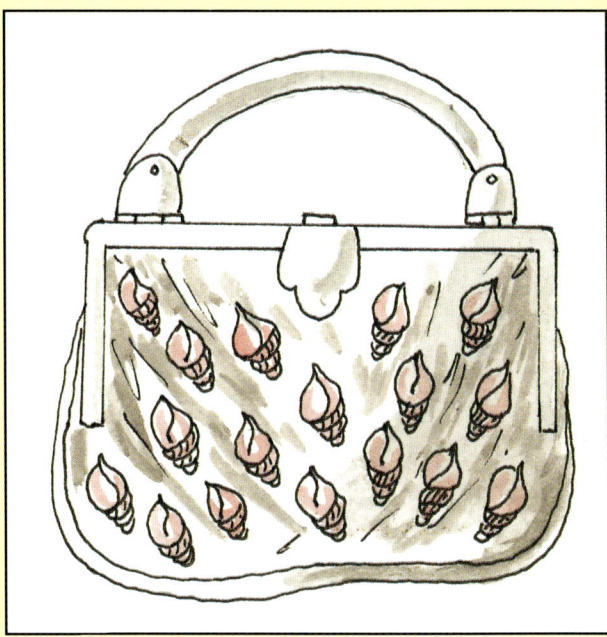

A novelty for the young: transparent plastic handbag, dotted with plastic shells on a solid plastic frame.

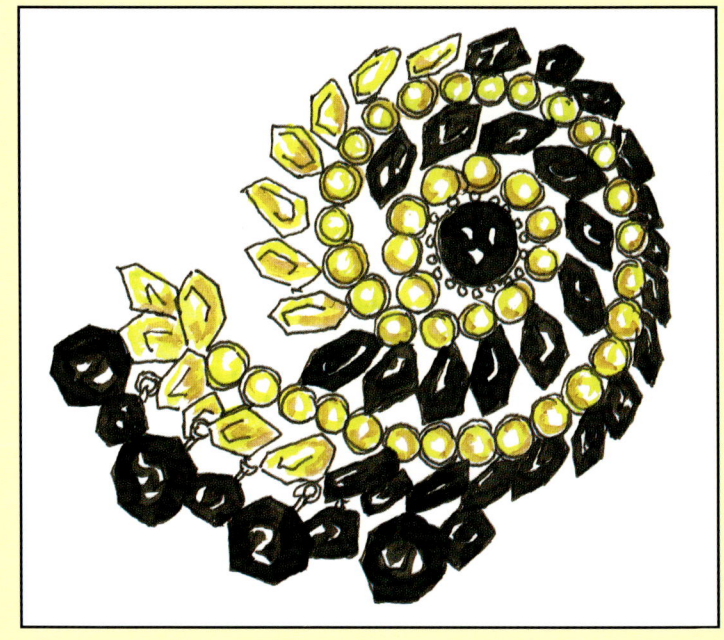

A spiral of Tyrot stones make up this costume jewelry brooch.

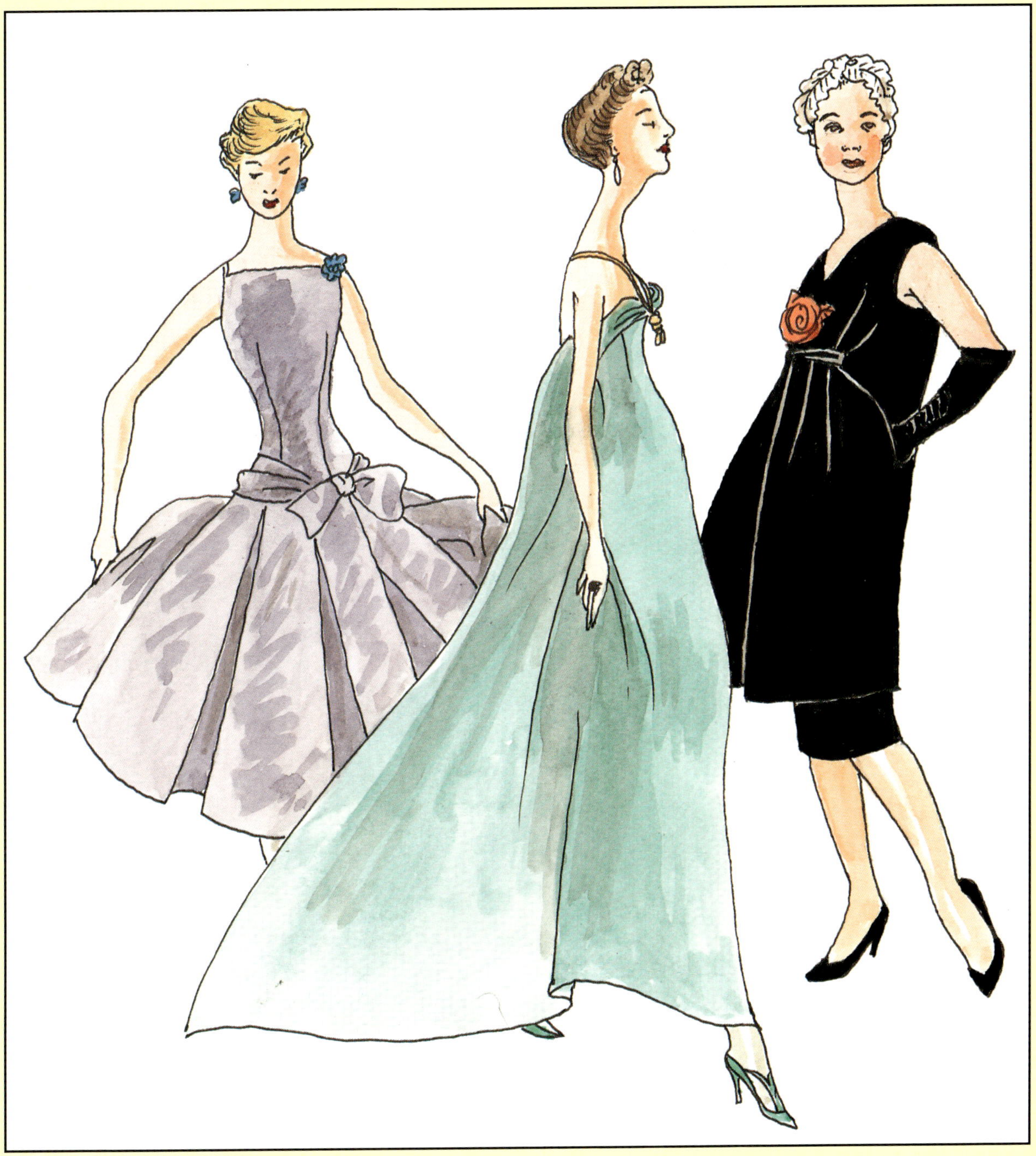

1955-1960 Evening Wear

Glamour still prevailed after 6:00 p.m. Dresses could have simple bodices with very full skirts (left) or be long and swirly (center). For cocktail parties, the ubiquitous "little black dress" (at right) was a fashion "must," worn with a striking hat.

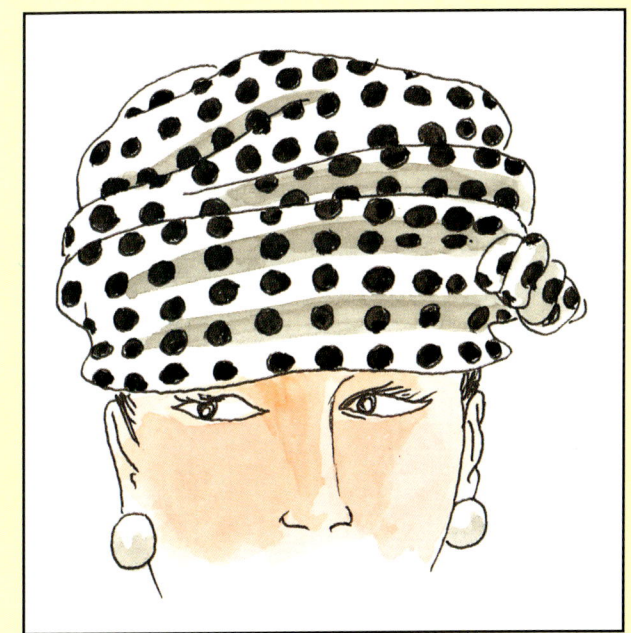

An organza turban for cocktail parties or for those London restaurants which allowed this French fashion.

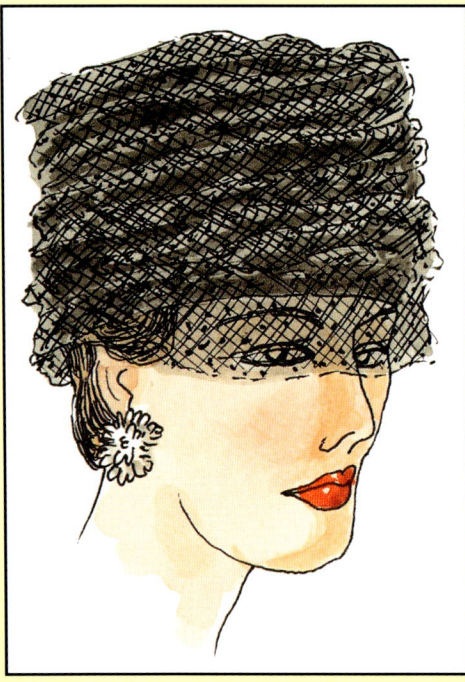

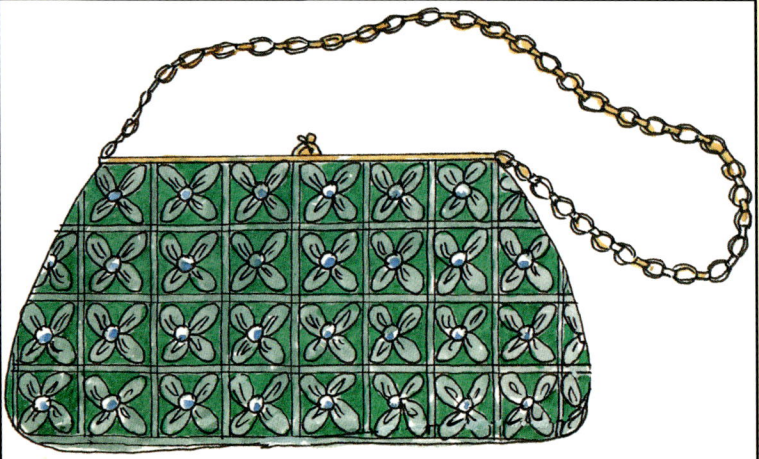

Two tones of silk, studded with beads and with a long gilt chain constitute this evening bag.

Layers of silk and a veil make up this cocktail hat.

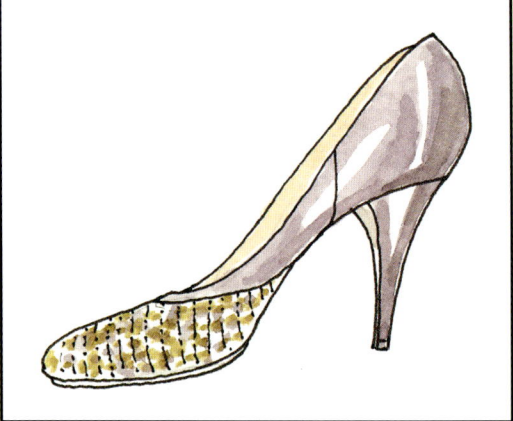

Padded silk, an artificial rose, and a veil for an "after-six" creation.

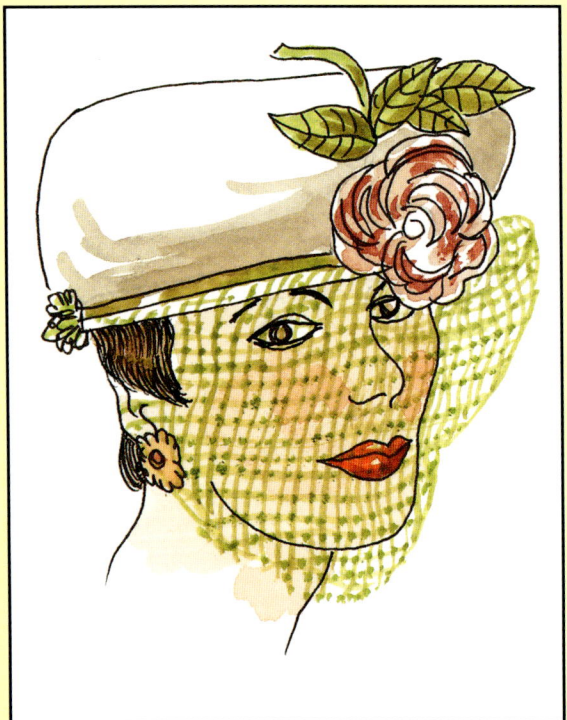

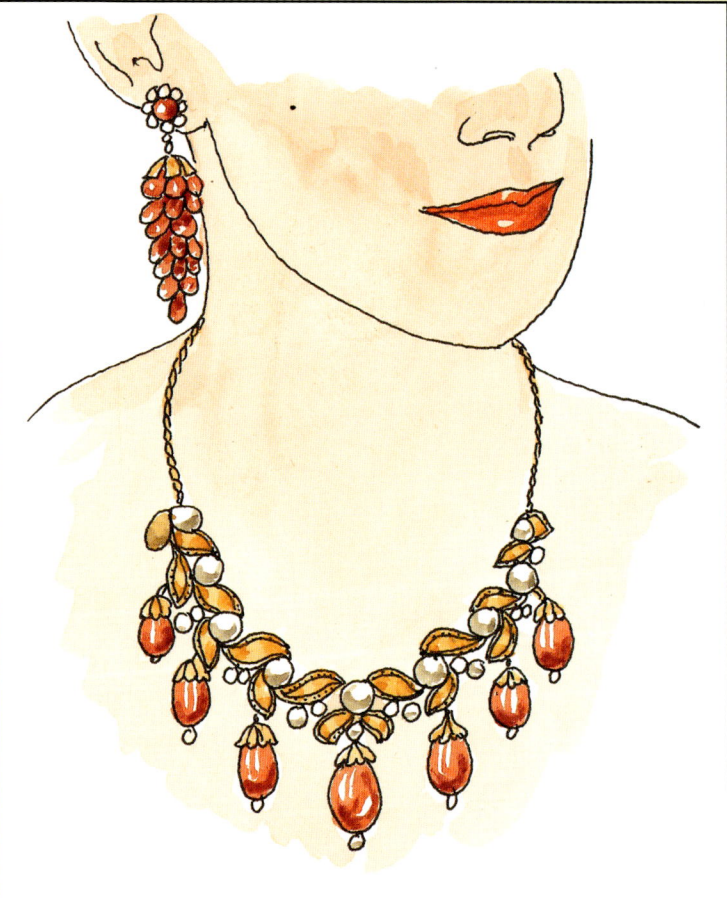

An unusual combination for evening: tweed and leather.

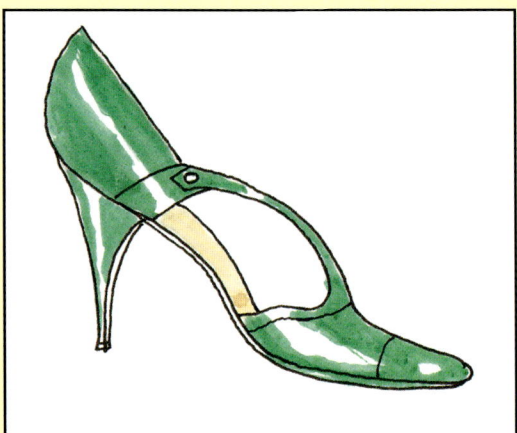

A silk sandal. Having shoes dyed to match an evening dress was popular.

A gold, pearl, and ruby necklace complemented by a "bunch of grapes" earring.

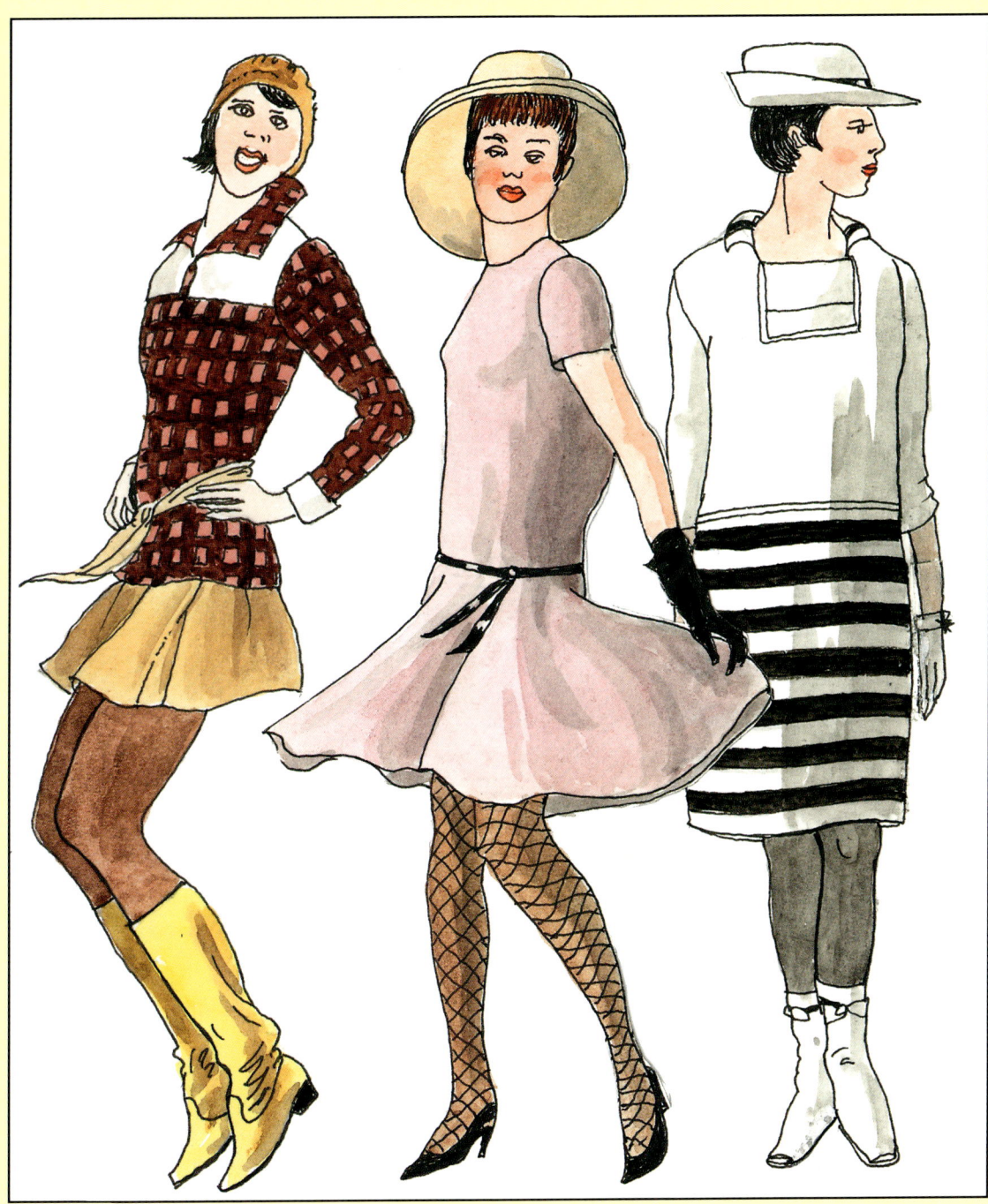

1960-1970 Day Wear

Swinging London! The Beatles! Pop Music! The Pill! Permissiveness! Mary Quant! Carnaby Street! Peace in Vietnam! Riots in Paris! Landing on the Moon! Youth! Youth! Youth!

The exclamation marks emphasize the great change that came over society and fashion during this decade, although change did not really make itself known until approximately 1963. The era was also remarkable in that, for the first time, fashion originated and permeated from the bottom strata of society to the top, with even the staid Queen of England wearing a mini skirt.

The 1960s began quietly, with women still wearing late 1950s clothing and accessories, but change was in the air. The fashion designer Mary Quant, with her husband Alexander Plunket, is credited with having created the "Chelsea Girl," although she denies it. Even though some short skirts were seen in Paris in about 1960, Quant certainly "invented" the mini, which reached its shortest in 1965—being a mere "bandage" between waist and mid-thigh. (Its brevity was said to be the cause of sexual permissiveness.) It was, however, adopted all over Europe and in America. Also new was the great number of boutiques, selling "way-out" clothing and serving coffee to the sound of pop music, such as Barbara Hulaniki's "Biba" on London's Kensington High Street. Models Jean Shrimpton and skinny Twiggy, photographer David Baily, along with pop stars and country singers in Britain and America, became symbols of the age.

The girl (at left) shows the craze at its most extreme: a scrap of mini skirt, a tight, brightly-colored top, tights, and boots. The girl in the center wears a less-exaggerated version in her low-waisted, short pink (a favorite color) dress, patterned tights, and huge hat. The girl (at right) wears the "space-age" look, which was the French couturier André Corrèges' answer to the "London look," which he launched in 1964. Although often modified, it was very popular with young women.

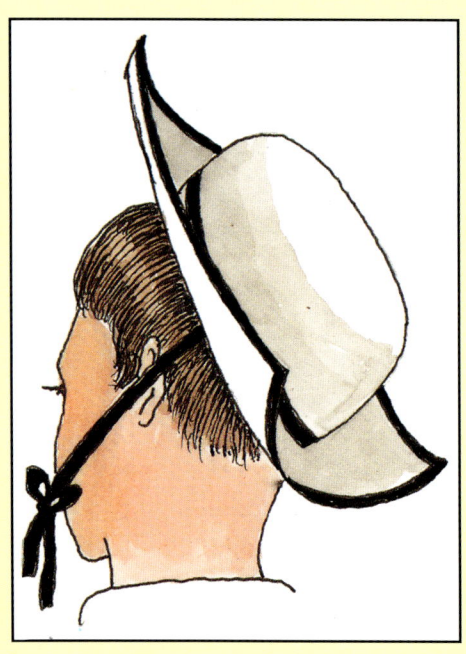

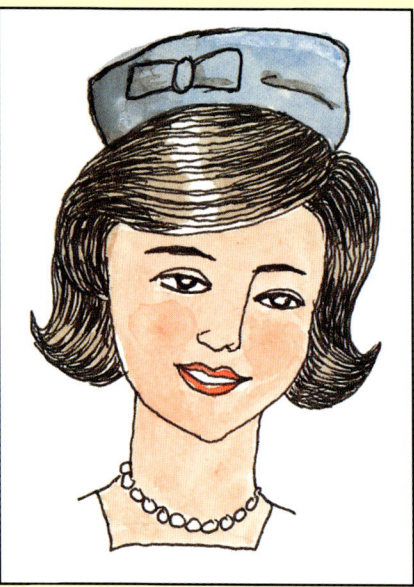

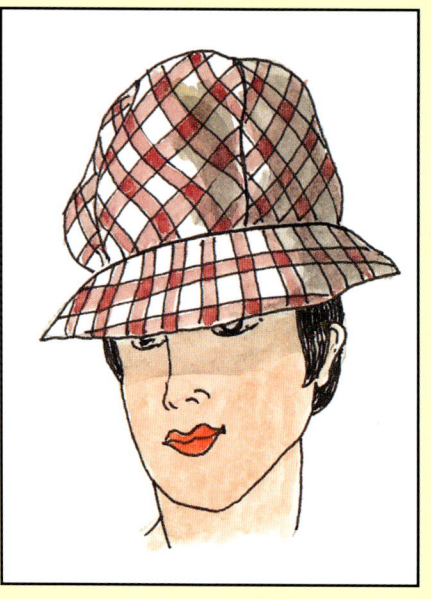

A cotton pull-on hat for the more conventional.

A cheeky braid-edged felt hat, tied on with ribbon.

Jacqueline Kennedy's famous pill-box hat, copied the world over.

A felt creation of *My Fair Lady* proportions.

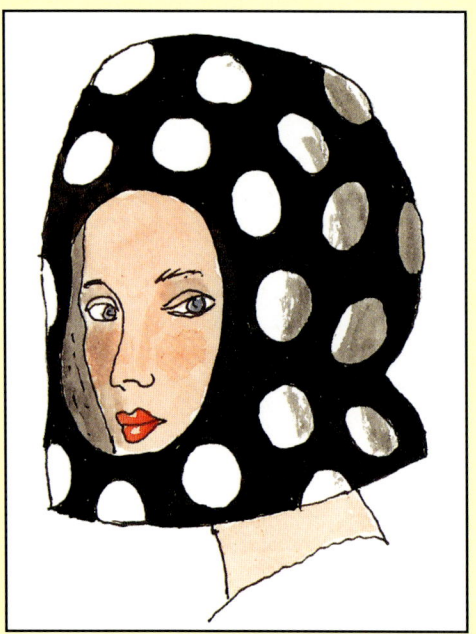

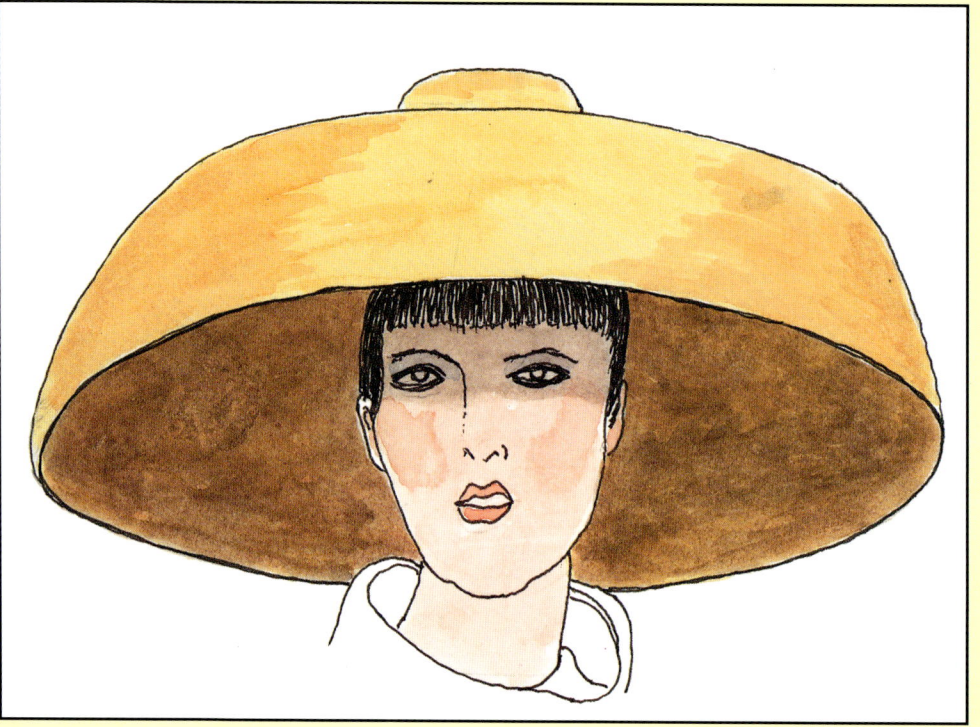

An eccentric hood for those who dared to wear the full "space-age" look.

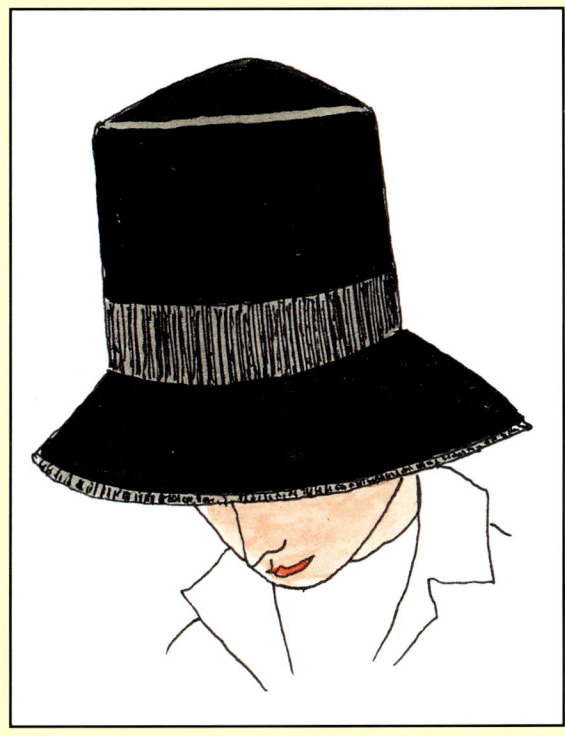

Bucket-shaped velvet trimmed with petersham ribbon.

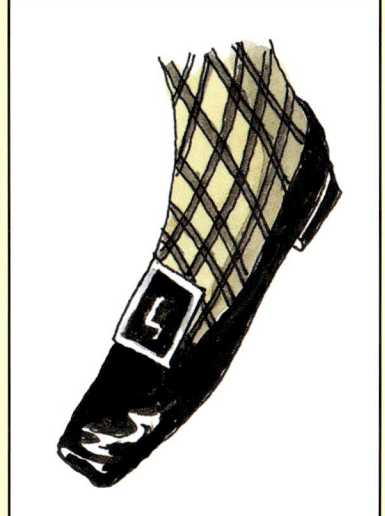

An almost pre-First World War patent-leather shoe with a large buckle, worn with checkered tights.

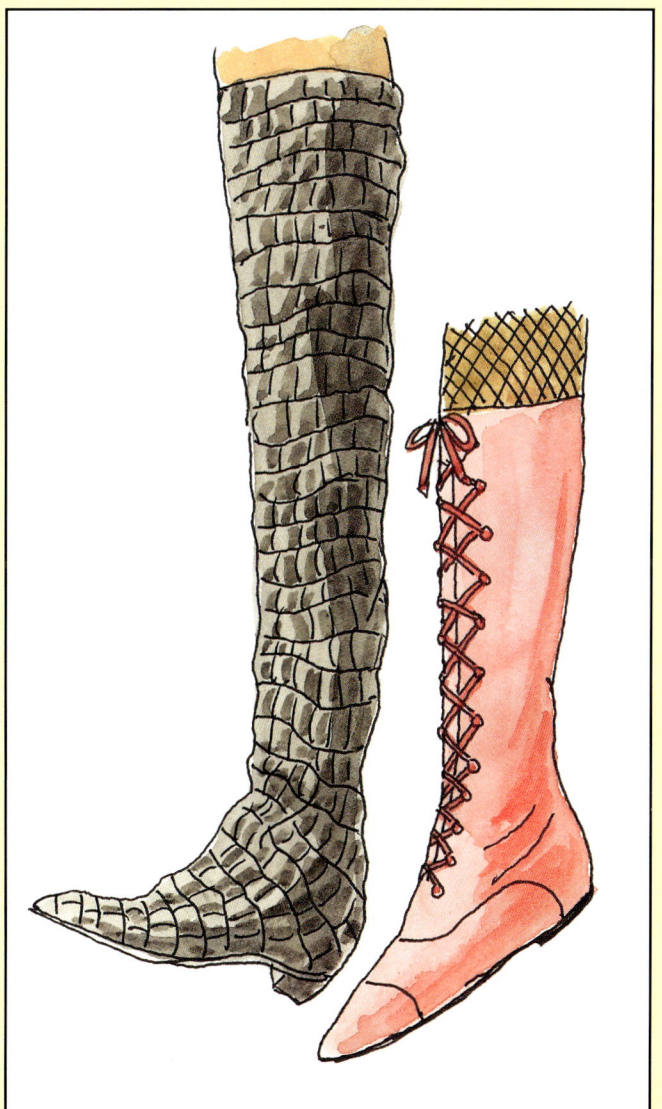

Boots came in all lengths, materials, and colors. *Left:* real or fake crocodile. *Right:* suede boots, tied up the front in Medieval fashion.

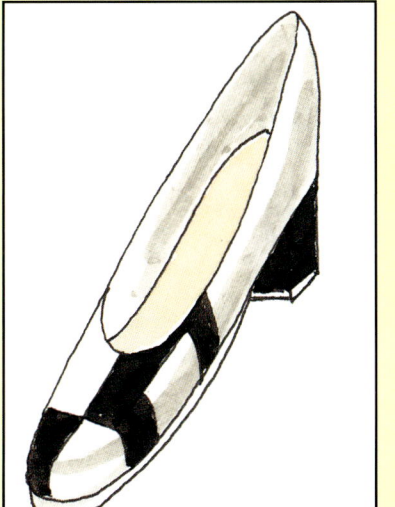

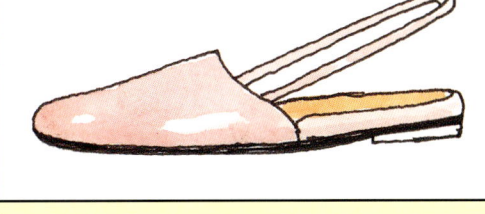

A slip of a sandal in a popular 1960s color.

Op-Art decorated, slipper-like, shoe.

A Second World War style of a heavy suede sandal with padded, extra-high heel.

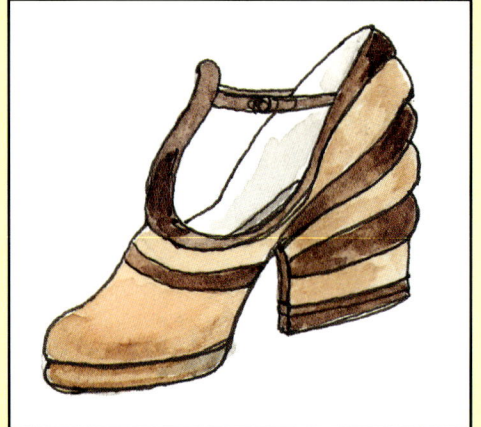

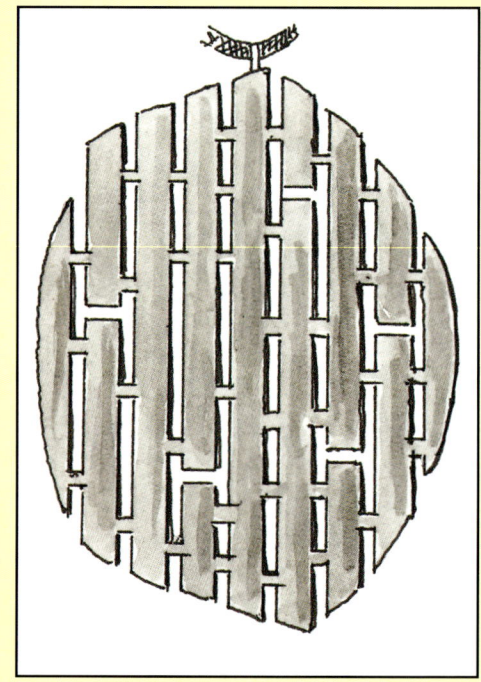

A metal "futuristic" pendant.

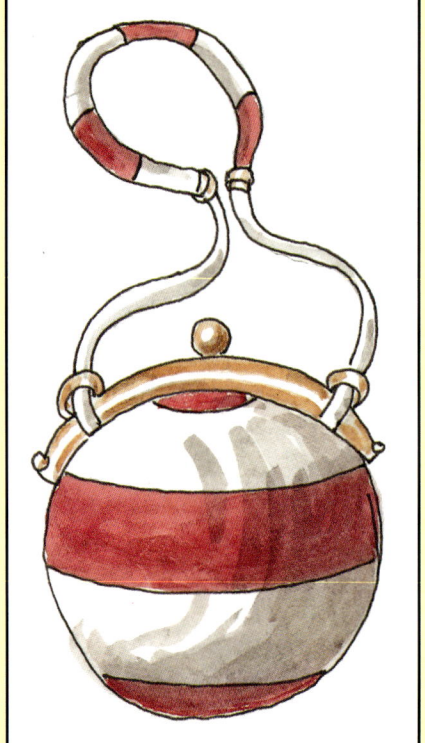

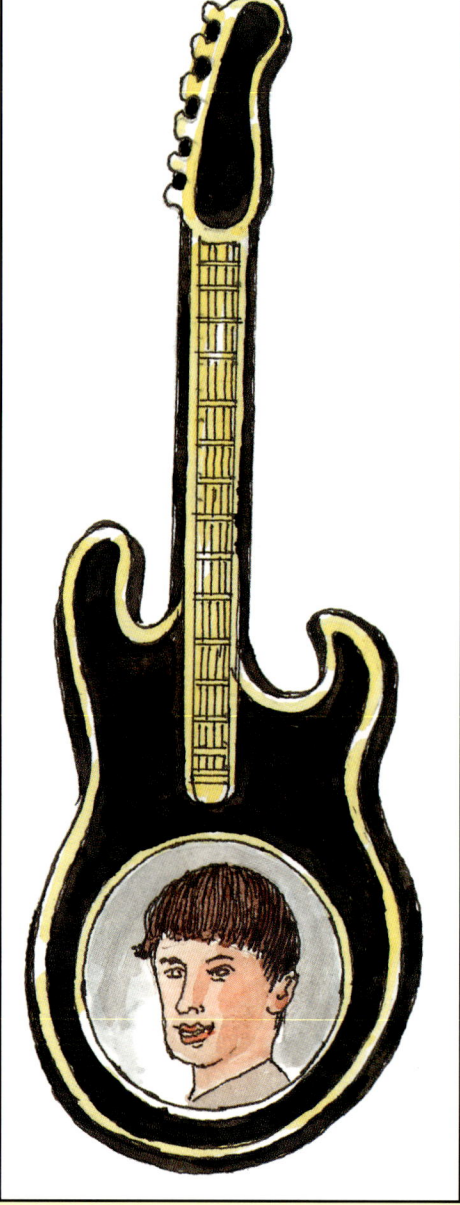

☞ The Beatles, naturally, inspired a wealth of fashions and souvenirs, such as this plastic guitar-shaped brooch with a photograph of Ringo, one of a set of the "Fab Four."

☞ On a Saturday morning in London, this was just the bag to carry down the King's Road in Chelsea, the fashion parade center of the "Swinging Sixties."

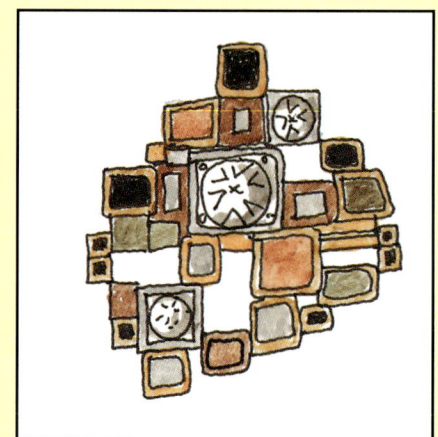

Many different stones and glittery objects make up this "weird" brooch.

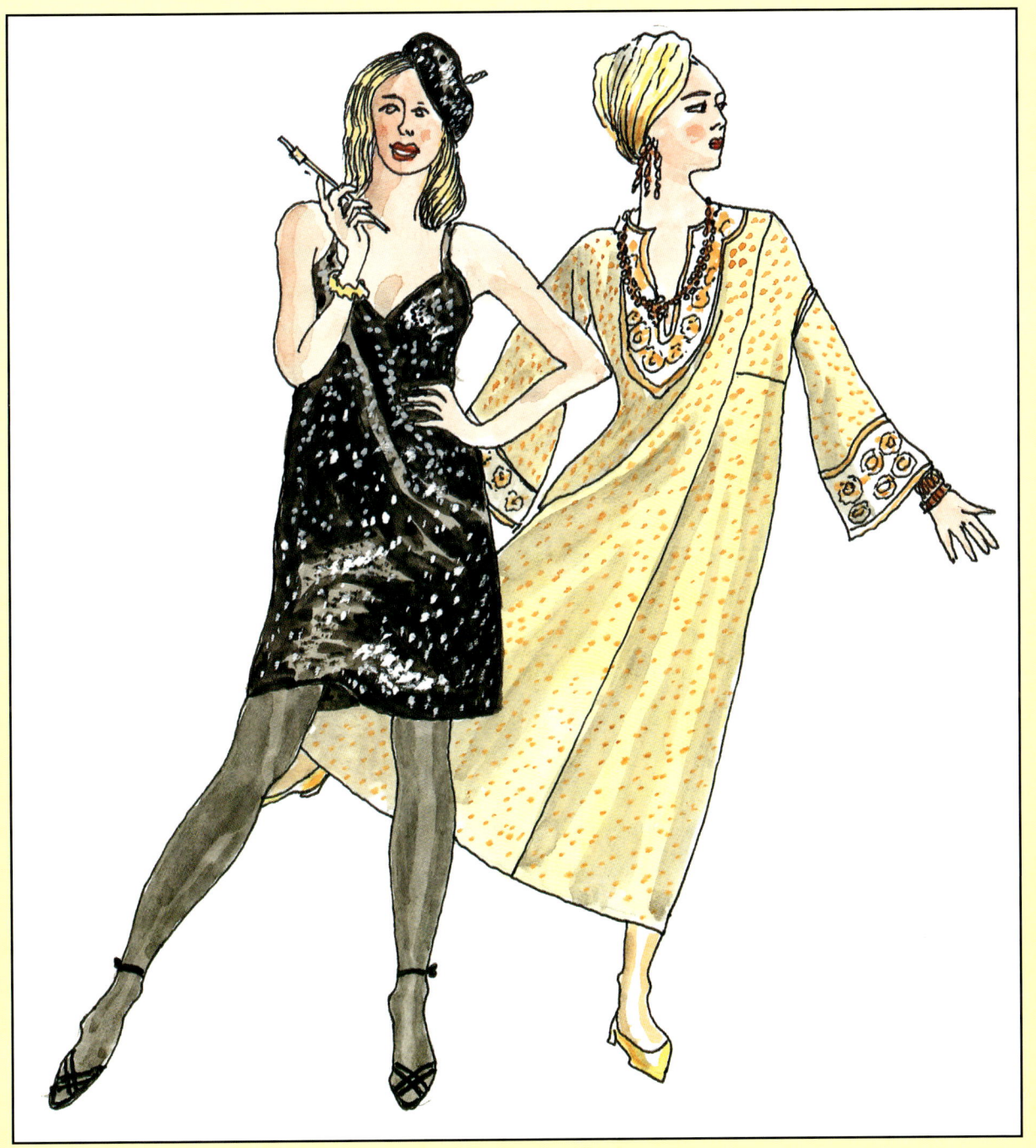

1960-1970 Evening Wear

To be swinging on a 1960s evening, women were seen wearing either a very short, slip-like, very often sequined dress (at left) or a long, caftan-like dress, richly embroidered and beaded, together with a turban and African-style jewelry (at right).

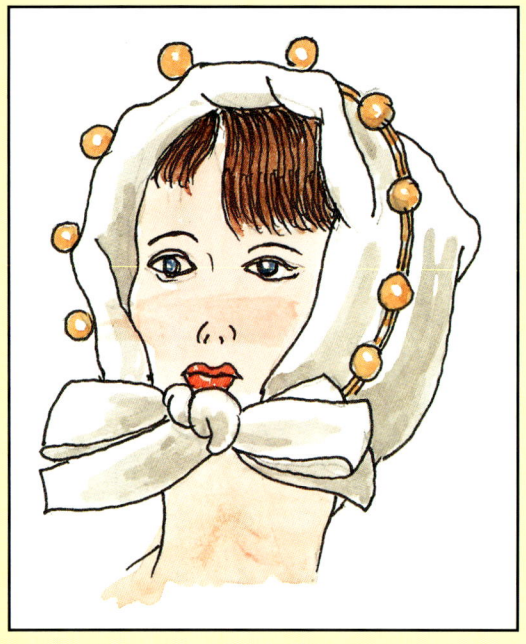

A French padded silk, gilt-trimmed hood.

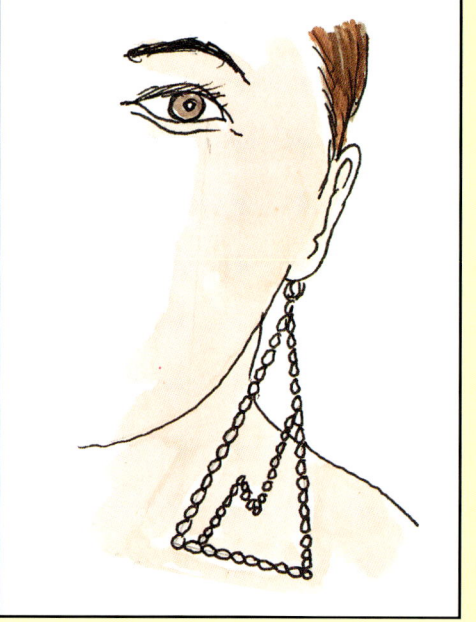

Weird beads for a daring earring.

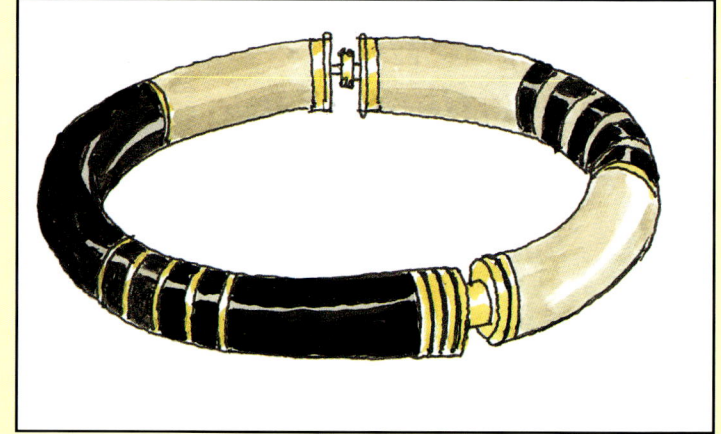

An African-style acrylic and plastic bracelet.

Glitter for evening predominated: a silver leather-and-bead sandal worn with silver thread stockings.

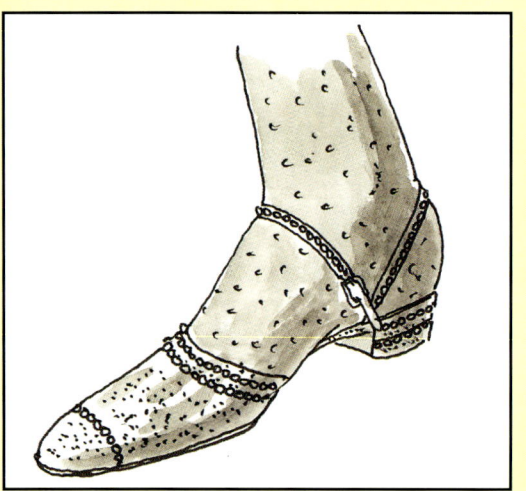

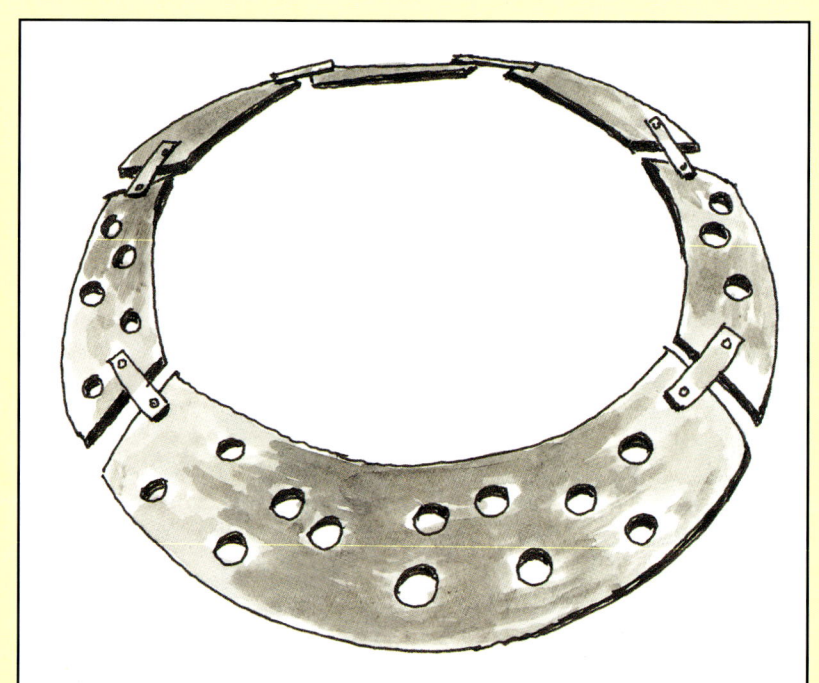

A metal collar necklace, which looks like a piece of ancient armor.

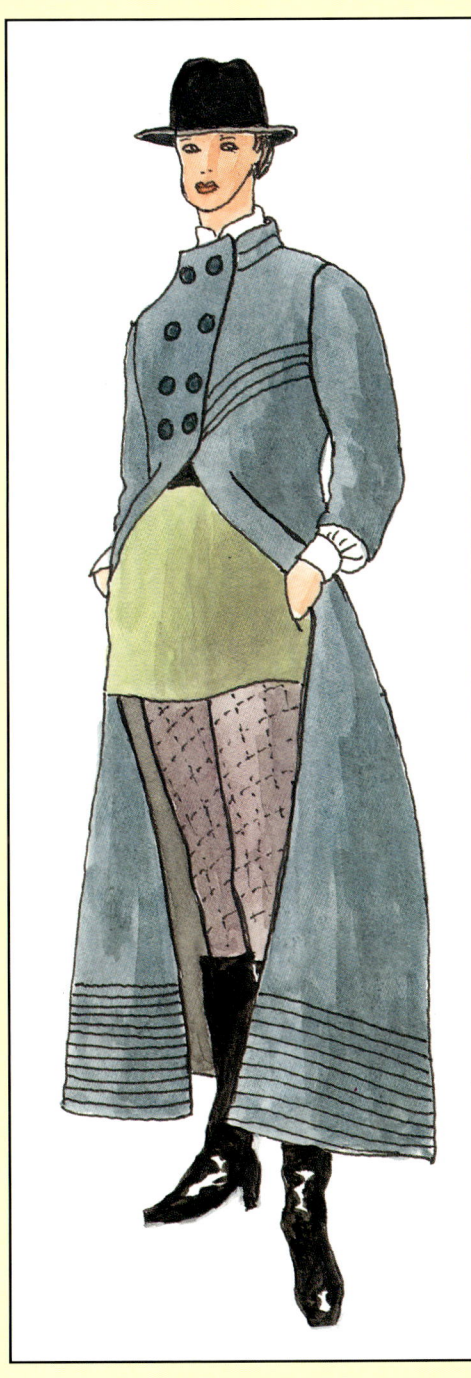

1970-1980 Day Wear

The "anything goes" fashion era when women had too many styles to choose from and when, as British *Vogue* put it in 1972, "Women are dressing to amuse themselves, not to improve their status or to attract men." It was bewildering for those women who still wanted to be told what was smart to wear, what was seductive to men, what would cause jealousy in other women.

Skirt length: mini, middy, maxi, or two at once? Boots or shoes? A slim or a bulky coat? A silk or denim blouson jacket? Tight jeans or "Oxford bags?" Twenties cloche, 1930s hat, or none at all? A hood or a scarf? The Japanese bulky, many-layered silhouette? Laura Ashley's nostalgic country style: long dresses, pinafores, and aprons in small flower or check prints? The ethnic look? "Street Punk" with its non-fashion image, and safety pins its trademark? Punk Chic, Zandra Rhodes' sophisticated version: embroidered dresses and gold safety pins? It was all too much.

Apart from relying on its prét-á-porté and perfumes, Paris had lost its grip; London couturiers had to do likewise, with their ready-to-wear lines in clothing and accessories.

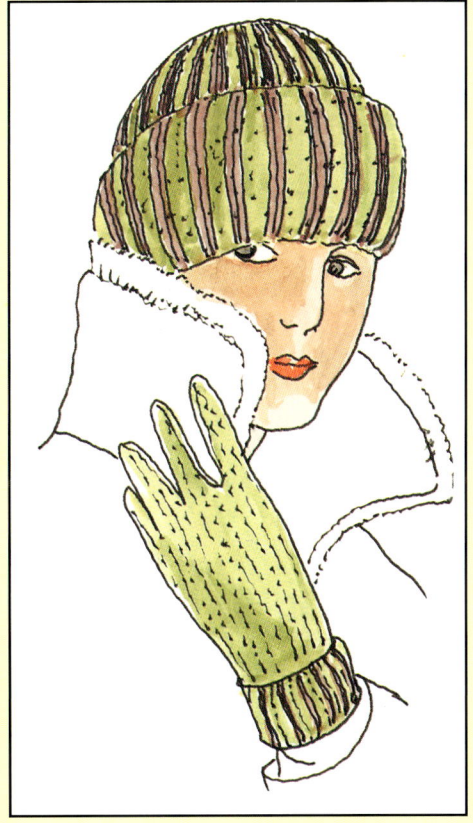

Real or machine knitting was very popular. In either, a cloche-like hat with matching gloves.

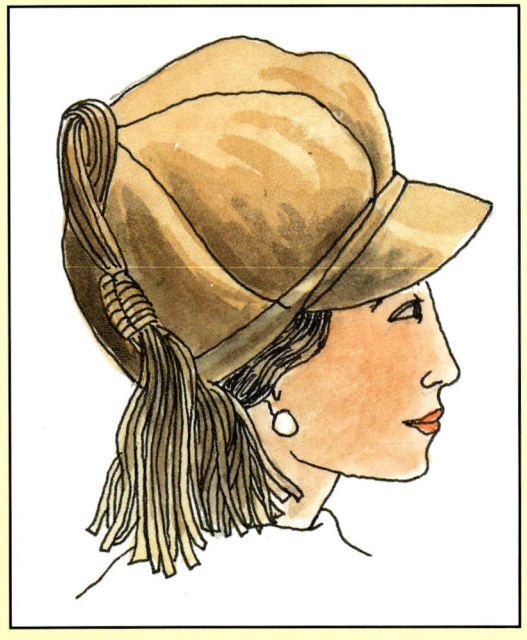

A felt jockey cap adorned with a twisted thong tassel.

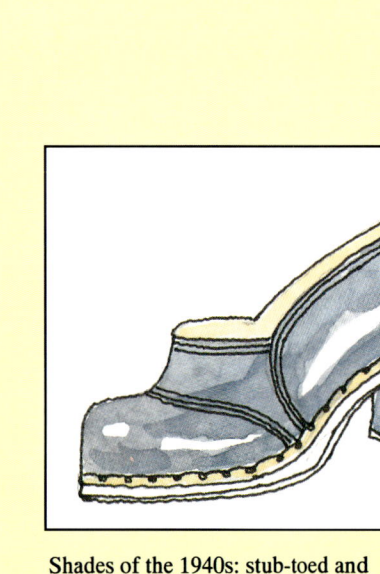

Shades of the 1940s: stub-toed and heavy-heeled.

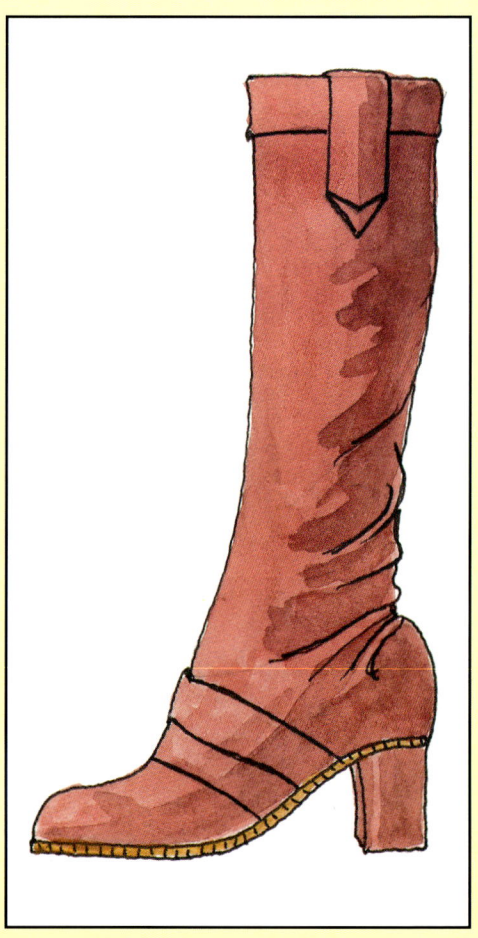

Boots were still very much around: here in suede with the minimum of decoration.

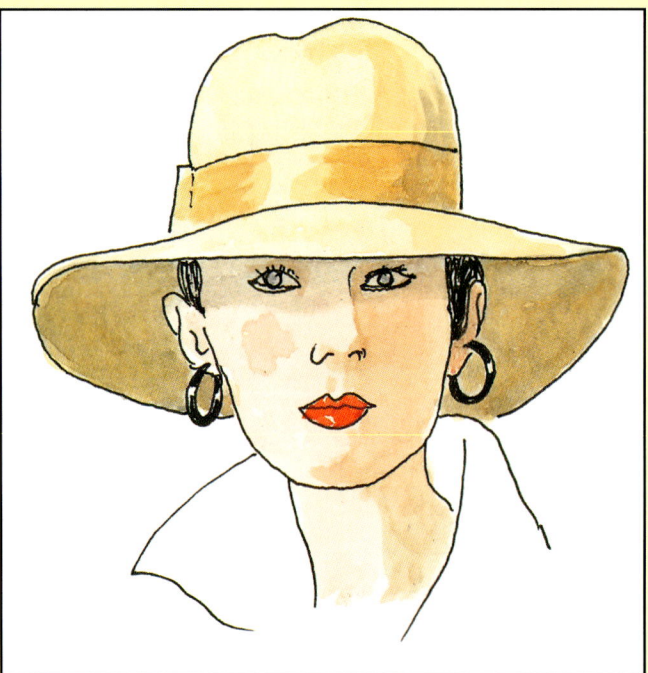

This felt 1930s-style hat is worn with plastic earrings.

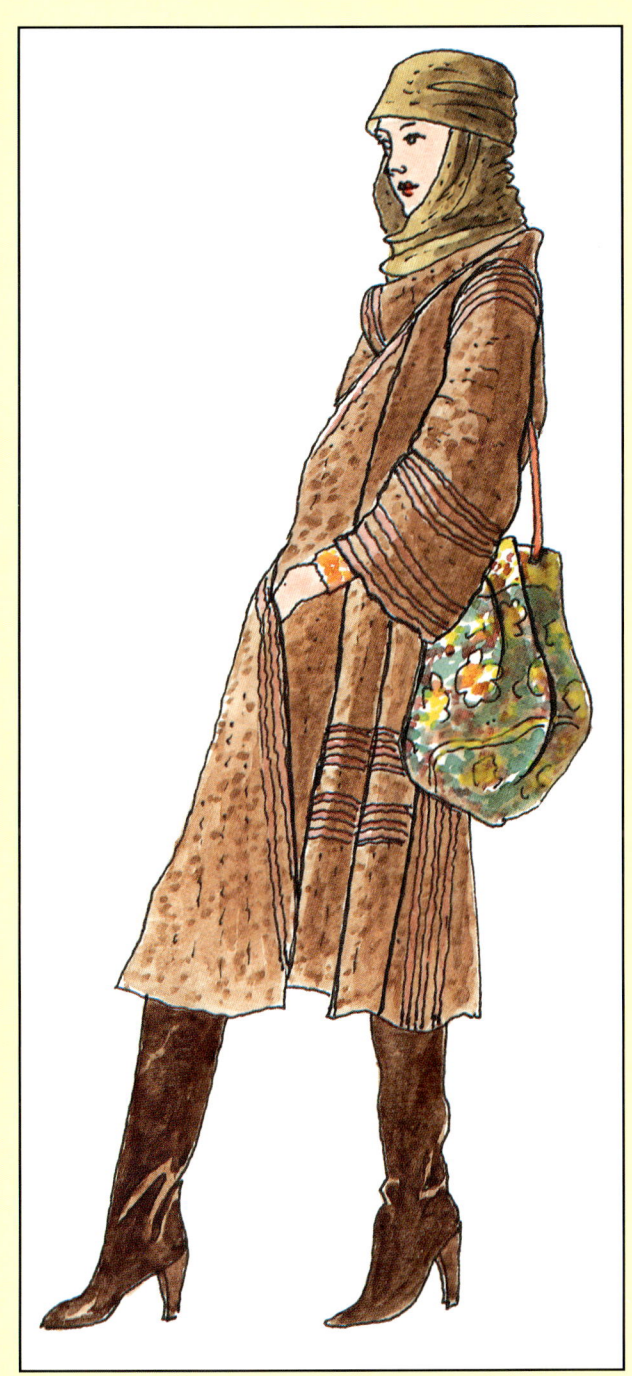

1970-1980 Day Wear

Out of all the alternatives I have singled out the ethnic look. Using ideas from the mainly peasant strata of society in many countries, there was a wealth of clothing and accessories from which to choose. The basic garment was either a middy or maxi rough woollen coat, or a maxi dress in a flowered print worn with a padded Chinese-style jacket. There were hoods, long boots, and shoulder-bags made out of pieces of old, preferably oriental or middle-eastern, carpet.

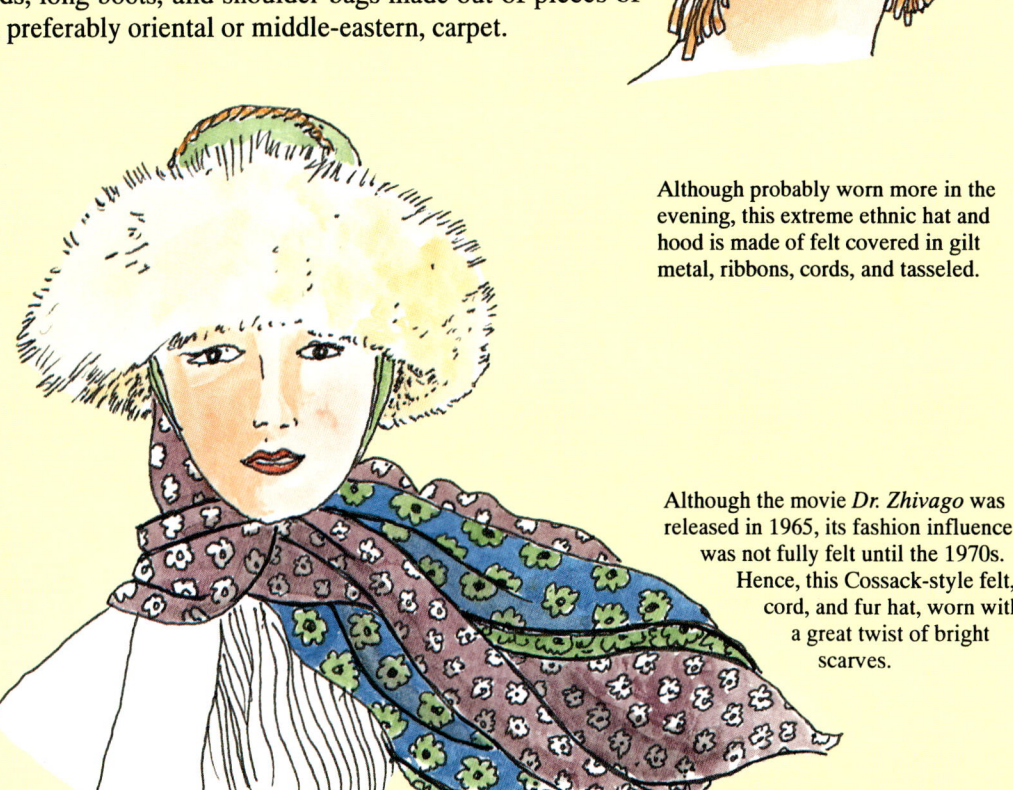

Although probably worn more in the evening, this extreme ethnic hat and hood is made of felt covered in gilt metal, ribbons, cords, and tasseled.

Although the movie *Dr. Zhivago* was released in 1965, its fashion influence was not fully felt until the 1970s. Hence, this Cossack-style felt, cord, and fur hat, worn with a great twist of bright scarves.

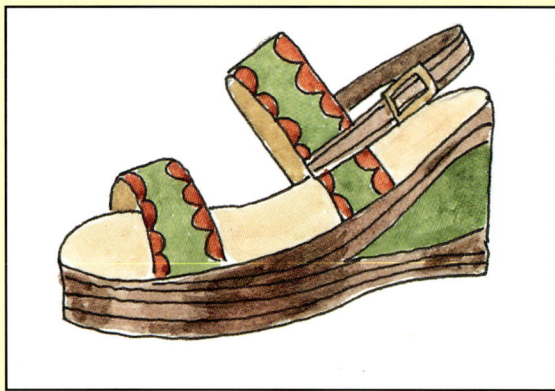

A felt peasant-like sandal with wedge heel.

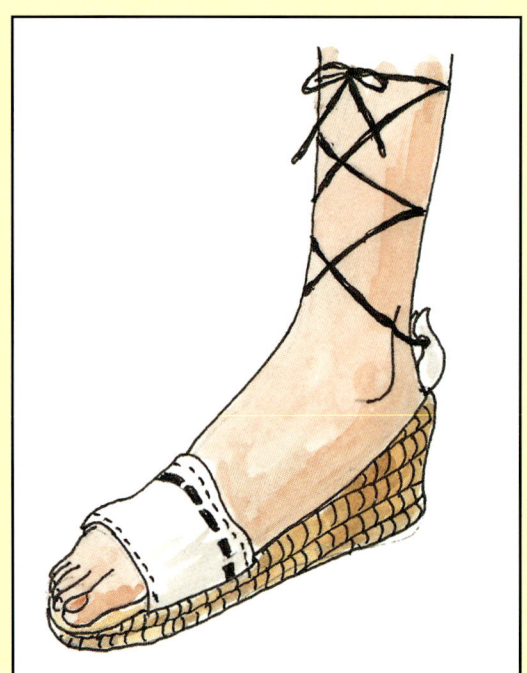

With its rope sole, minute cloth upper, and ribbon fastening, this sandal could have been worn in the country, on the beach, or even in the evening.

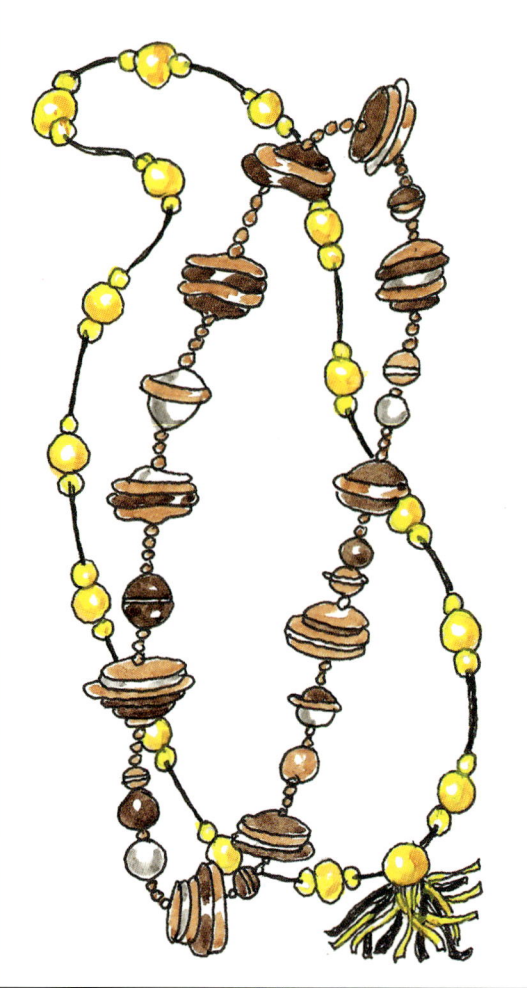

An African-influenced wooden earring.

Real or imitation African beads, which were popular with "hippies," "flower-children," and those who were ethnically-minded.

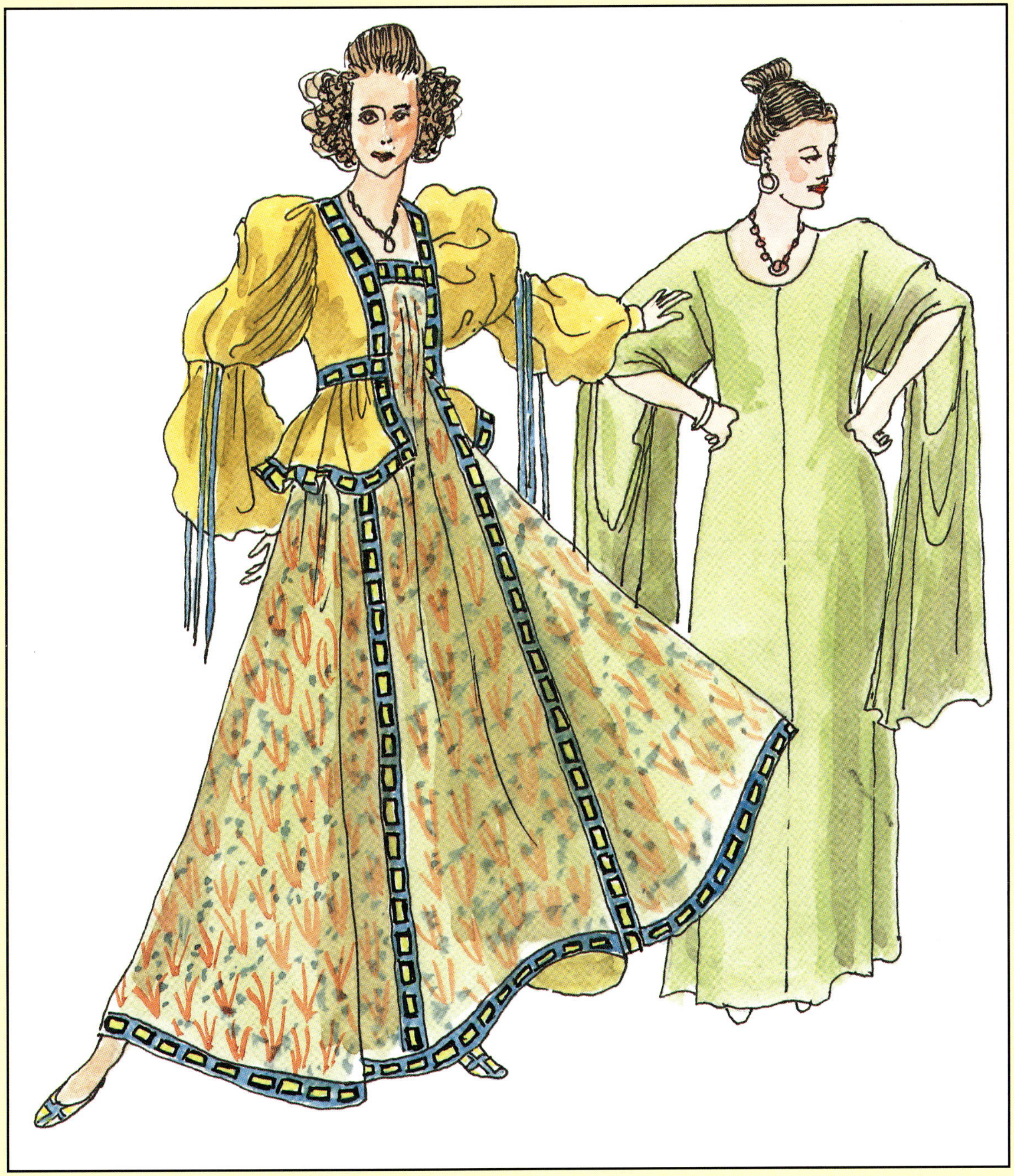

1970-1980 Evening Wear

There was either a vaguely ethnic-looking dress (at left), with its puff-sleeved jacket and full, maxi skirt or one in svelte 1930s-style (at right) to choose from; whichever, as British *Vogue* advised, "amused" you.

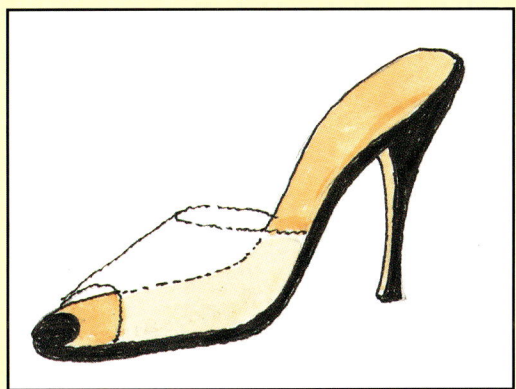

A mere sliver of leather and transparent plastic.

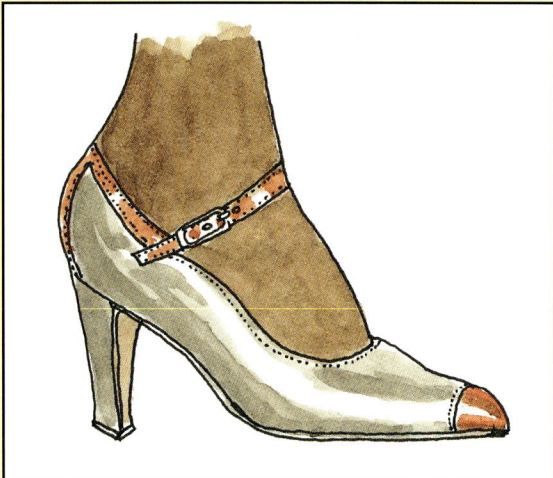

For the more conventional: a 1920s-like silver kid shoe, with contrasting strap, back and toe decoration.

Gold lamé for a floppy bag.

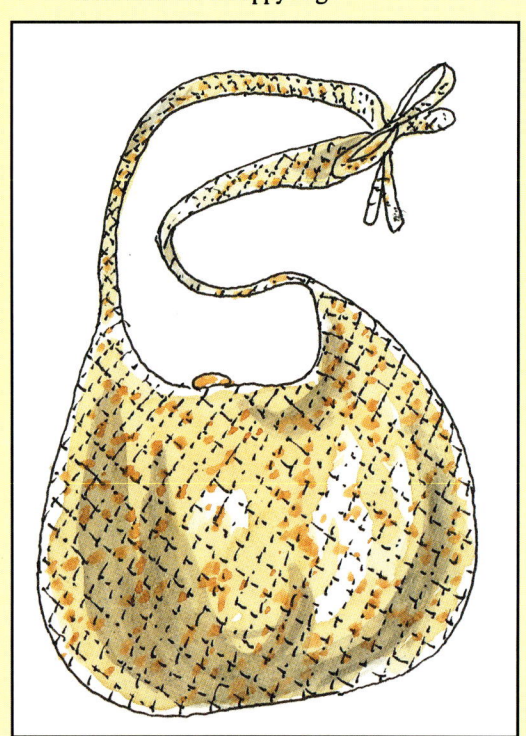

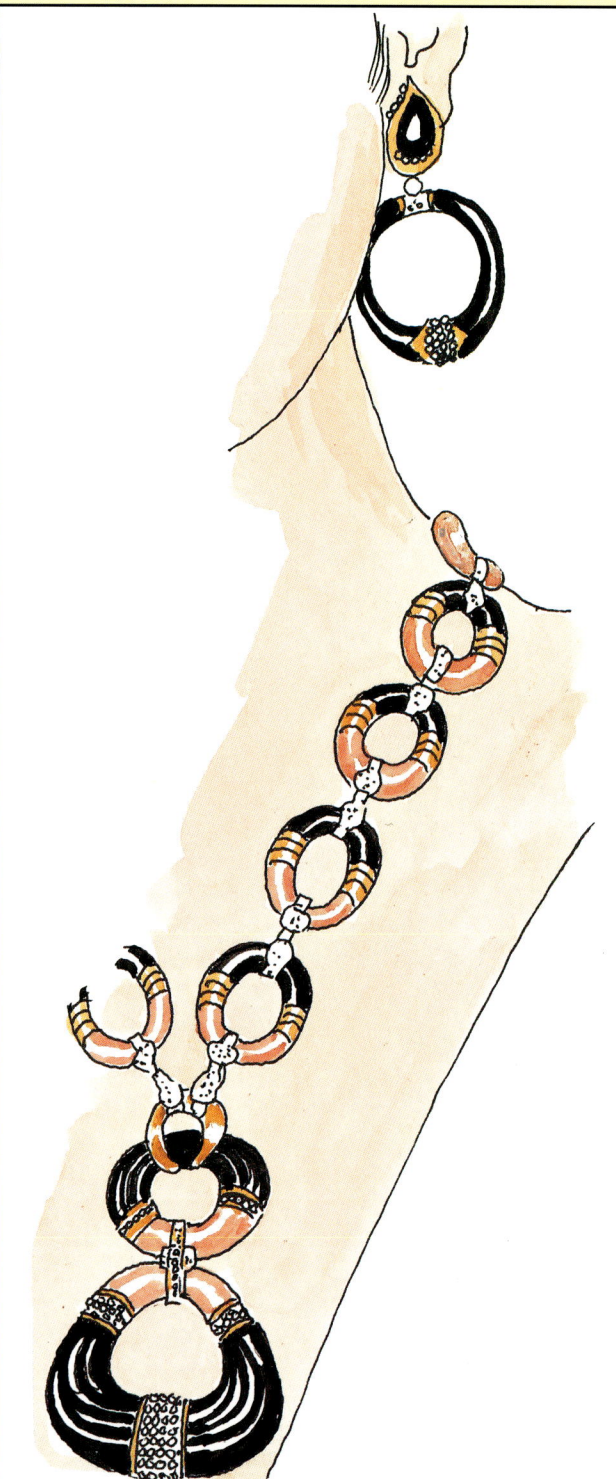

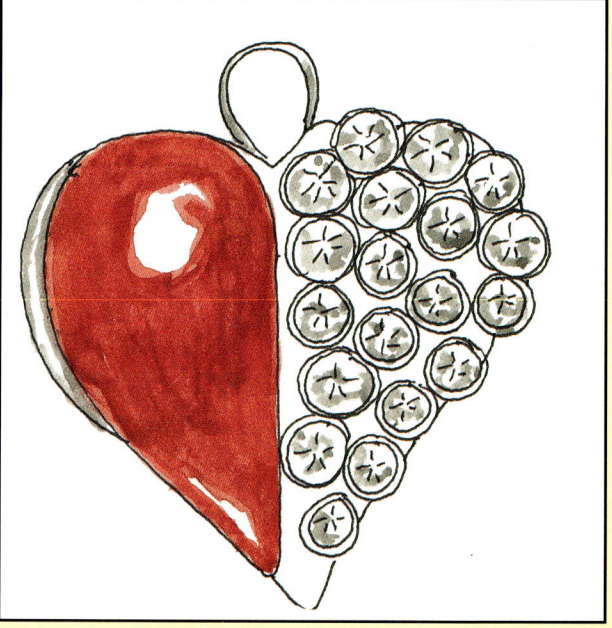

An echo of nineteenth-century sentimentality: a heart-shaped pendant locket, one side enamel, the other plastic, studded with brilliants.

A gilt and rhinestone-encrusted pendant.

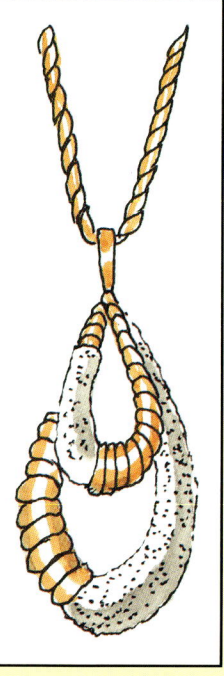

Magnificently barbaric matching plastic, onyx, and gilt necklace and earrings for the ethnically-minded or even conventional woman.

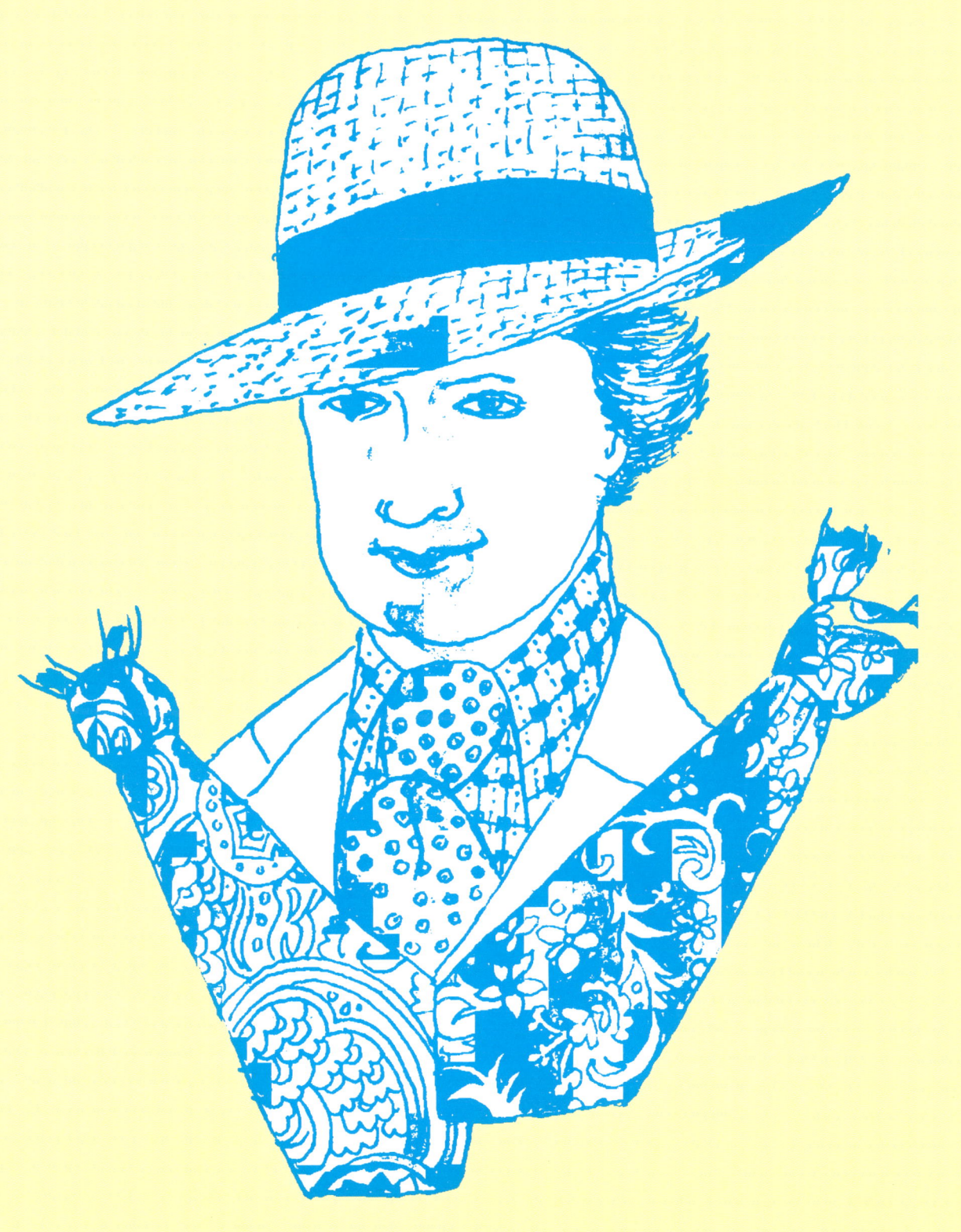

Men

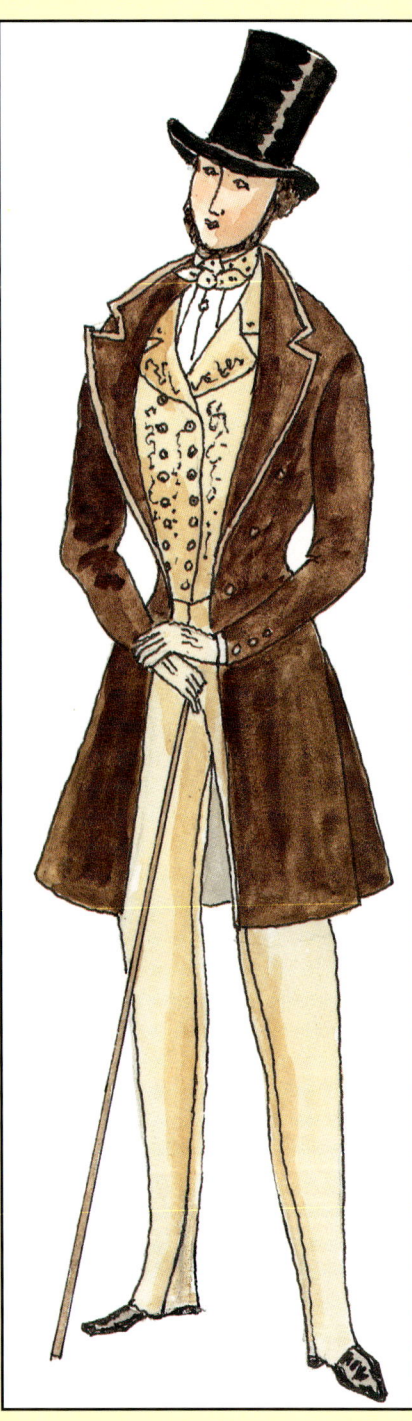

1840-1850 Day Wear

Although the women looked overly feminine, men did not look overly masculine, apart from mustaches and whiskers; in fact, they appeared almost effeminate. Their frock coats, in brown, green, or blue cloth, were full-skirted, with nipped-in waists and sloping shoulders. Vests could be plain but were often richly embroidered. Trousers were narrow, with or without straps under the shoes. A man would carry an ebony or bamboo cane or a short thick walking stick.

The "Oxonian" patent leather half-boot which was to become standard daywear for many years.

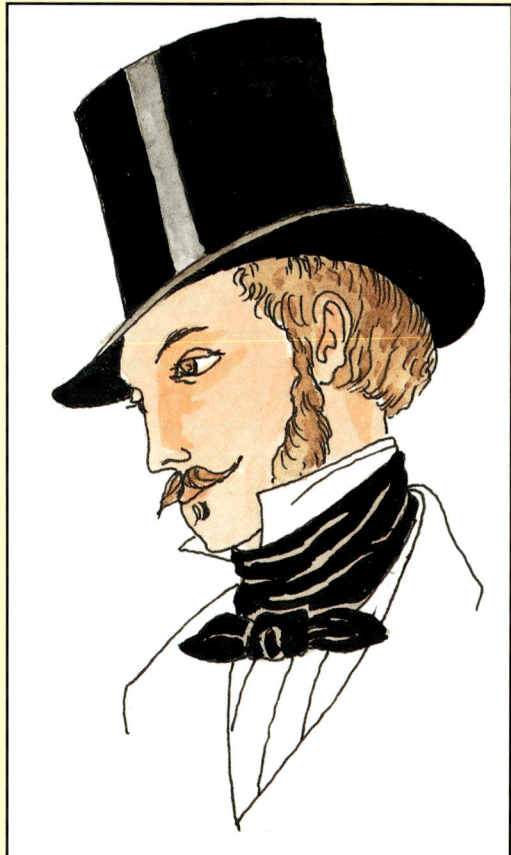

As in the full-length figure, men were still wearing tall, "stove-pipe" beaver top hats, but shallower versions, more usually made of French silk, were becoming more fashionable in the early 1840s. Although a few neck-to-vest neckcloths were still being worn, they were more often replaced by this kind of silk cravat, tied in a bow.

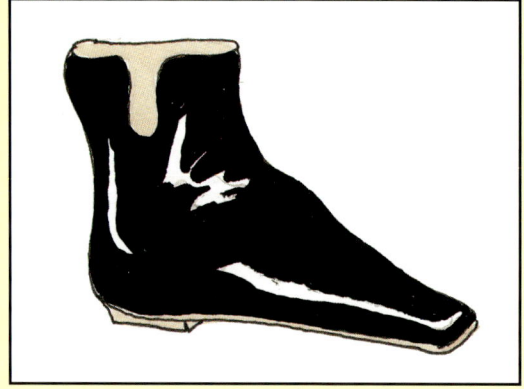

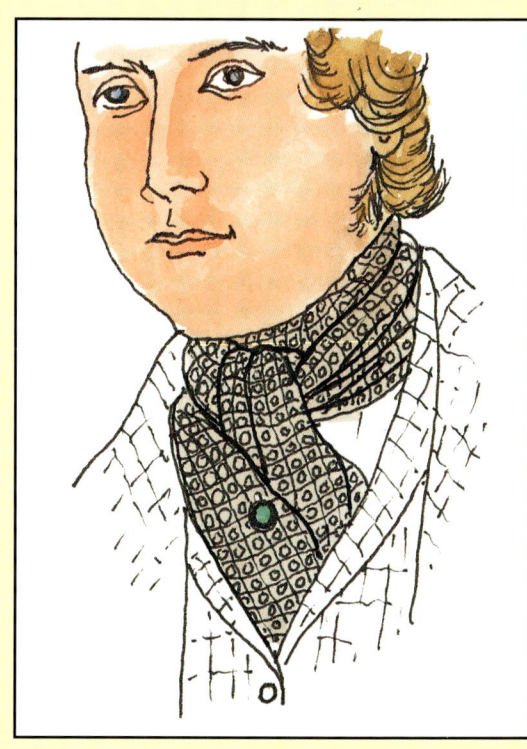

Worn with a casual tweed suit, this young man sports a silk scarf neckcloth fastened with a tie pin.

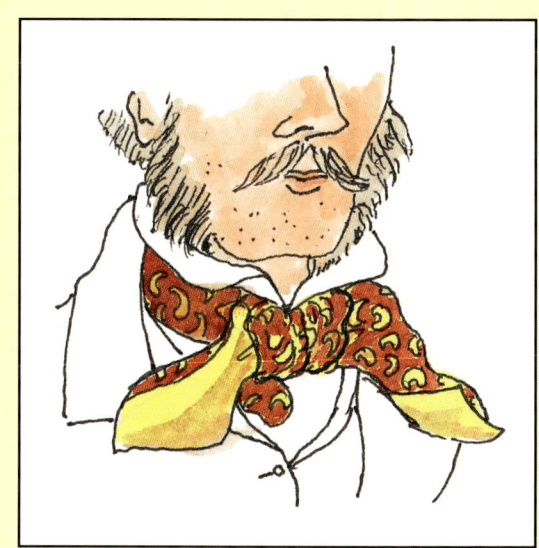

A casually-dressed man wears a semi-stiff collar with a loosely tied, brightly-colored scarf-like cravat.

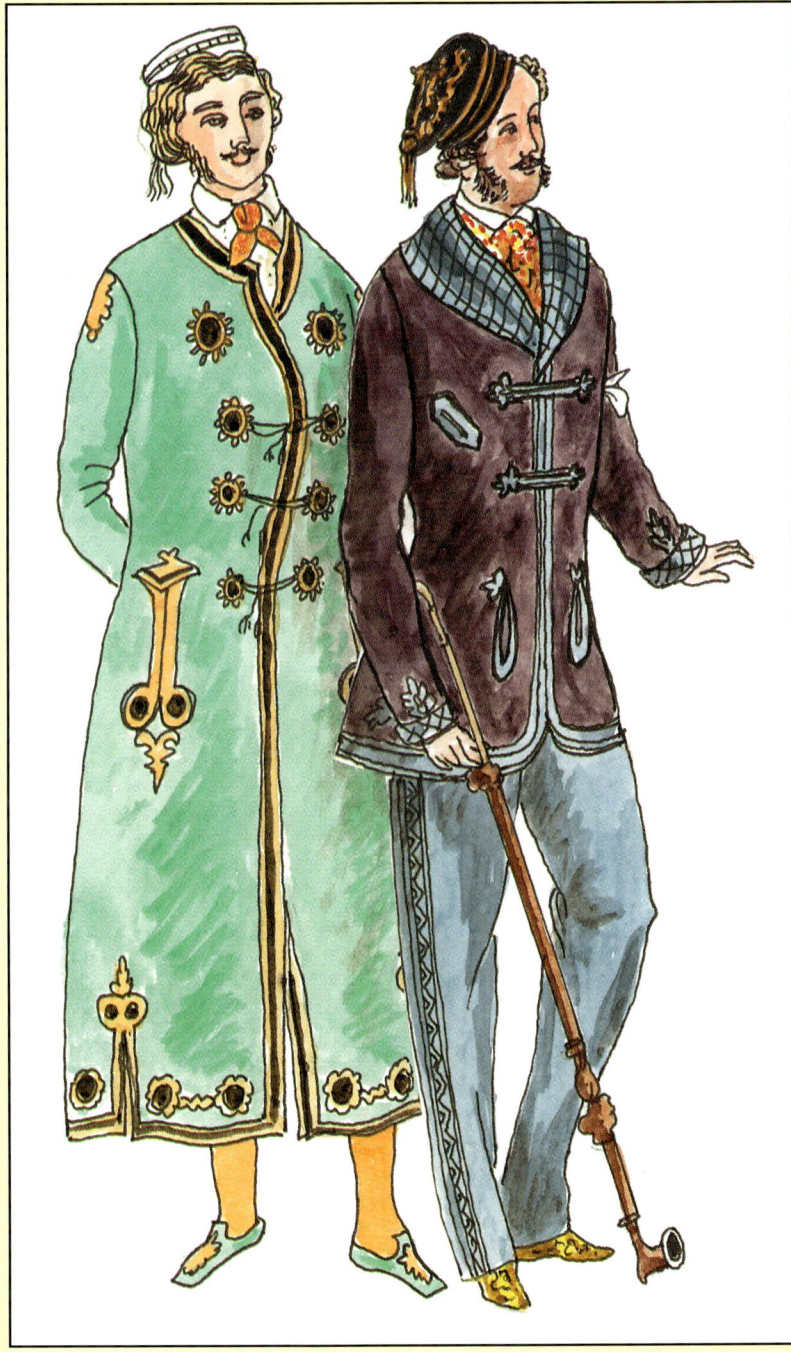

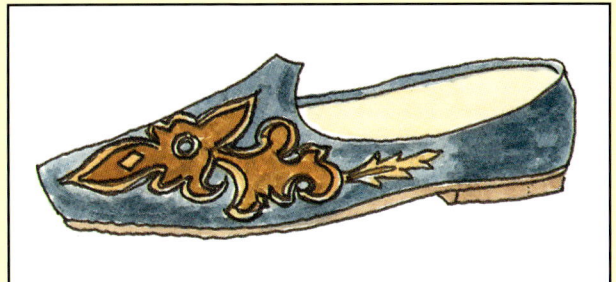

1840-1850 Day and Evening Wear

A gentleman could look like a "peacock" at both ends of the day. In the morning, he could wear a silk or cashmere, highly decorated robe de chambre or dressing-gown (at left), and in the evening he could wear a velvet, quilted, and equally highly decorated smoking jacket and "fancy" trousers (at right), which he wore in his study or smoking room, because it was impolite to smoke in front of ladies. Such an outfit was also worn in the billiard room.

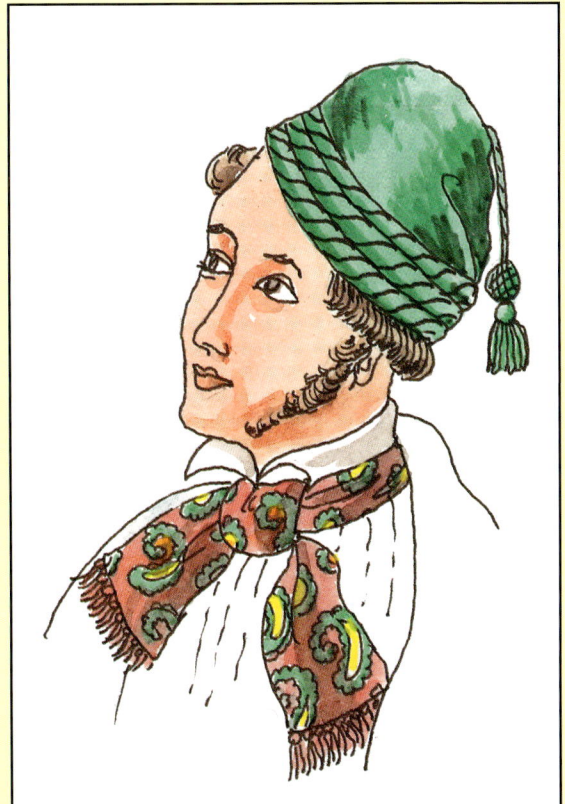

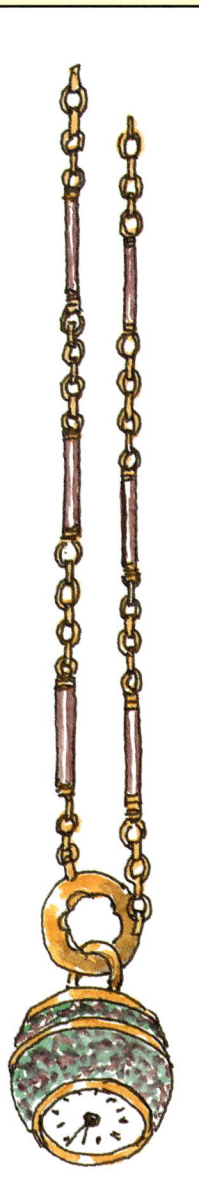

Above: A silk morning or evening slipper decorated with appliqué. The making of such slippers, also embroidered or carried out in Berlin woolwork, was a favorite occupation for a gentleman's women for most of the nineteenth century.

Left: A silk morning or evening smoking cap with a tassel, worn with a paisley-patterned silk "joinville" scarf, named after Prince de Joinville who wore one when visiting Queen Victoria at Windsor Castle in 1843.

Right: Before pocket watches were worn on chains, this style of gold and enamel watch on a matching chain was hung around the neck during the day and in the evening: a fashion dating back to approximately 1650.

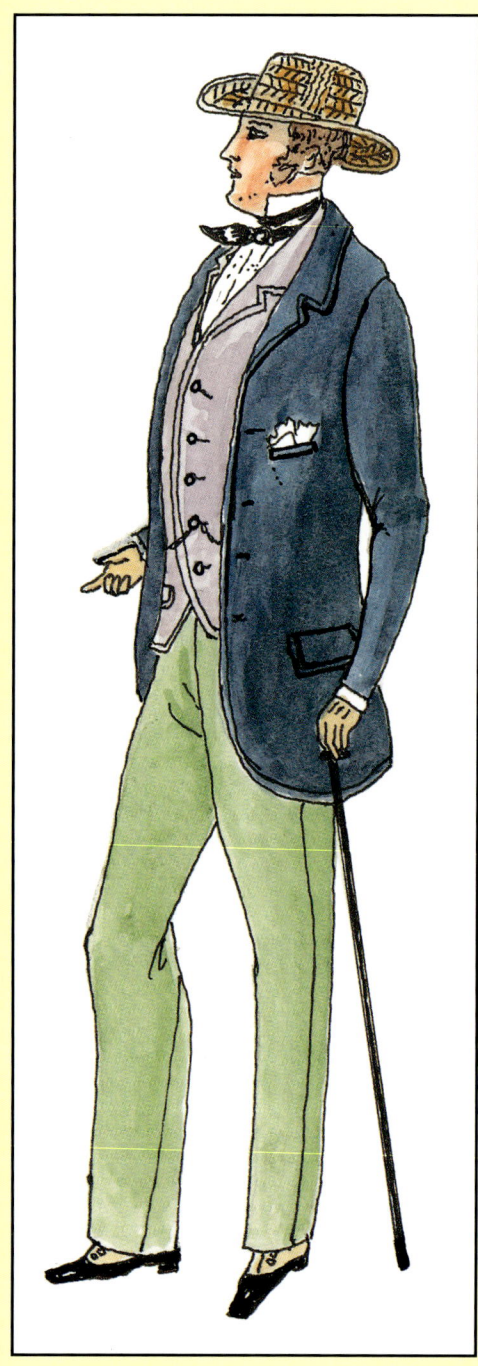

1850-1860 Day Wear

This gentleman is wearing one of the new "lounging" jackets, a vest, and fairly loose trousers. From 1850 to 1855, the jacket and vest were usually made of the same material; later, they would be made of different materials, such as wool with tweed. A mixture of colors for all three garments was very fashionable.

As the century progressed, more and more different hats appeared for casual occasions and for various sports, such as this hard felt "widewake;" a similar one in straw can be seen in the full-length figure.

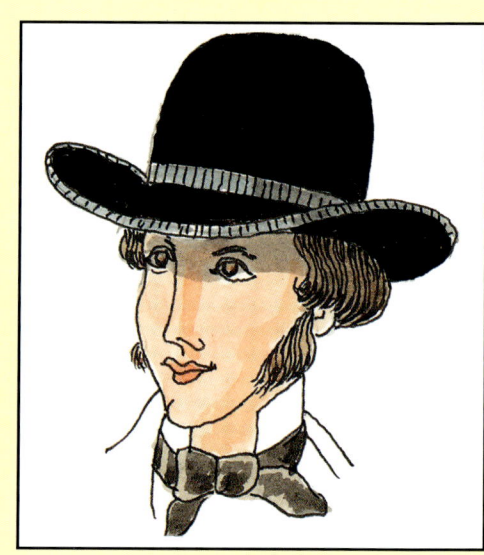

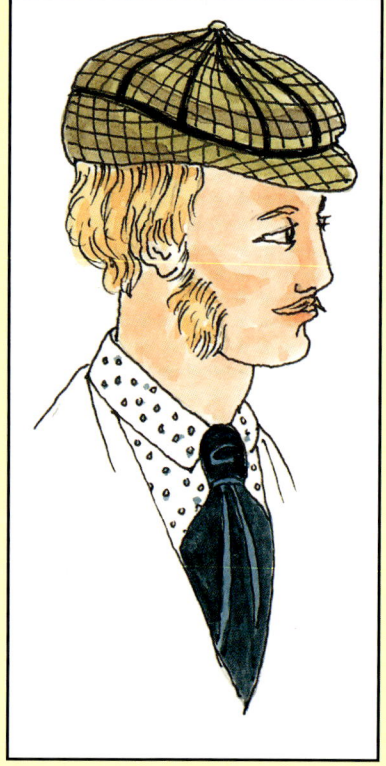

Tweed caps were worn only in the country, often with soft shirts and loose neckties.

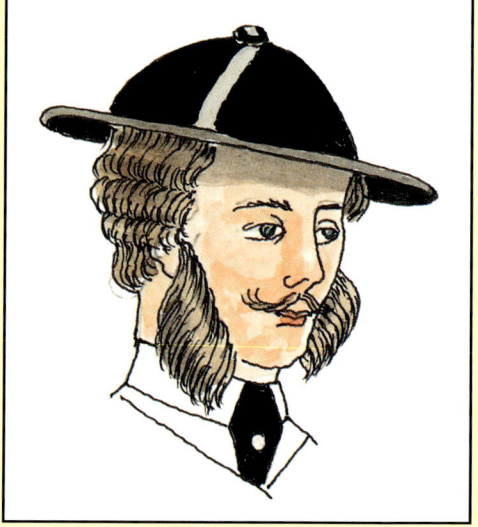

Even harder, a domed hat call a "Bolinger."

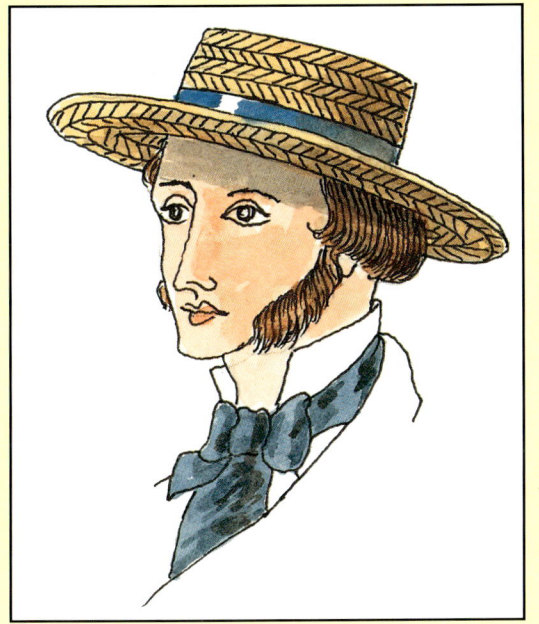

Straw hats were for the country or the seaside.

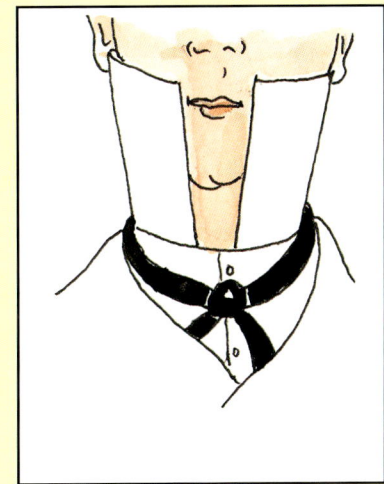

A "shoe-string" necktie. Because this is taken from a cartoon, the excessively high shirt collar is probably a satiric exaggeration, but it shows how high collars could be.

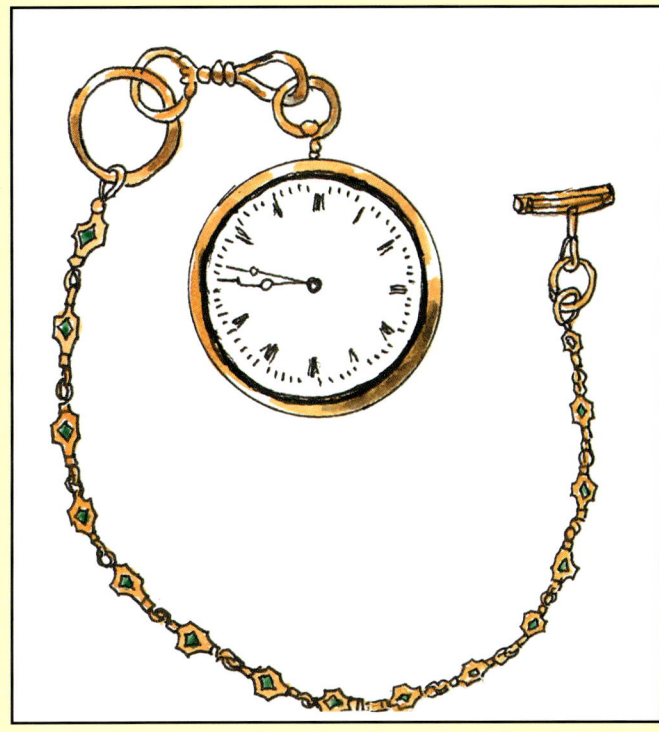

Hitherto men kept their pocket watches only in their pockets, but in 1849, the "Albert" watch chain appeared by means of which the watch could be suspended between one vest pocket and its opposite. This style was called the "Albert" after Queen Victoria's husband, the Prince Consort. This early example is made of enameled gold; "Alberts" continued to be worn well into the twentieth century, particularly by older men.

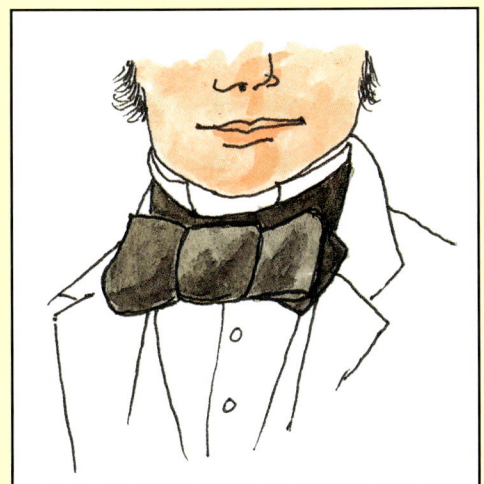

A barrel-shaped necktie called an "Osbaldiston."

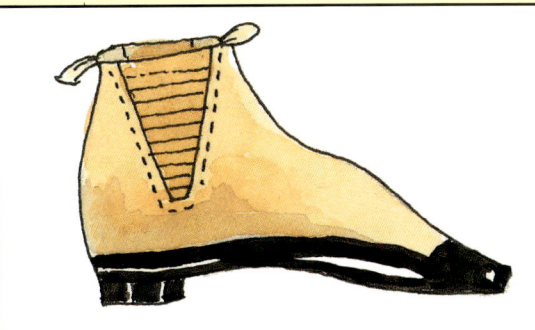

Patent leather: its cloth upper has elastic gussets.

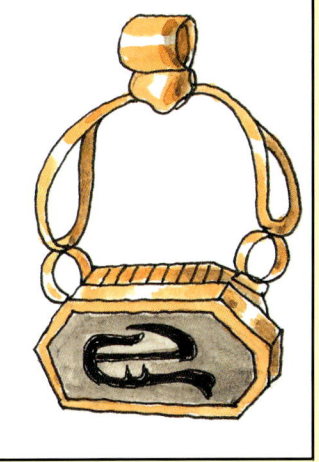

A gold seal. A man's initial, monogram, or crest would be engraved on the steel face, with which he would stamp the sealing-wax on the envelope of his letters or on documents. Along with other trinkets, seals were often hung on watch chains.

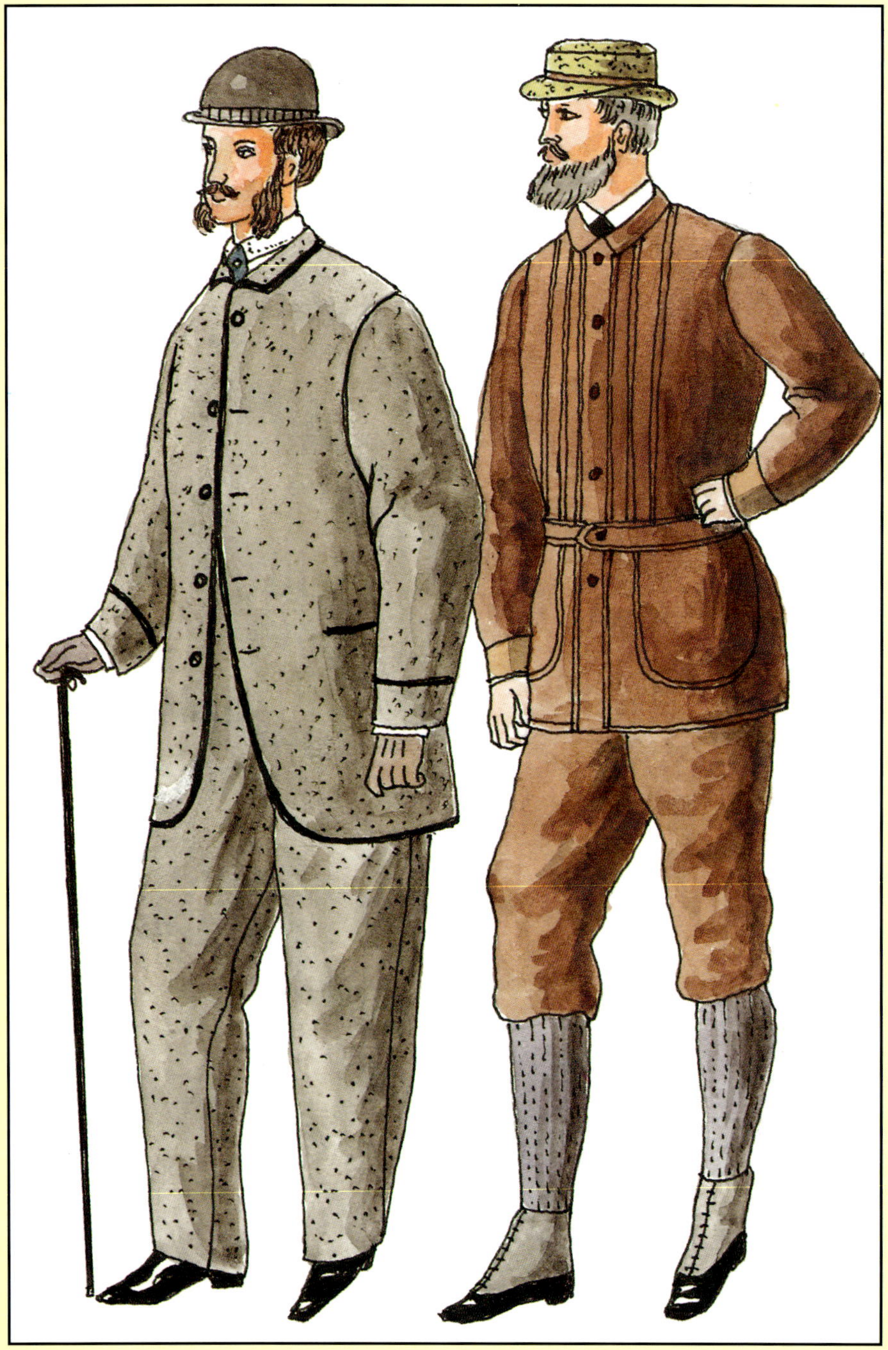

1860-1870 Day Wear

I have chosen only two outfits to represent this period, because by the 1860s, there were so many informal garments from which men could choose, such as the Reefer, the Pea, and the yachting jacket. A tweed or cloth lounge suit (at left), with its full, long jacket and wide trousers, was for general wear. For the country, 1886 saw the first Norfolk shirt (at right) in tweed, with matching knickerbockers, woollen socks, and cloth and leather shoes.

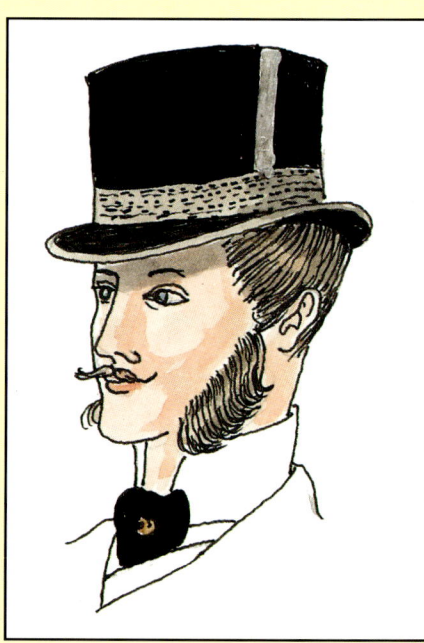

After 1865, the height of top hats was very much reduced in Britain but remained tall in France.

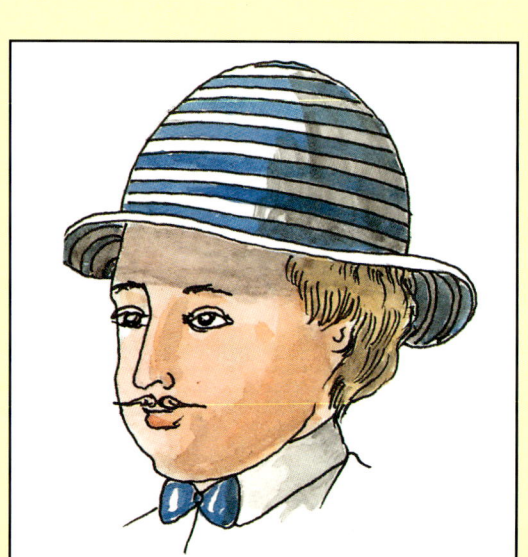

A felt bowler (derby), correct for cricket.

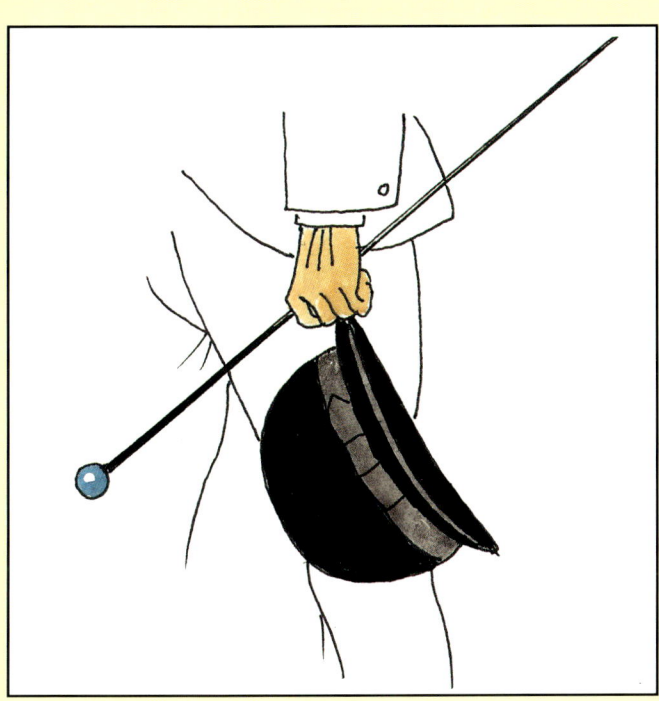

☞ The first bowler (named after a Mr. Bowler and called "derby" in America) appeared in the 1860s but was worn with only informal suits. The cane in the illustration has a lapis lazuli knob.

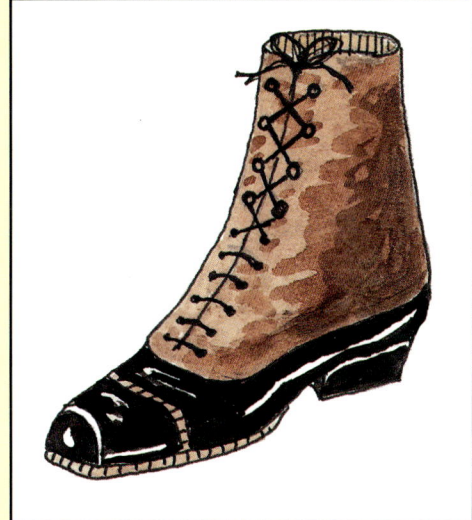

A patent leather half-boot (full boots, up to the knee, had gone out of fashion) with a cloth, laced upper.

Neck cloths were giving way to neckties.

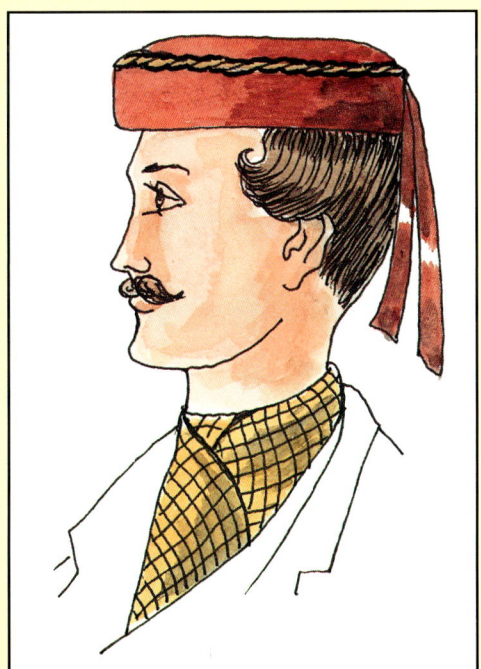

A velvet and cord morning or smoking hat called a "muffin;" similar ones were made in straw for outdoor wear. The man also wears a folded silk neck scarf.

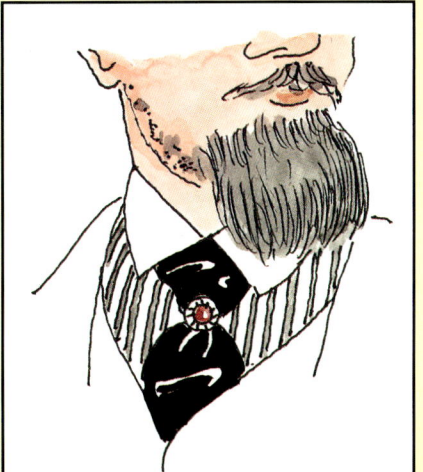

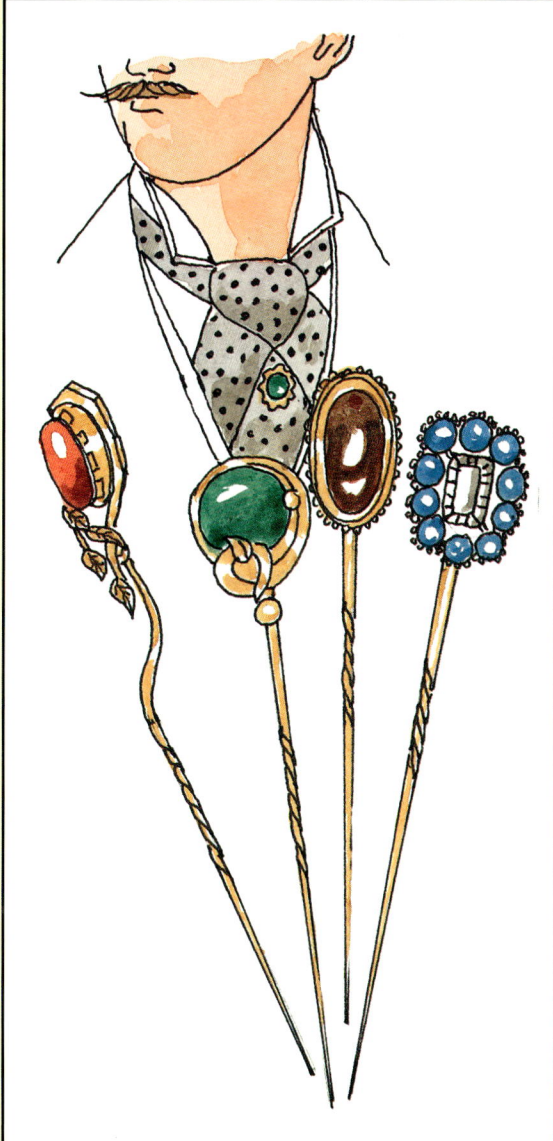

An elaborately folded necktie fastened with the ubiquitous tie pin. Tie pins are still worn today, of course, if only for formal weddings and at grand race-meetings, so they have a long history. Shown is a selection of this period, all gold with gems. *Left to right:* decorated with tiny leaves and set with a ruby; an emerald resting in a strap; an onyx; a diamond surrounded with turquoises set in tiny pearls.

149

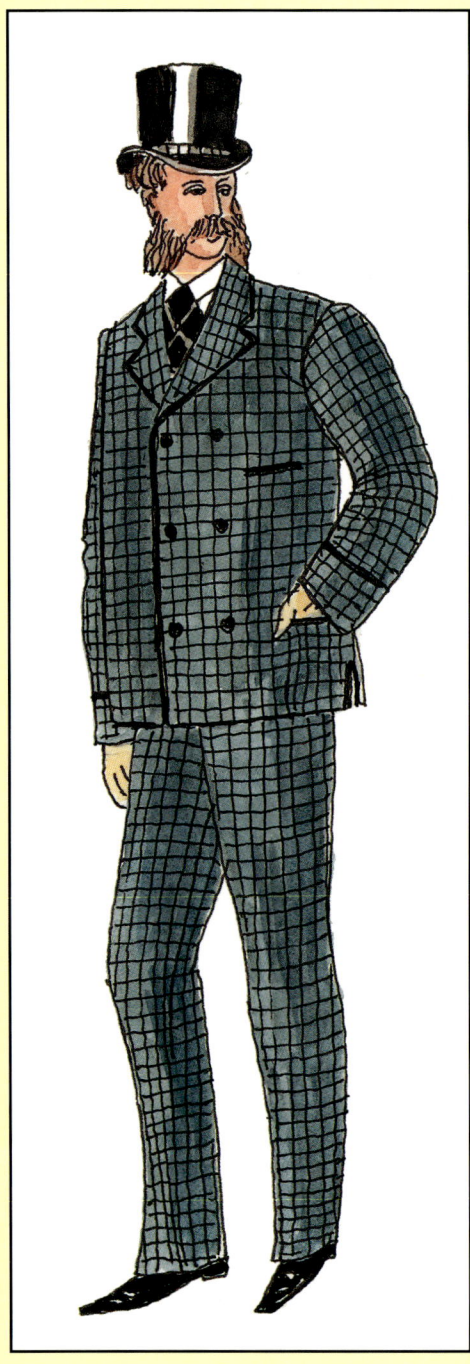

1870-1880 Day Wear

Although wearing a formal, shallow top hat, this man is clothed in a lounge suit with a shorter, double-breasted jacket and slimmer trousers in checked tweed, described by a contemporary as a "business suit for all occasions, especially as a yachting suit or as out-of-town wear and in blue diagonal for the seaside." However, another critical contemporary observer noted that "gentlemen are not so well dressed as they were."

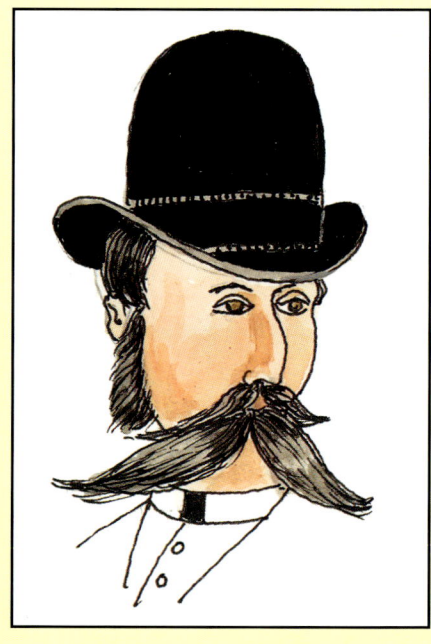

A high bowler (derby).

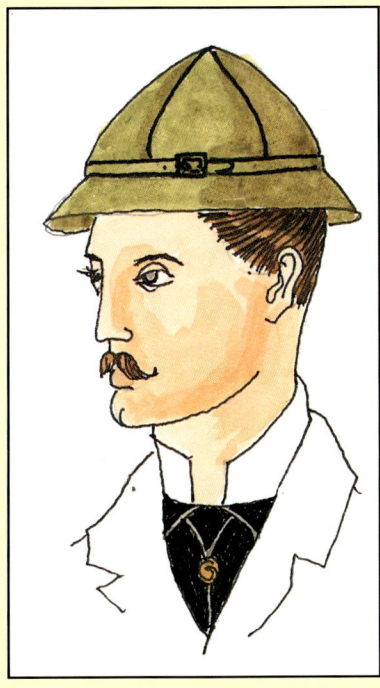

This felt "helmet" was for country wear.

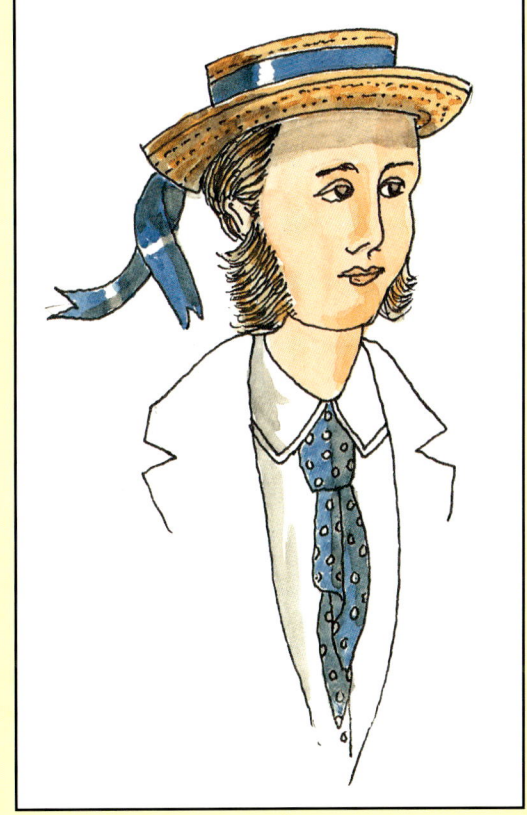

A dashing straw hat, with extra-long ribbons worn with a scarf-like necktie, were fashionable for rowing and yachting.

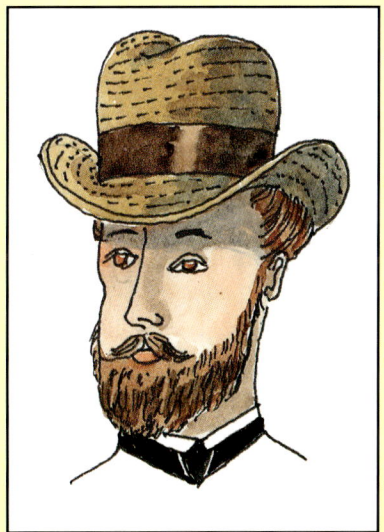

This tweed, ribbon-bound hat was mostly worn with a matching Norfolk jacket and knickerbockers.

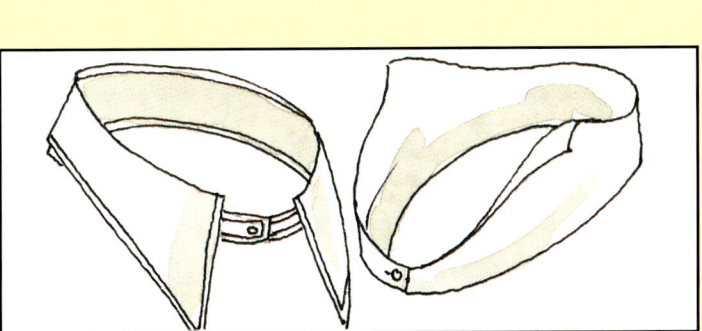

Stiff collars were detachable: a formal "Shakespeare" and an informal style.

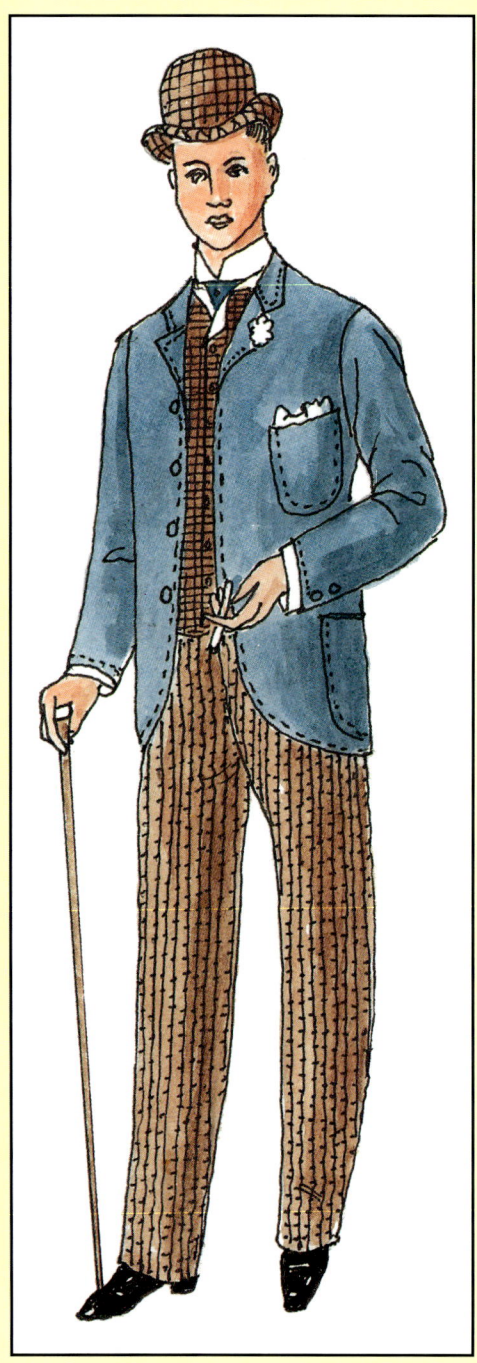

1880-1890 Day Wear

In 1884, the conservative British magazine *The Tailor and Cutter* noted disapprovingly that "Broad- or American-style shoulders in coats and suits are worn by the class known as Mashers." A typical one is shown here in his natty narrow jacket, check vest and trousers, and (rather vulgar) matching bowler (derby). Young or older men of all classes in evening dress who frequented music halls, hoping to pick up chorus girls (some of whom did marry into the peerage) were known as "stage-door-Johnnies."

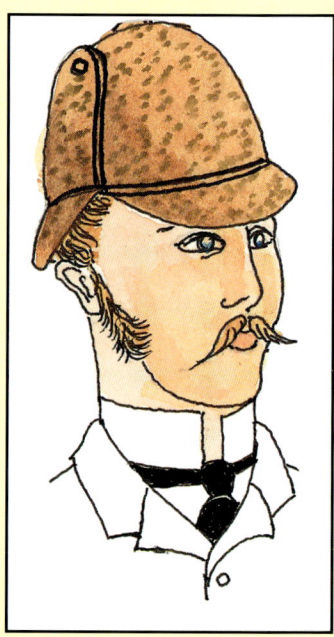

A tweed "deerstalker" with ear flaps, worn for hunting in the country or for cycling. Even in the country, it was obligatory to wear a stiff collar and necktie.

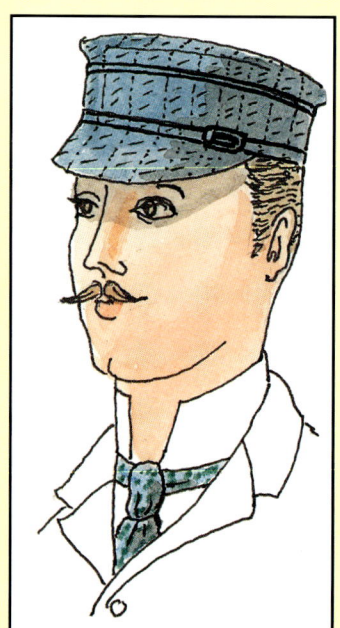

A cloth yachting cap.

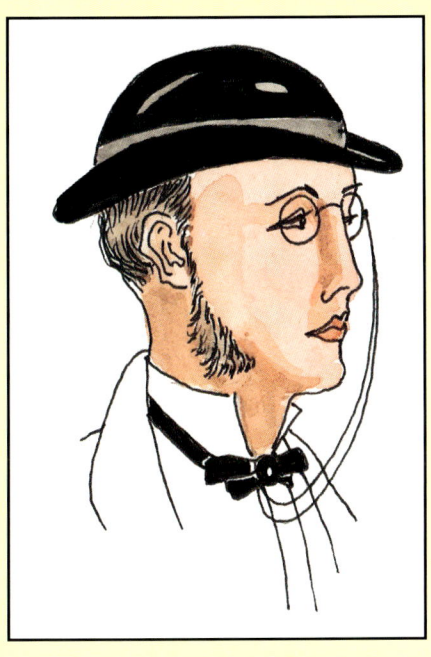

Worn more in Europe than elsewhere: a shallow bowler (derby) with a narrow bow tie and a pair of *pince-nez*.

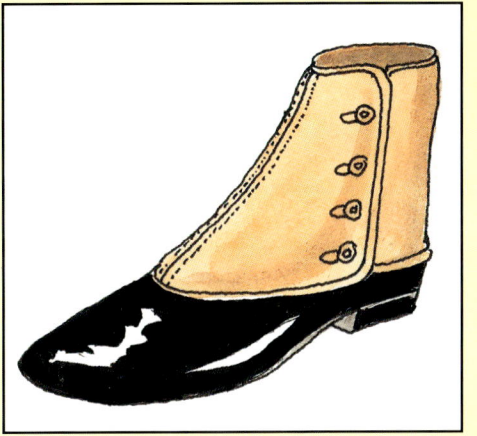

For town wear, a cloth spat over patent leather.

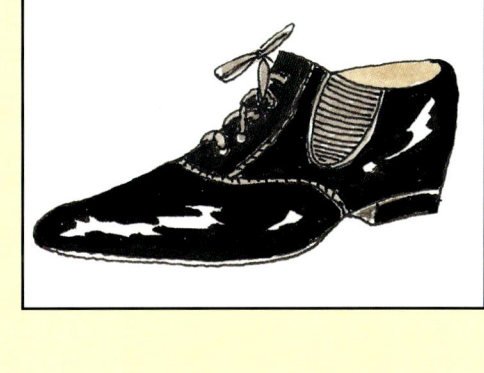

A patent-leather boot, which is laced as well as having gussets.

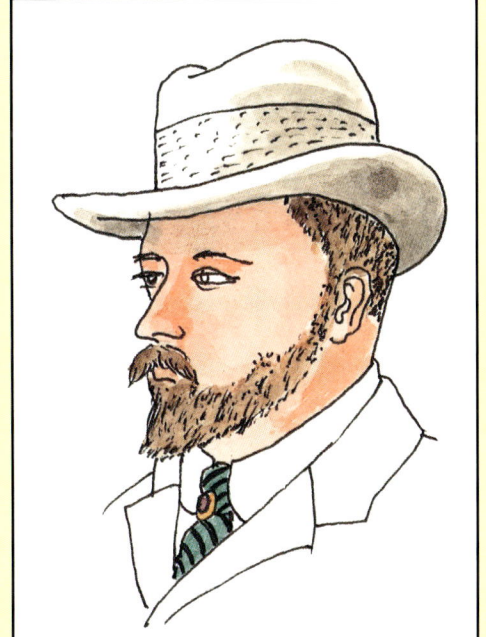

After visiting a hat factory in Hamburg Germany in 1889, the Prince of Wales, later King Edward VII, bought one of their hats, which he immediately made popular, as it was to remain, to a lesser extent, up until the Second World War.

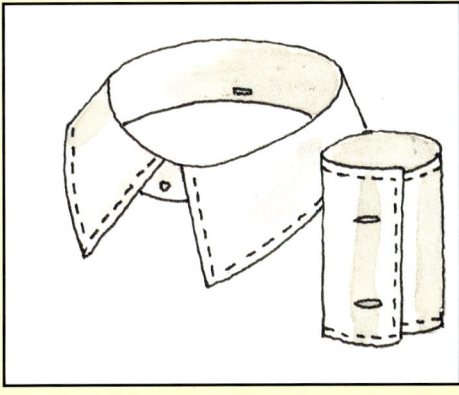

Although considered "bad taste" by smart men, for those who could not afford them to be laundered often, or for those who found them uncomfortable, stiff, starched lined collars and cuffs could be replaced by those made of celluloid.

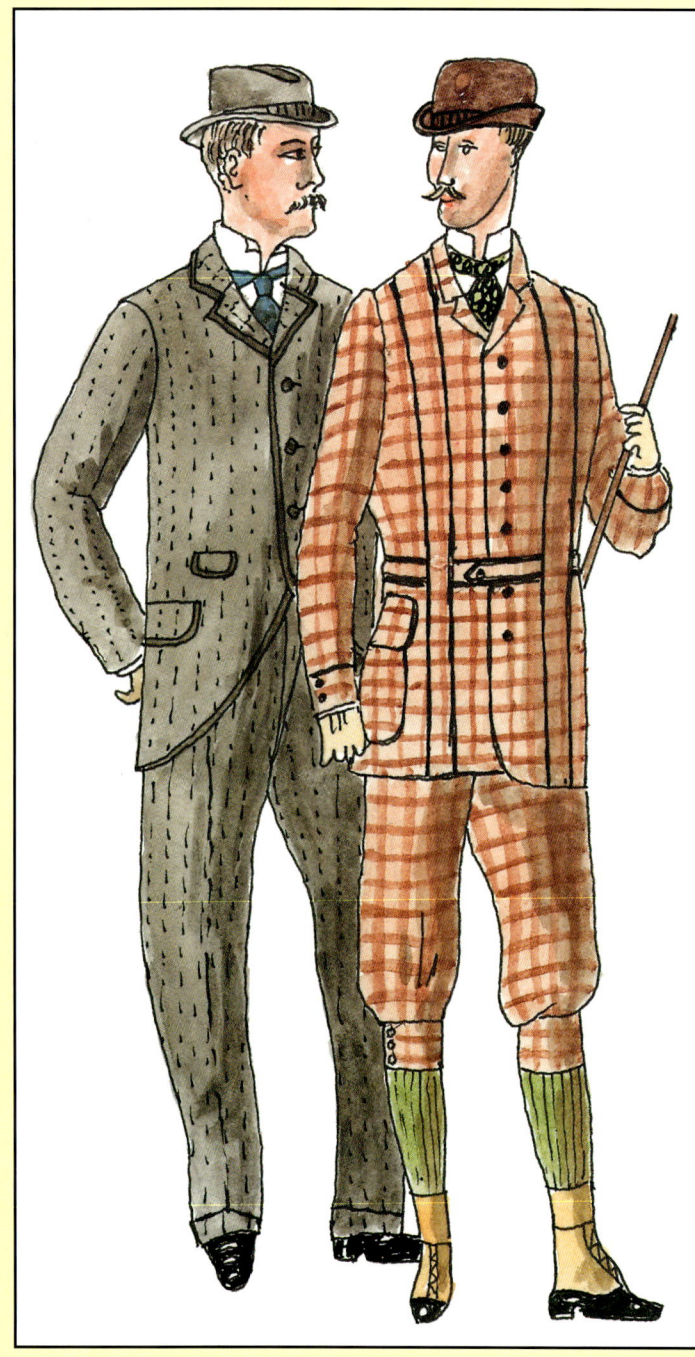

1890-1900 Day Wear

Fin de siecle: Oscar Wilde and his infamous trial; Sarah Bernhardt; Toulouse-Lautrec and low life; the Can-Can; Aubrey Beardsley and *The Yellow Book*; the British Empire at its peak; the flowering of Art Nouveau in Britain, Europe, America, and even in Australia. This was a rich and colorful decade indeed. The single-breasted tweed or wool lounge suit (at left) was still very popular informal wear, but for the first time, trousers were given front and back creases and cuffs, called "turn-ups" in Britain.

In 1890, *The Tailor and Cutter* grudgingly admitted that "The usual demand. . .for big loose and flowering knickers with the Norfolk jacket. . .shows the Englishman to be a lover of comfort." I make no excuse for showing it again, so general and so acceptable had it become for country and sportswear and also for wear by schoolboys well into the next century. George Bernard Shaw famously wore one until his death in 1950.

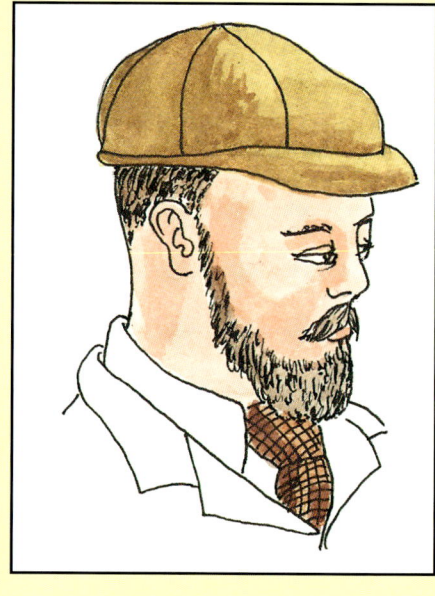

In Britain, a cloth cap has for long been a symbol of the working class, but from this period on, it was acceptable for gentleman and royalty to wear a cloth or tweed cap in the country.

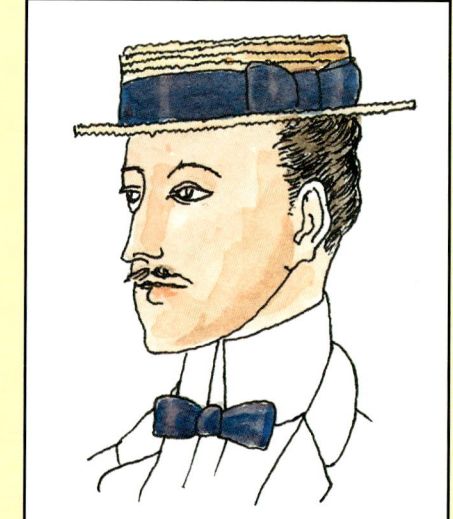

A straw hat for the seaside or the tennis court.

154

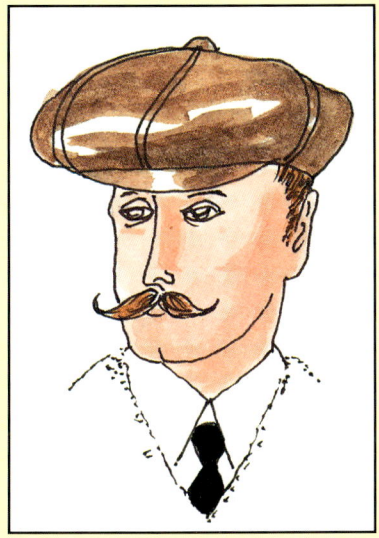

As with women's hats, the invention of the open motor car in 1896 inspired the creation of a special leather cap for men.

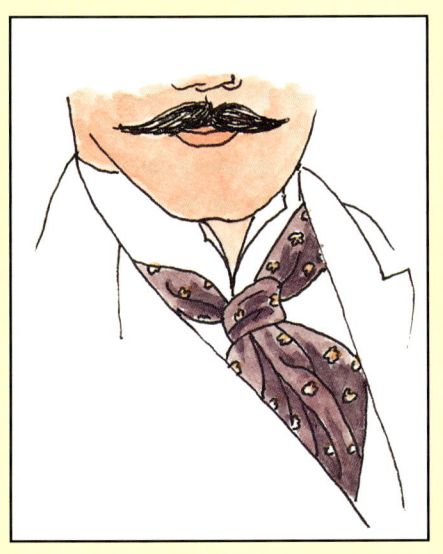

A loose, almost scarf-like necktie worn with a "Dux" collar.

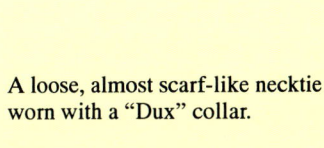

Looking like a character out of Proust, this Frenchman wears a "dog collar" with a cravat in fashionable French colors.

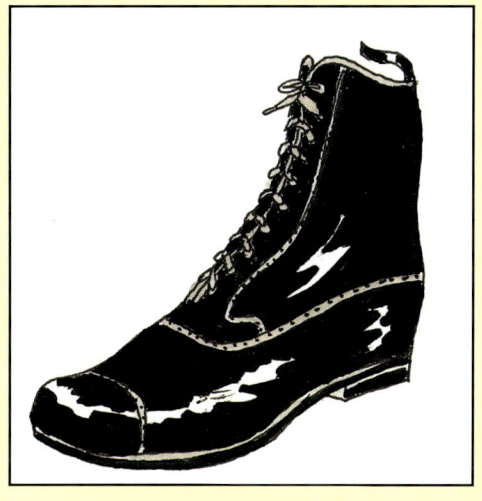

In 1898, this type of boot prompted a contemporary to forecast that "laced shoes will dominate the next century." He was not entirely correct, because, from the 1930s onward, the slip-on shoe would become just as "dominating."

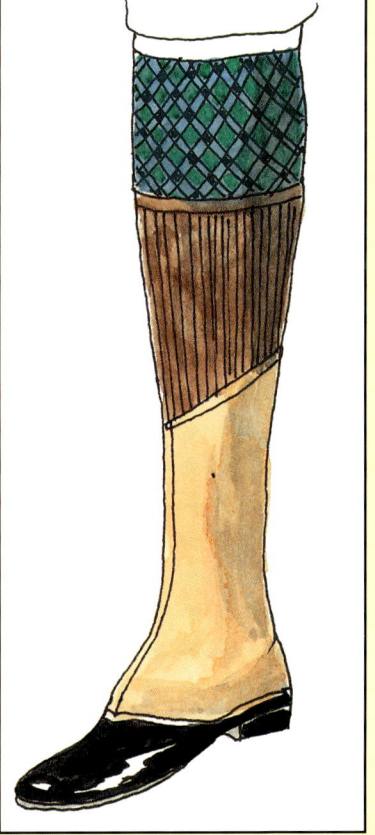

Worn with a Norfolk jacket and knickerbockers: ribbed woollen socks with tartan-patterned top, cloth gaiters and a patent leather shoe.

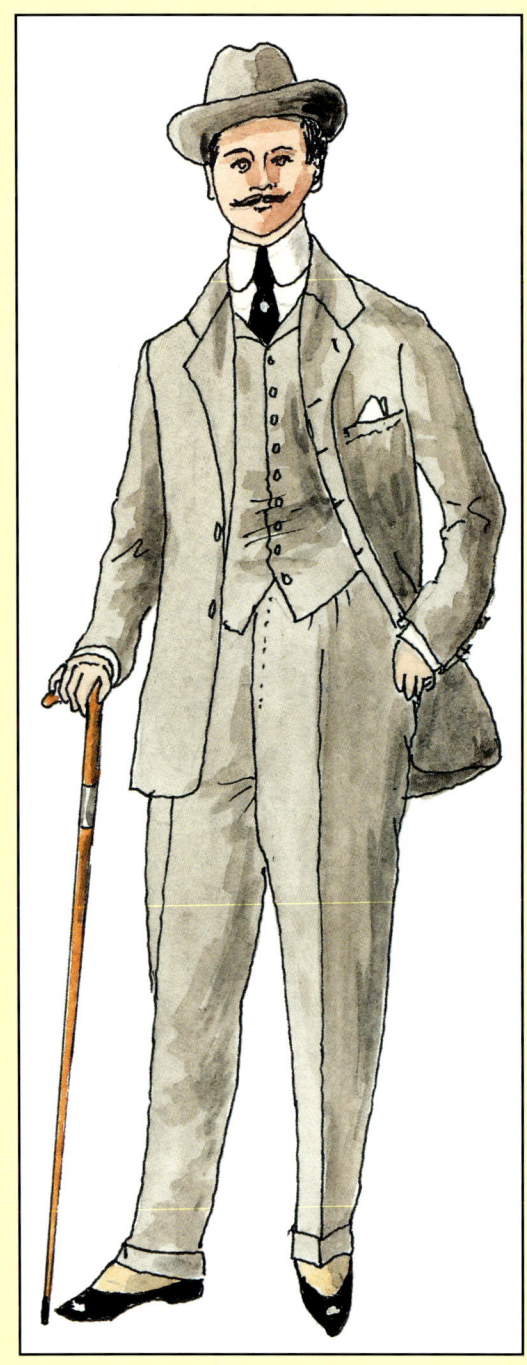

1900-1910 Day Wear

A new century but not much of a new look. Suits could be either single or double-breasted with long, fairly loose, slope-shouldered jackets. A general "natural" style which complimented Poiret's "freeing" women from "S" bend bondage. Canes and walking sticks were still very fashionable, swung with élan down Piccadilly, the Champs Elysées, and Fifth Avenue.

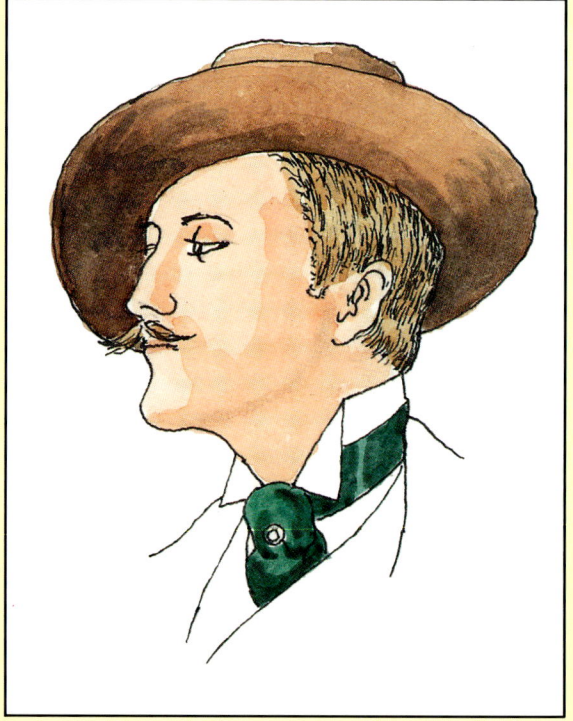

Other hats were making their appearance, such as this wide-brimmed felt hat, worn with a wing collar and luxuriant cravat.

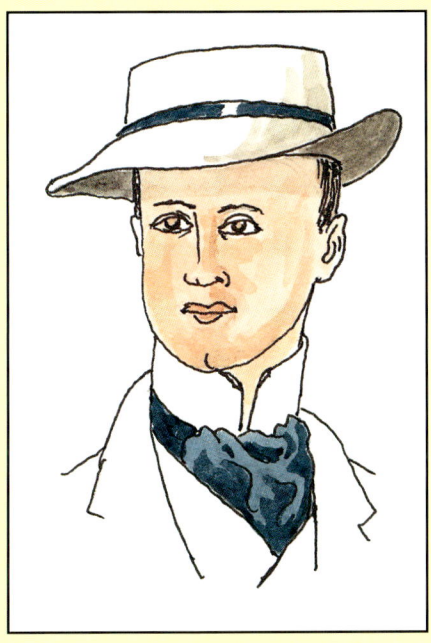

Probably for the seaside, a felt hat worn at a rakish angle; with a high, slightly turned-down "dog collar" and full necktie.

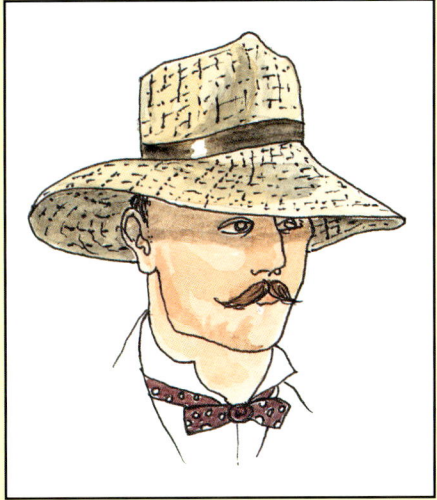

Very finely woven and soft straw Panama hats were very popular for country, seaside, and for watching sport. The hat, in fact, came form Ecuador and was made fashionable by the Emperor, Napoleon III of France, as early as 1855 as a summer dress hat. It is still worn today; it saw a particular revival among the young in the 1970s - see page 00.

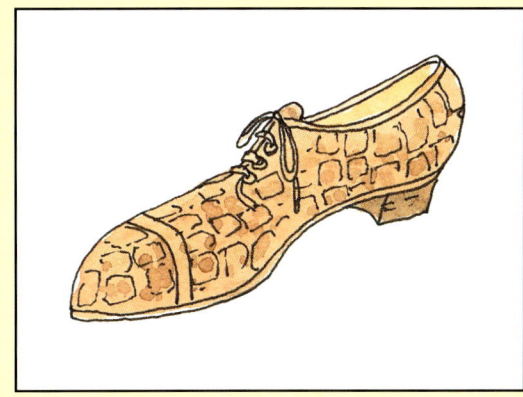

An alternative: an elegant, crocodile "Derby".

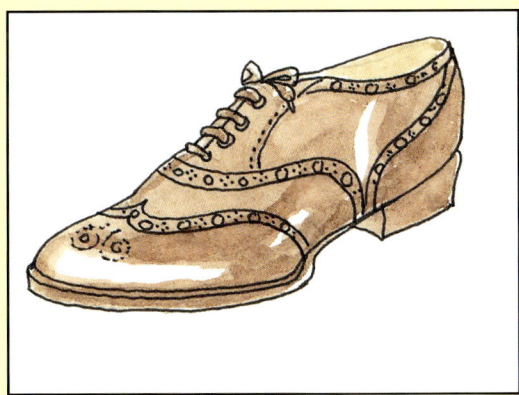

The prototype of today's "Oxford" or brogue shoe, stitched, punched, and pierced, which made its first appearance between 1900 and 1905. At first, men of high fashion thought the style to be vulgar.

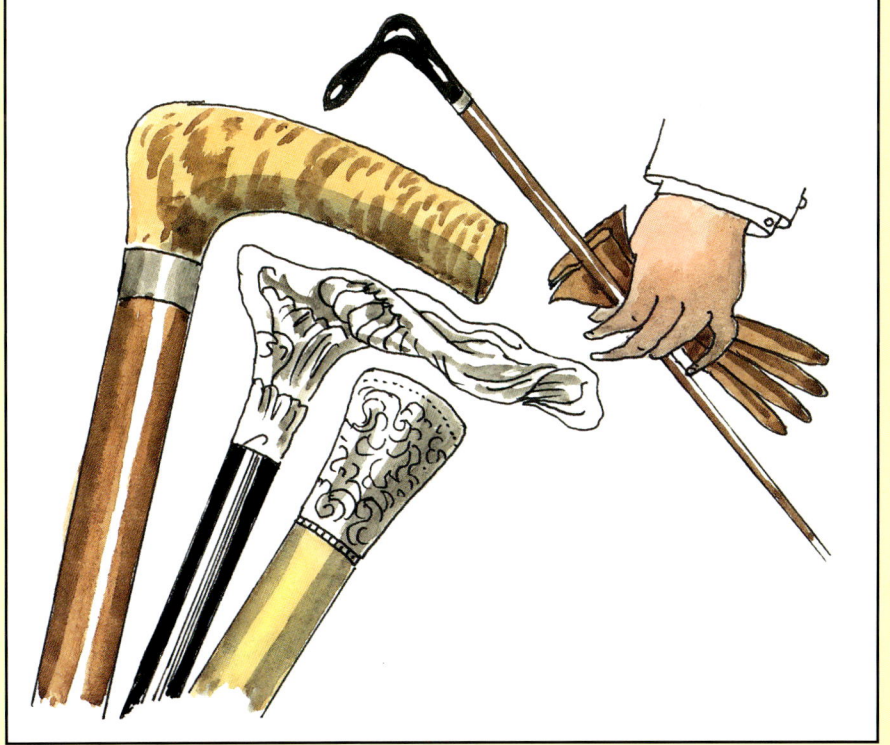

Canes and walking sticks have, of course, a long history. This is a selection of some of those of this era. The man in the picture carries an ebony-handled stick. *Left to right:* a stick with a tortoiseshell handle and silver band; a stick with a silver handle in Art Nouveau style; a cane with a repoussé silver knob.

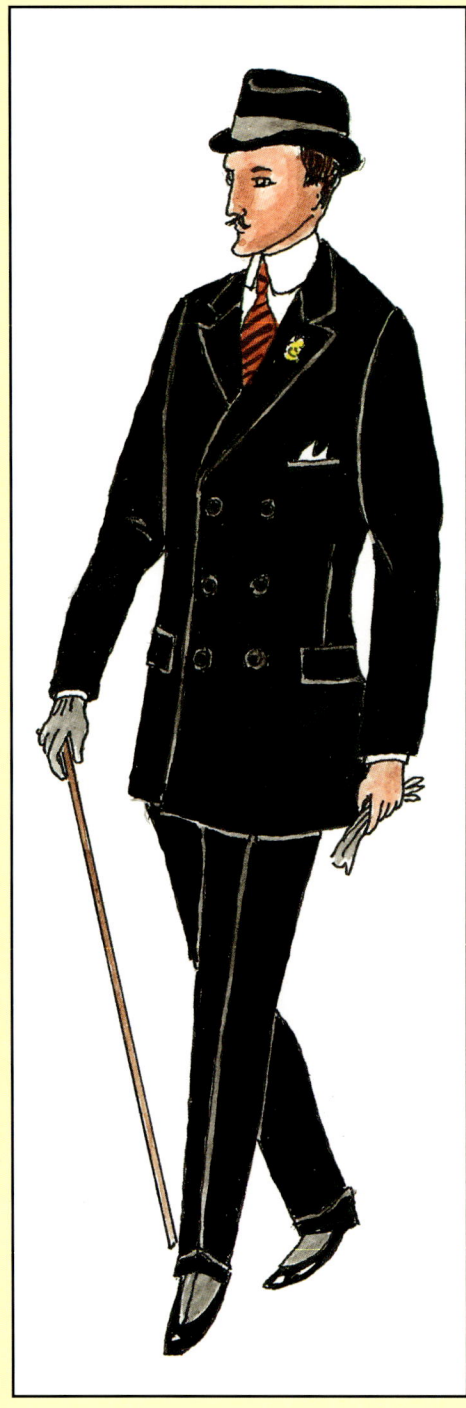

1910-1920 Day Wear

Unless, of course, he were in uniform, on both sides of the Atlantic during the First World War, there were very few changes in men's fashion, except for a certain formality creeping back and much black coloring, in tune with the times perhaps. Suits were still single- or double-breasted with long jackets and narrow trousers. For town, spats were the inevitable choice. The man depicted here offsets his semi-formality by wearing a homburg.

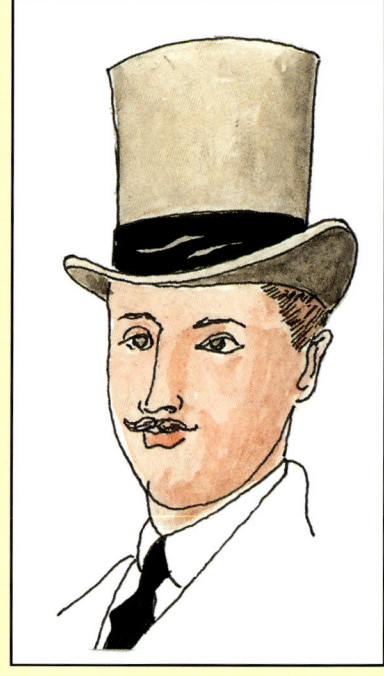

For those men not fighting in the First World War, elegance in fashion continued as strong as ever. "Swells" wore gray top hats, which are still correct wear (although less tall) for formal weddings and Ascot.

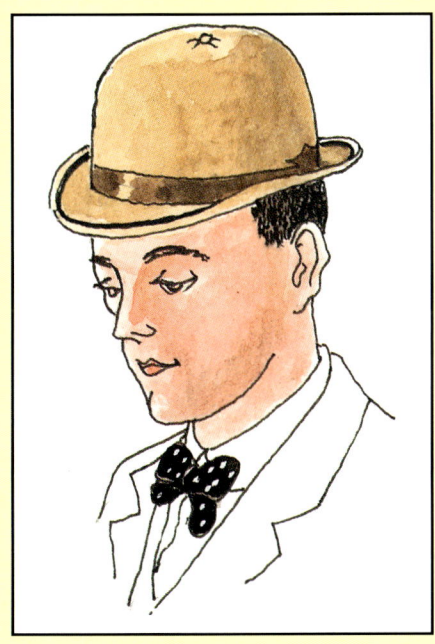

Upper class and upper middle class men frowned on "Brown in Town" ("Town" meaning London in particular), but those men not so far up the social scale, or those men who did not care for convention, sported brown bowlers (derbies). This young man also wears a probably made-up bow tie, which was also frowned upon by "gentlemen."

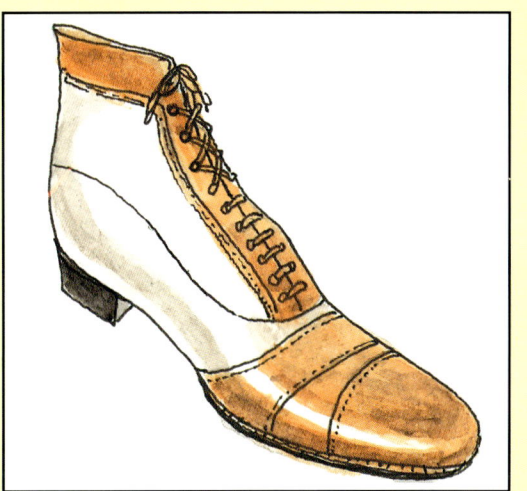

Two-toned leather shoes are associated with the 1920s and 1930s, but this French example was made in 1913.

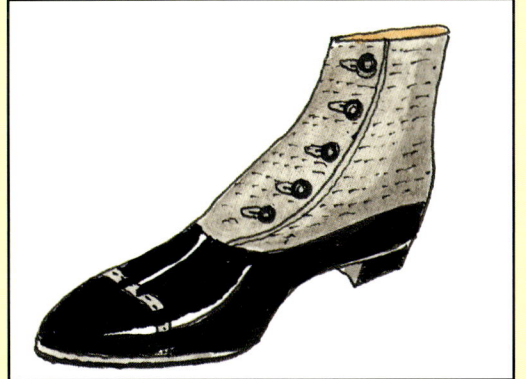

Patent leather with a spat-like tweed upper. Varnished buttons were being replaced by more fashionable horn or mother-of-pearl buttons.

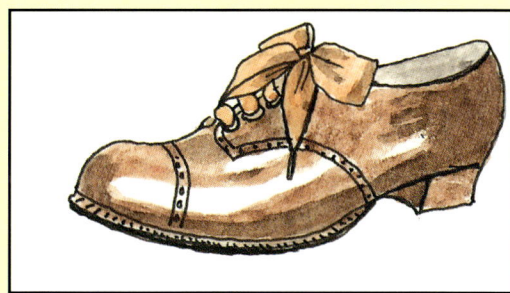

Some American shoes, admittedly, were rather less elegant; hence, this blunt-toed, heavy example, with a singularly wide ribbon lace.

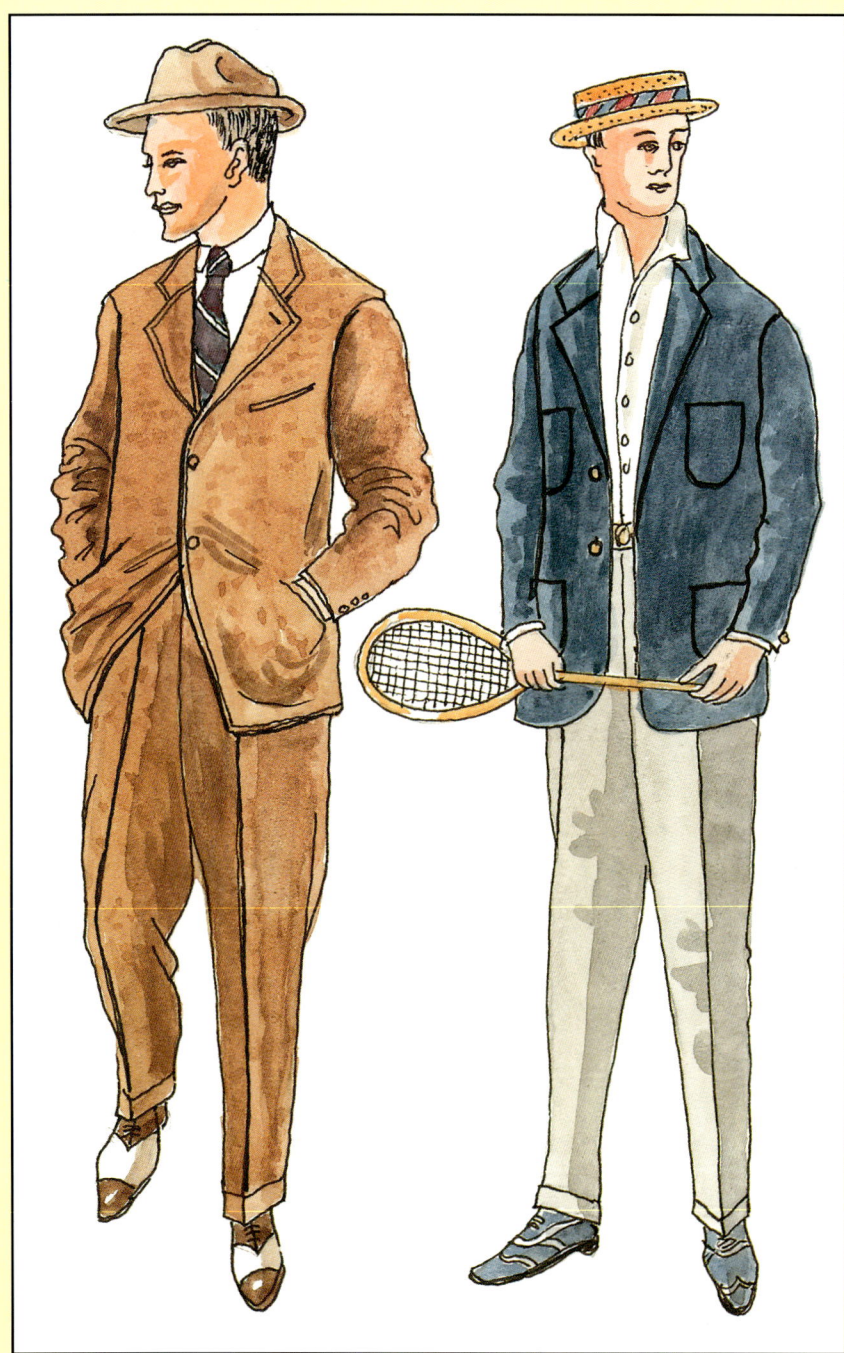

1920-1930 Day Wear

As with women, youthful styles predominated, especially among the young men who wanted to forget the horror of the war trenches. Only older and conservative men still clung to formal clothing. The young instead chose easy-fitting lounge suits (at left) and sport-inspired casual garments such as blazers (at right) with flannel or linen trousers, influenced by America, soft-collared shirts, often worn without neckties. "Oxford bags"—very wide trousers named after the British University—were something of a minor fashion in Britain but also were adopted by some American young men. "Bags" did, however, have an influence on the width of trousers from the late 1930s to the early 1950s.

During this time, the most eligible bachelor in the world, the young Prince of Wales (later King Edward VIII and the Duke of Windsor), exercised his good looks and charm as an "Ambassador for Britain" and also became a leader of fashion, with his Fair Isle sweaters and golfing plus-fours. The Prince's father, the very conventional King George V, believed his son and heir's liking for loud colors and mixing stripes with checks to be in "bad taste"; the Prince and other "Bright Young Things" cared not a jot. The British style, with its tailoring considered the best in the world, was fashionable in France and America as were Scottish homespun tweeds.

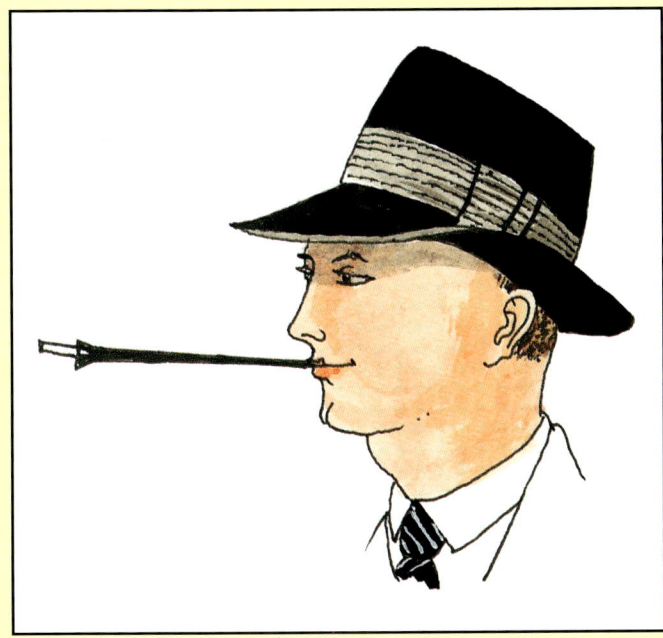

The new felt "trilby" became very fashionable at this period and for long after, in gray, black, dark blue, and dark green. Sophisticates, copying Noël Coward, favored very long cigarette holders.

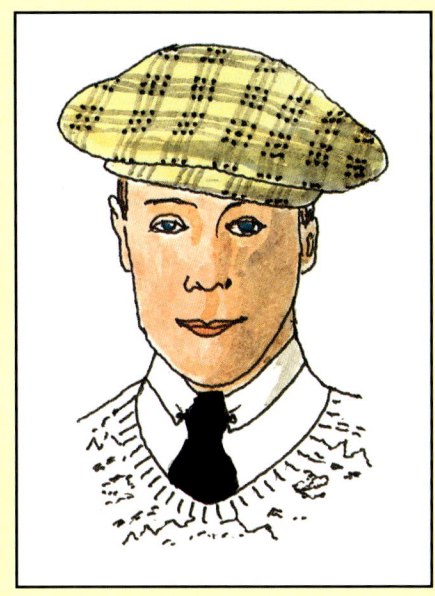

A flat tweed cap, as worn for golf by one of the leaders of men's fashion, the glamorous, universally popular Prince of Wales (later King Edward VIII and the Duke of Windsor).

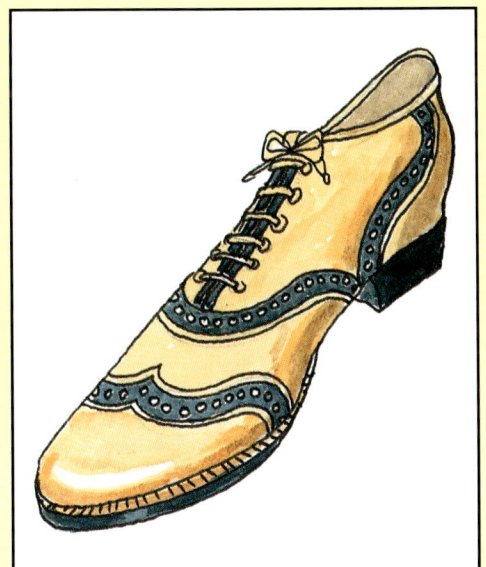

Two-tone leather brogues came into their own, often nicknamed "co-respondent" shoes.

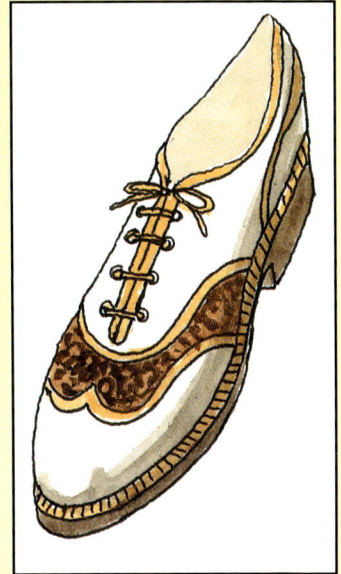

An unusual three-toned brogue, consisting of pale bands outlining snakeskin.

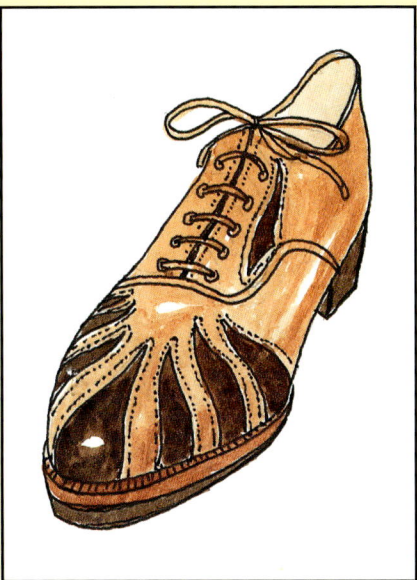

Two shades of brown leather. Most brogues had heavy, thick soles.

1930-1940 Day Wear

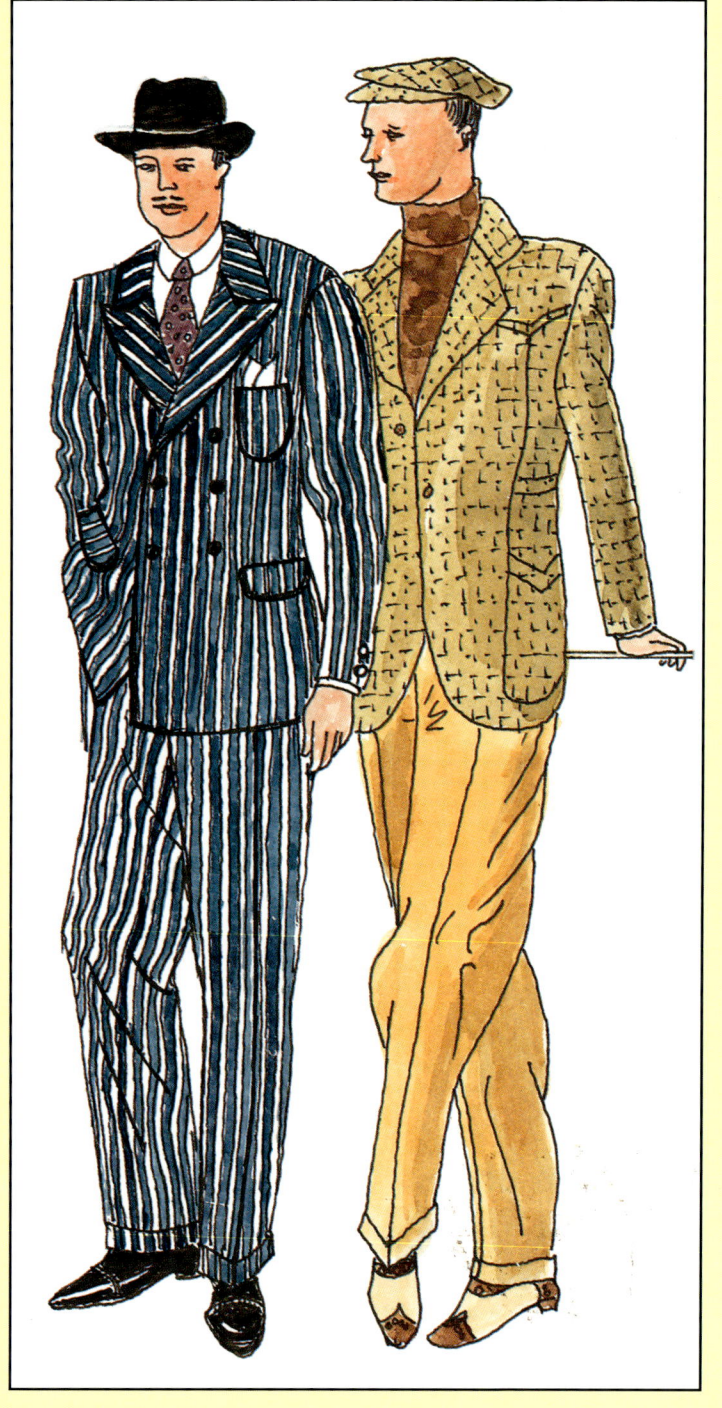

Continuing its good tailoring tradition, Britain's "London Cut" or the "Drape Cut" (at left), in fine wool with a double- or single-breasted jacket and large pointed lapels, often in pin-stripe with fairly wide trousers, was popular, smart town wear. With it, this man wears a black homburg called the "Anthony Eden," after the Head of the British Foreign office during this period, who made it popular. For the country or when dressing informally in town, a tweed sport jacket (at right) with flannel or linen trousers, a polo-necked sweater, and a flat cap were the things to wear.

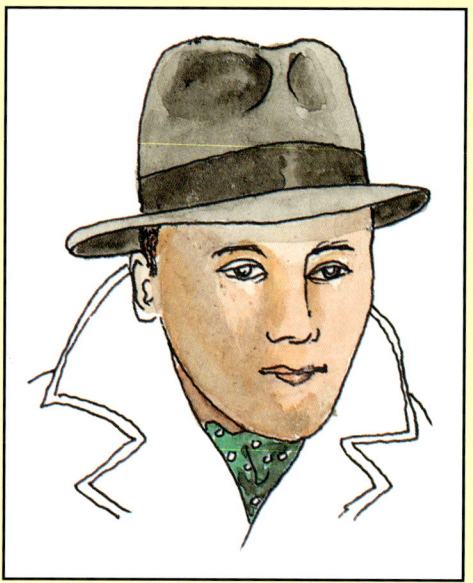

In general, in Britain the trilby was relatively shallow. Very few men went without hats up to the Second World War.

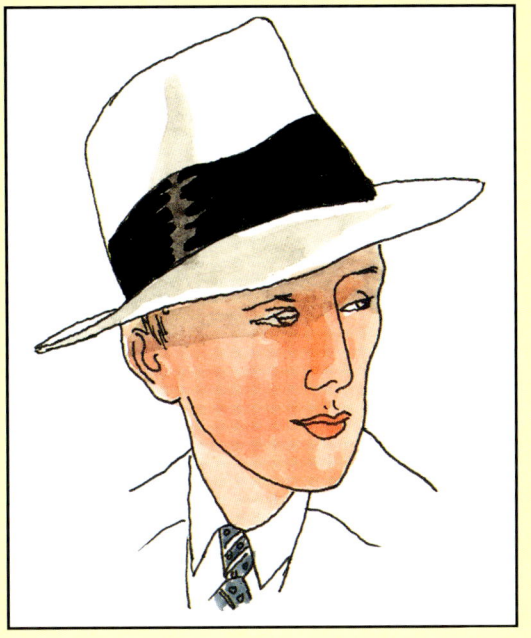

The American trilby tended to be taller with a wider brim.

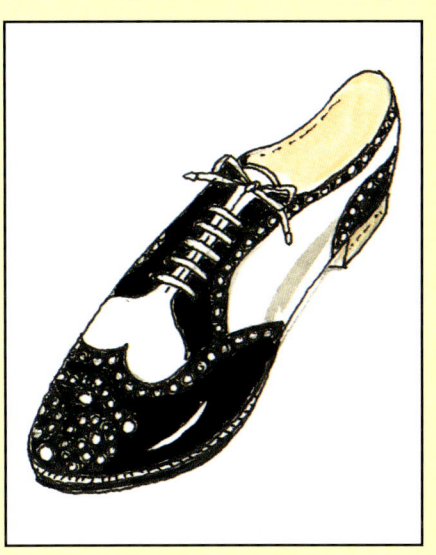

A heavily-decorated two-toned brogue.

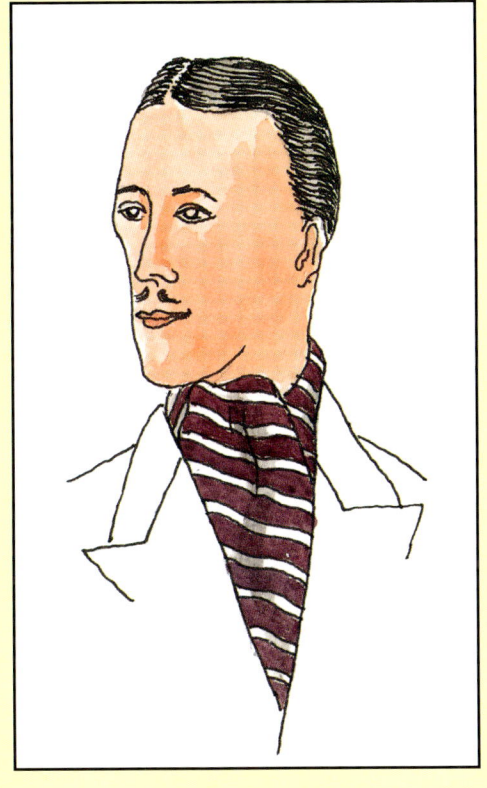

Striped or spotted silk scarves were much worn with casual wear, especially blazers. Showing the great influence of Hollywood, this man sports a "Ronald Coleman" mustache.

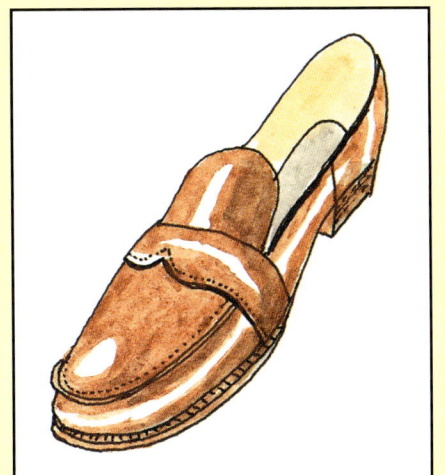

By the mid-1930s, laced shoes were being supplemented by leather slip-ons.

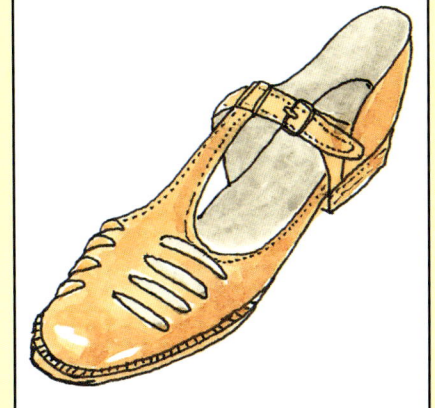

Leather sandals for the beach were new and popular.

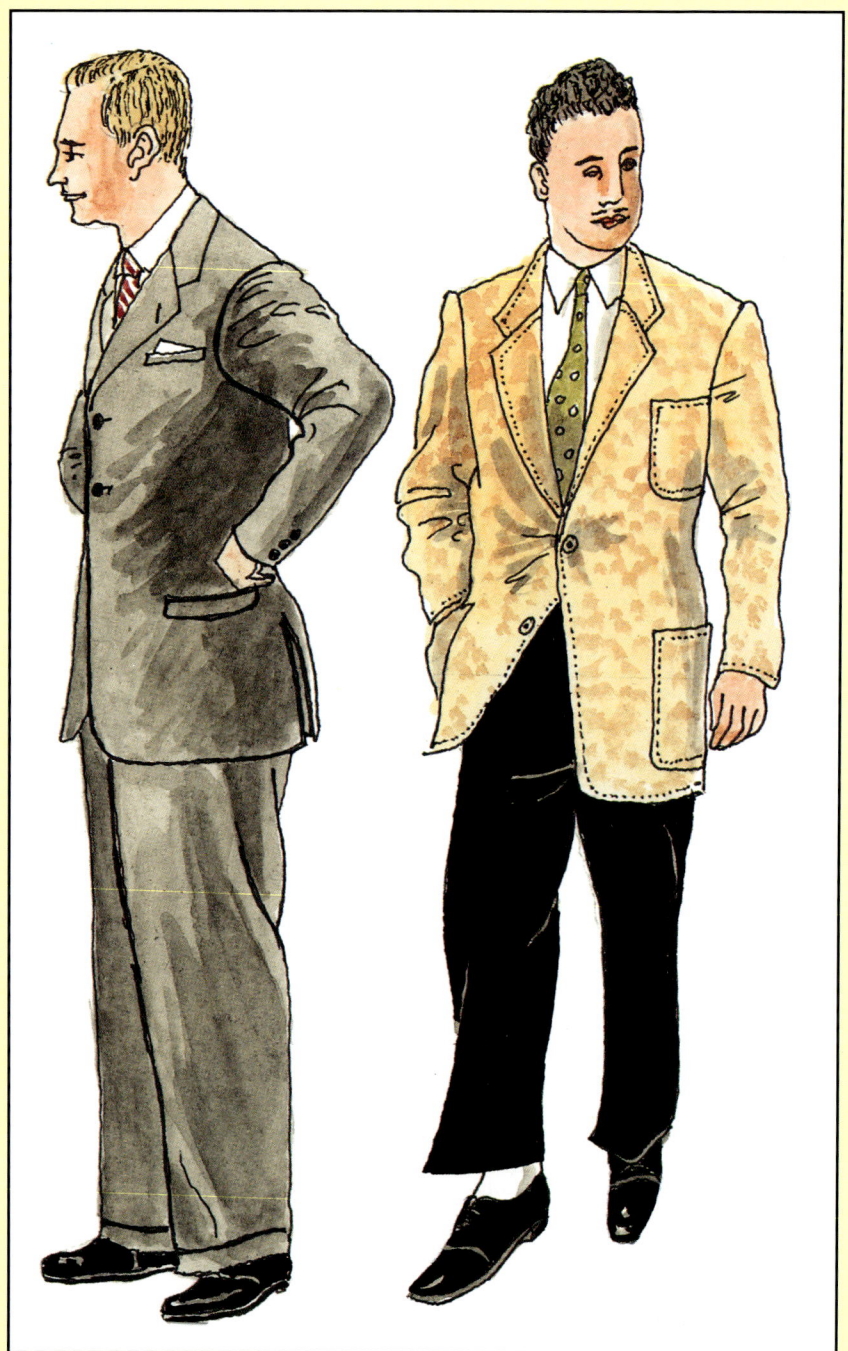

1940-1950 Day Wear

During the Second World War and for some years thereafter, men's fashion came virtually to a halt. In late 1939, it was already said that men's clothiers should do away with "all ornament, all extravagant personal touches." The typical suit (at left) in flannel or tweed had a two-buttoned, slightly waisted jacket with one or two back vents and wide trousers and was worn by many men into the 1950s. Along with jive, American fashions came to Britain after the War, such as the Zoot suit with its long, tapered waist and padded shoulders. Multicolored sports shirts were fashionable on California beaches in the 1940s. A not particularly elegant style emerged from Italy just after the War which consisted of a loose, low-buttoning usually tweed jacket with patch pockets (at right), worn with short black cloth trousers. All that could be considered at all elegant were the shoes.

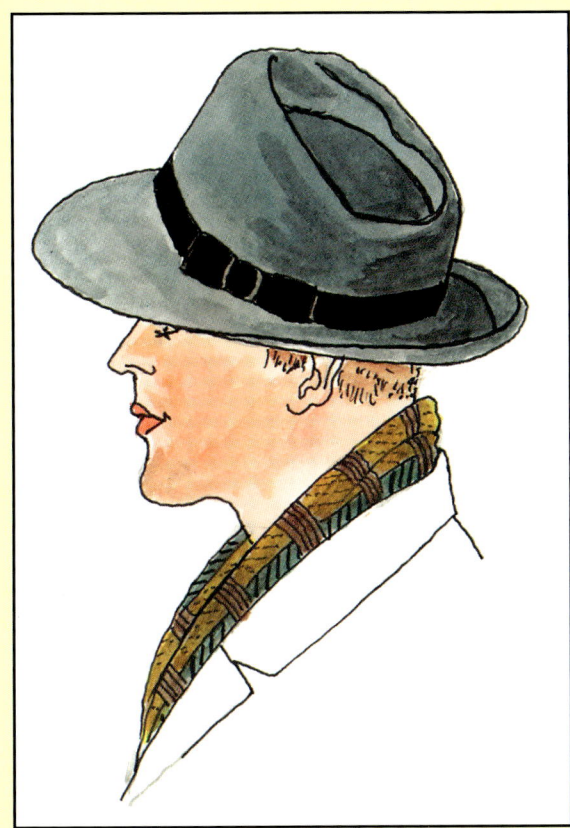

A deep, crushed-in American trilby, worn with a woollen scarf.

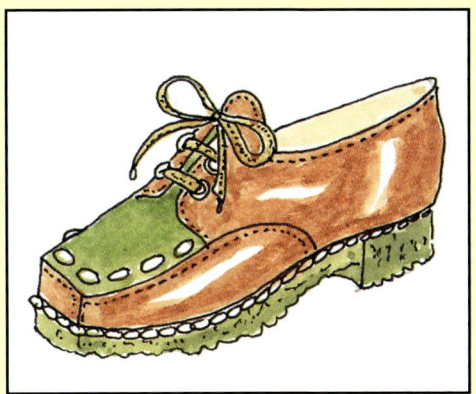

As with women's footwear during the Second World War, especially in Britain, shoes were blunt-toed and clumsy-looking; this two-colored example has a deep crêpe sole.

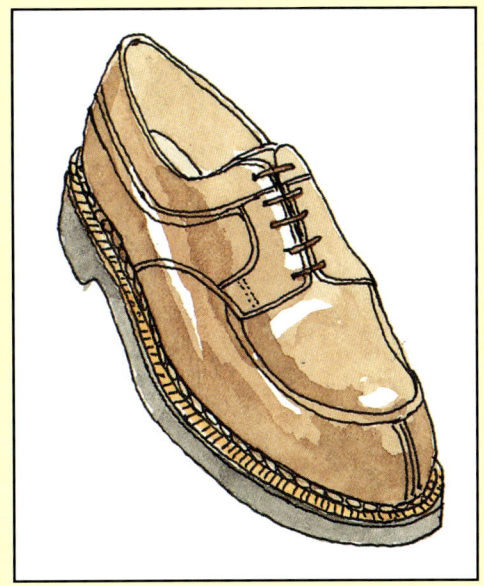

A leather derby with a thick crêpe sole.

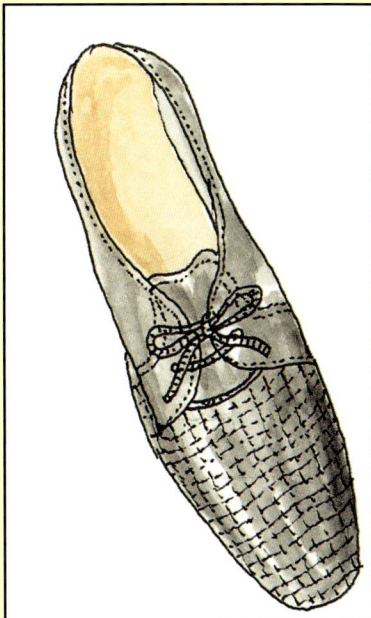

The only elegant kind of shoe to appear shortly after the War was an Italian leather, narrow and sleek, with a plaited front.

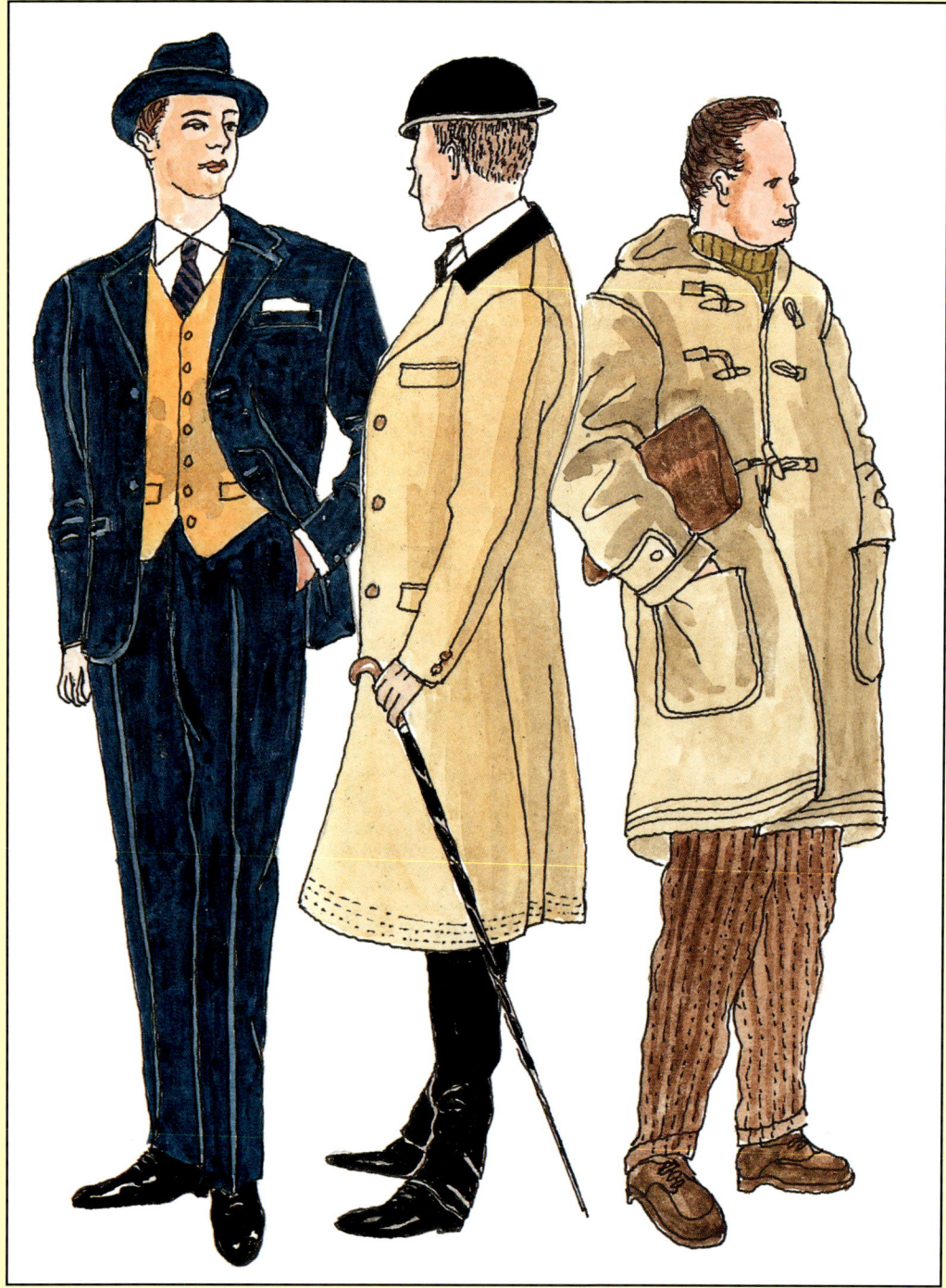

1950-1960 Day Wear

The man on the left wears the standard, smart (if conventional) suit, made in various dark colors in wool, tweed, or the new lightweight, man-made fabrics. Trilbys were worn by a few men, and in Britain, the bowler (derby) was favored by the "city gent" and especially by the unconventional, usually upper-class British men who adopted the "New Edwardian" style of the early 1950s (at center). Their suit jackets were high-buttoned, tight-waisted, and slope-shouldered with velvet collars and were worn with "drainpipe" trousers. Striped shirts with stiff white collars, a "British warm" cloth overcoat (also with a velvet collar), and a furled umbrella completed the nostalgic picture.

In complete contrast to these two styles was the "student" style (at right), featuring a toggle-fastening and hooded duffle coat, which had been beige-colored in the Army and dark blue-colored in the Navy during the War and could be bought cheaply at post-war Government Surplus Stores in Britain. Similar stores opened in America. Such young men wore polo-necked woollen sweaters, wide flannel or corduroy trousers, and heavy shoes.

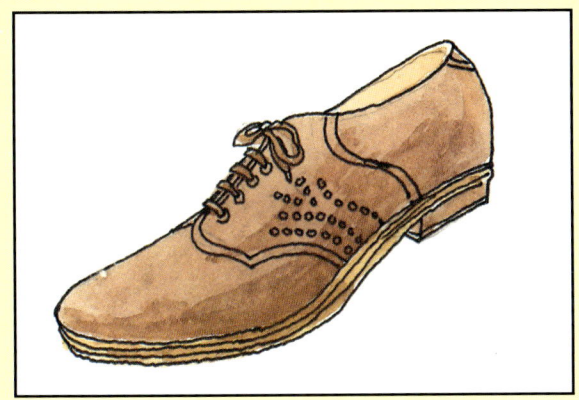

A leather "Oxford," restrainedly stitched and punched, worn with a smart suit.

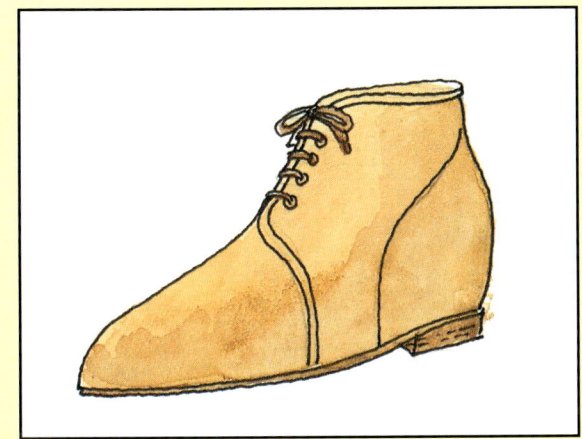

A suede "Chelsea" boot, much favored by the "New Edwardians," which was also made in leather and generally worn.

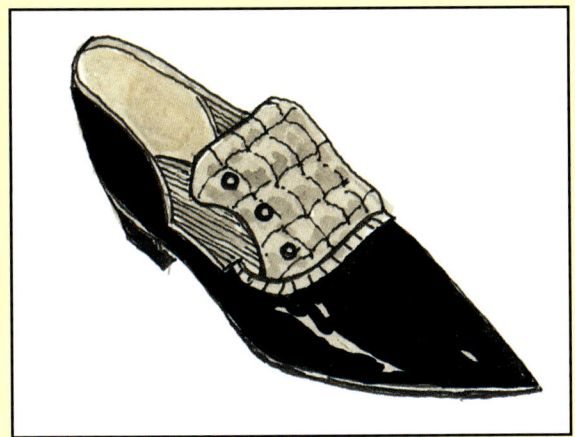

This "Winklepicker" in patent leather and imitation crocodile with elastic gussets was favored by the very young, lower-class, rebellious British "Teddy Boys" who mockingly aped the "New Edwardians."

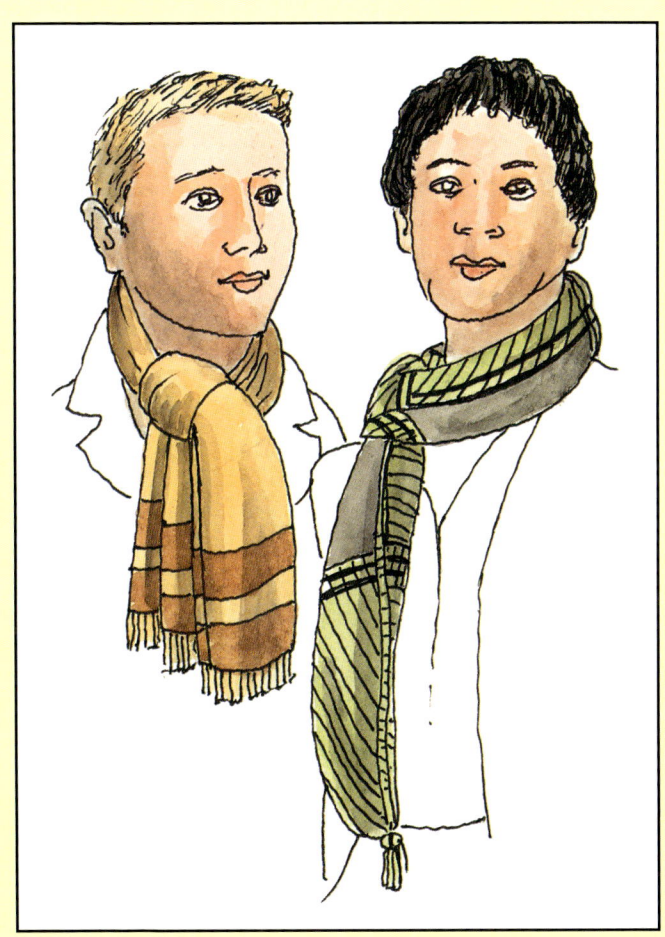

All types of long woollen scarves were a sort of trade-mark, worn by students everywhere in the 1950s, especially on the Left Bank in Paris, haunt of Jean-Paul Sartre, and home of Existentialism.

167

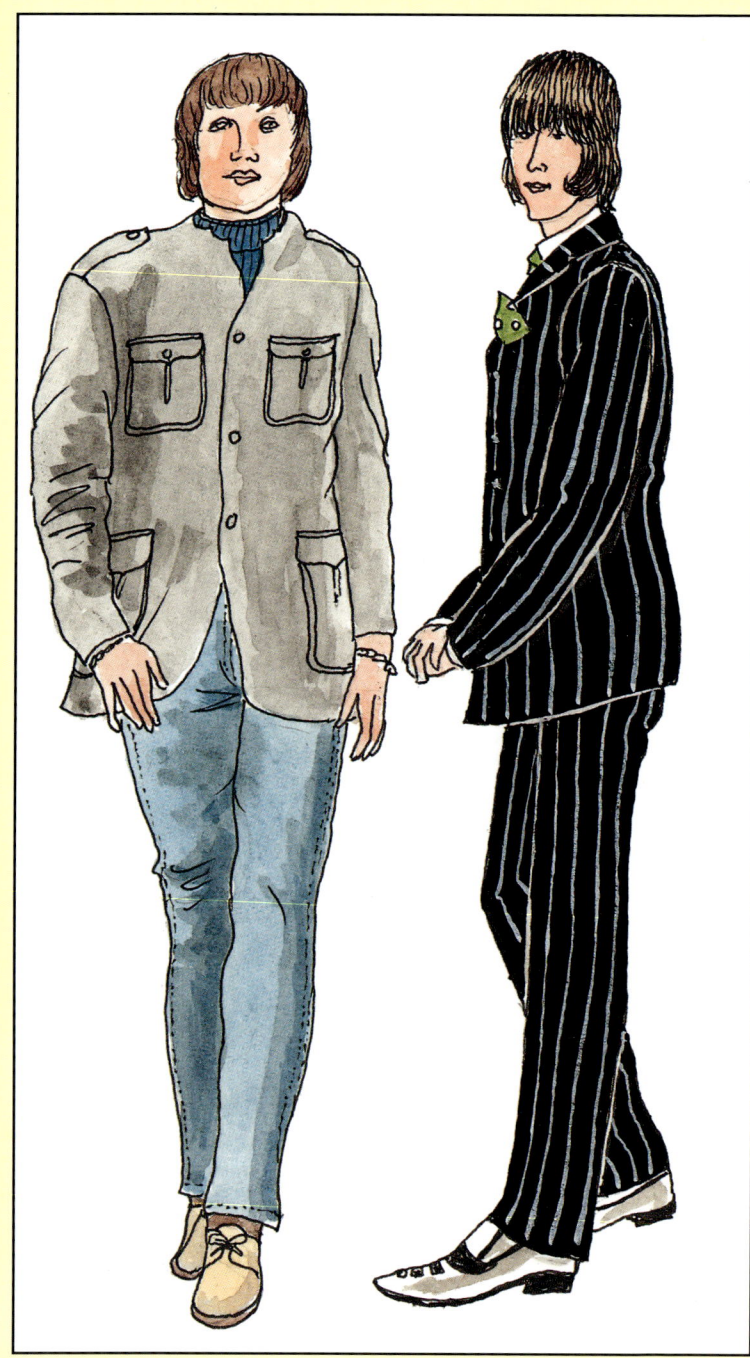

1960-1970 Day Wear

Many of the social and sexual factors governing women's clothing and accessories during this period also, of course, applied to men's fashions, particularly among the young.

Apart from those worn by passionate devotees, the Beatles-inspired jackets with their shallow, stand-up collars and tight trousers were not much worn, although the young man (at left) wears a jacket influenced by this style. His jeans, which, as everyone knows, originated in America and are now worn worldwide, were becoming more and more popular, particularly if low-waisted. A formal suit (at right) had a long, high-buttoned jacket and narrowish trousers often made in a boldly-striped fabric. Long hair (worn very long by "hippies") was adopted by even older men, and there was a revival of sideburns (or sideboards).

The 1960s witnessed the "Peacock Revolution," when men of all ages and classes wore brightly colored, sometimes patterned shirts, with neckties to match. It was not unusual to see a man with long hair working on a building site, wearing a bright shirt, an identity bracelet, and a medallion around his neck; only a few years before, such men would have considered it all effeminate. With almost universally longer hair and more women wearing men's clothes, unisex fashions came in. In America, President John Kennedy's black, loose suits set a style for some years to come.

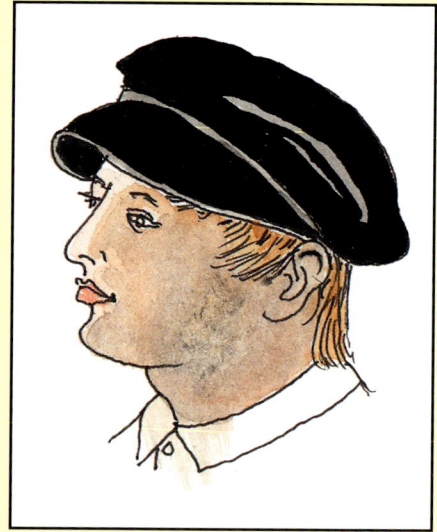

Headwear for men, especially the young, was becoming popular again. The really "trendy" wore a leather "Beatle" cap.

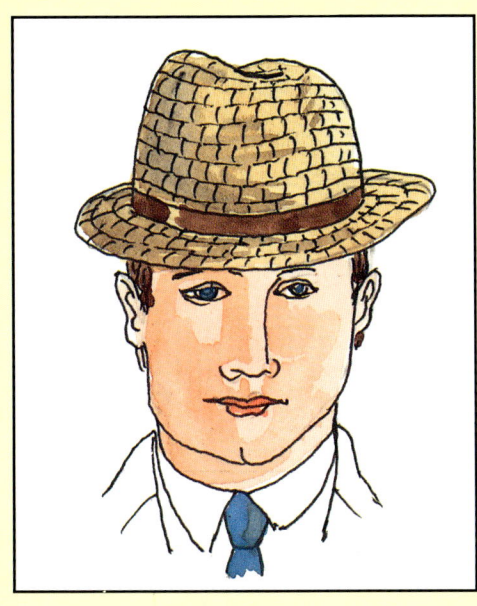

The more conventional young man wore a tweed trilby.

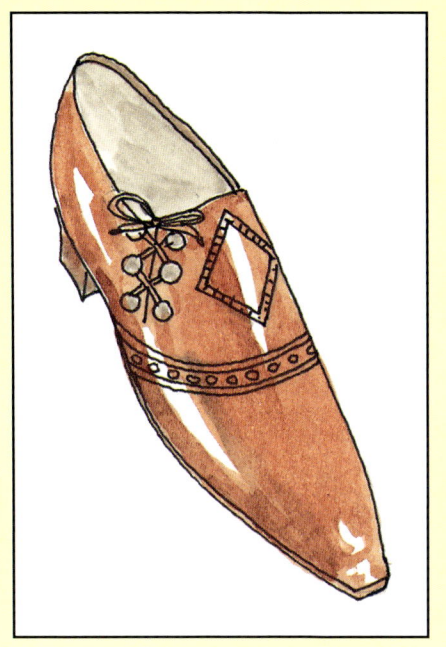

An Italian-style, somewhat overdecorated, leather "Winklepicker" with a blunted toe.

The famous "Beatle"-inspired boot, in leather with elastic gussets and a wooden Cuban heel.

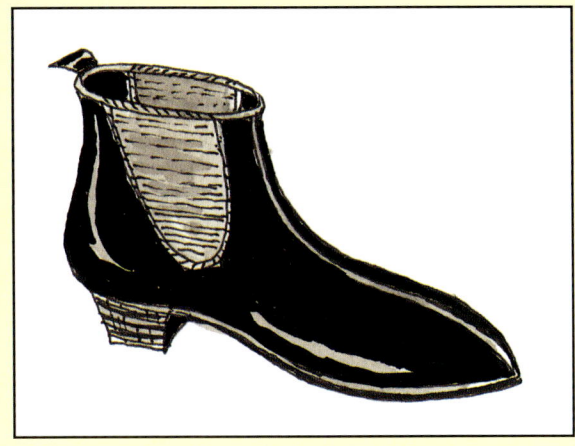

An eccentrically-patterned leather shoe with a very high, stacked heel and sole.

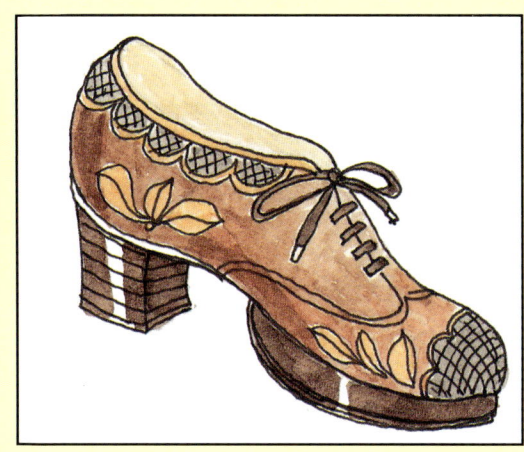

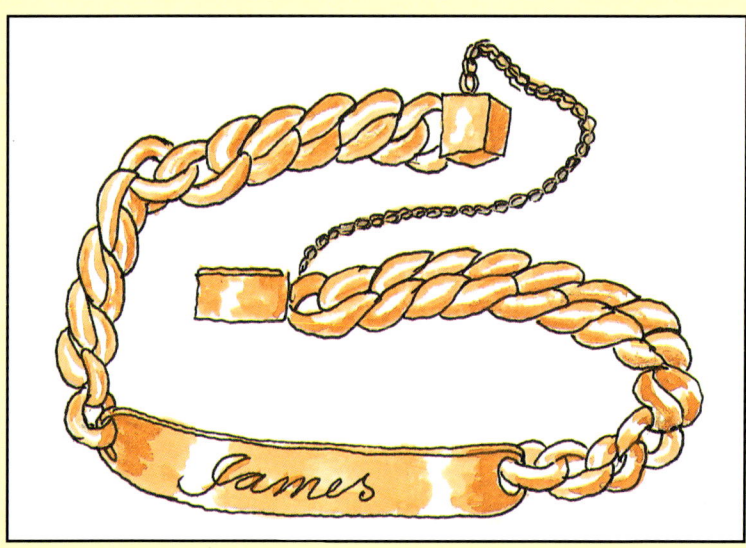

Heavy-linked in gold, silver, or base metal, identity bracelets became fashionable with all classes of men and continued to be so in the 1960s and 1970s. They are still worn by a few men today.

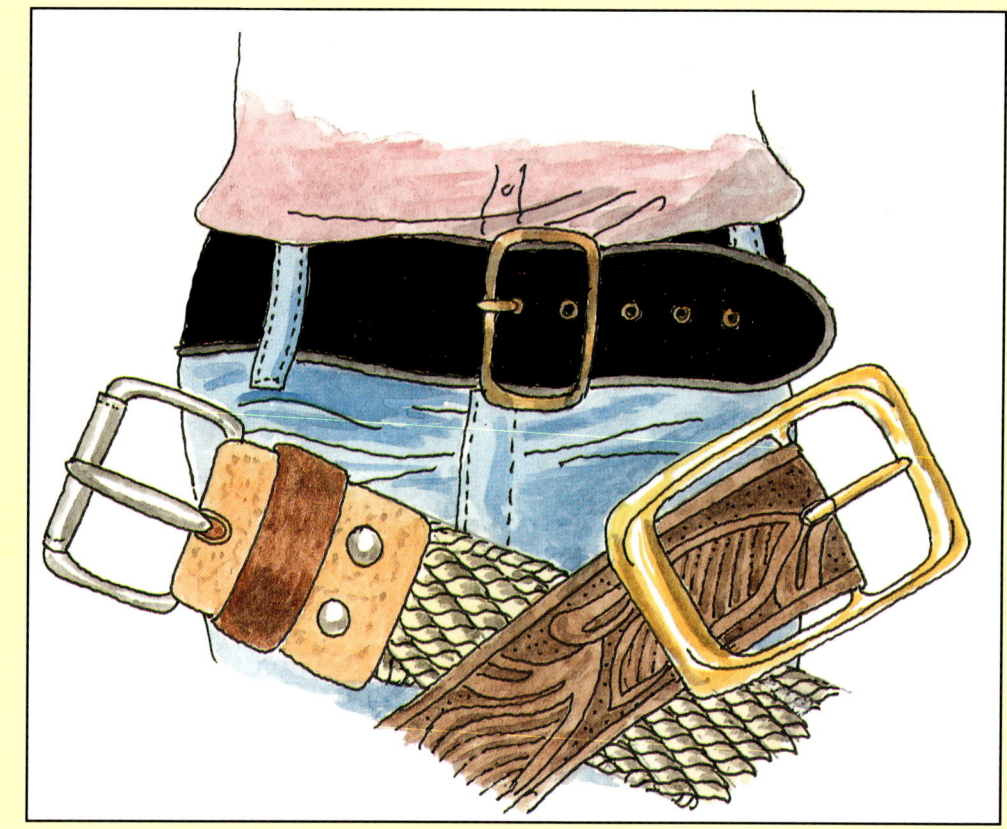

'Hipster" jeans, for those with slim hips and those without, were further accentuated by wide belts. *Center:* simple leather. *Left:* leather and plaited string. *Right:* Machine-embossed leather, imitating hand-tooled work.

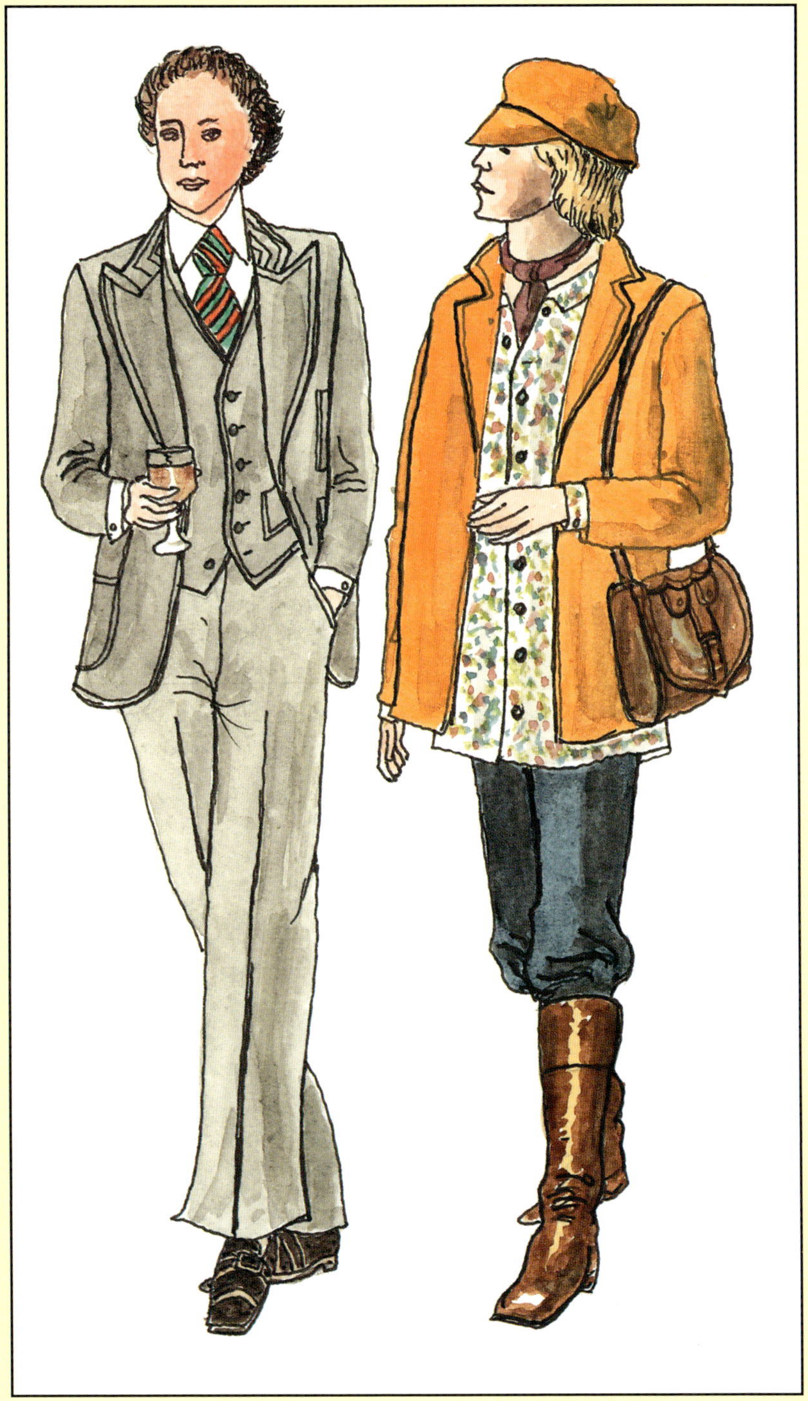

1970-1980 Day Wear

There were fewer styles for men to choose from than for women during the 1970s, but these styles could still be quite varied. Some authorities claim that this era saw the demise of the suit, collar, and necktie, but from my own experience and research, I would say that the formal suit made a comeback, especially for the professional man. The typical woollen (also made in denim) suit (at left) had a long, narrow-waisted jacket; very wide, pointed lapels; buttons low at a slim waist; a vest; and most significantly, a symbol of the age—flared or "bell-bottomed" trousers, which also appeared on men's and women's casual trousers and jeans. Shirts had high, wide collars and were still made in bright colors and were often highly patterned. For plain or checked shirts, cheesecloth was a favorite material. Very wide "kipper" neckties were tied in huge knots.

For casual wear, there was the linen "safari" suit and (at right) a mixed ensemble, with many jackets to choose from in leather, suede, or denim. The shirt, as here, was sometimes worn outside the trousers. Jeans, cloth, or woollen trousers, in bold plaid designs, were often tucked into the tops of high or low boots. Many men unashamedly wore much jewelry and carried small handbags or larger ones hung over the shoulder. This whole casual look, plus the rakish cap, was popularized in Britain by Rudolf Nureyev.

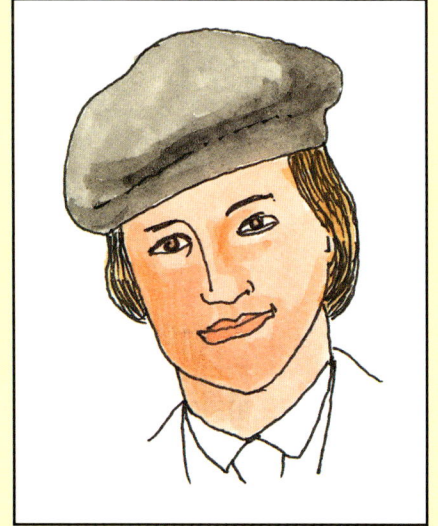

All kinds of headwear made a comeback in this decade, such as this cloth beret.

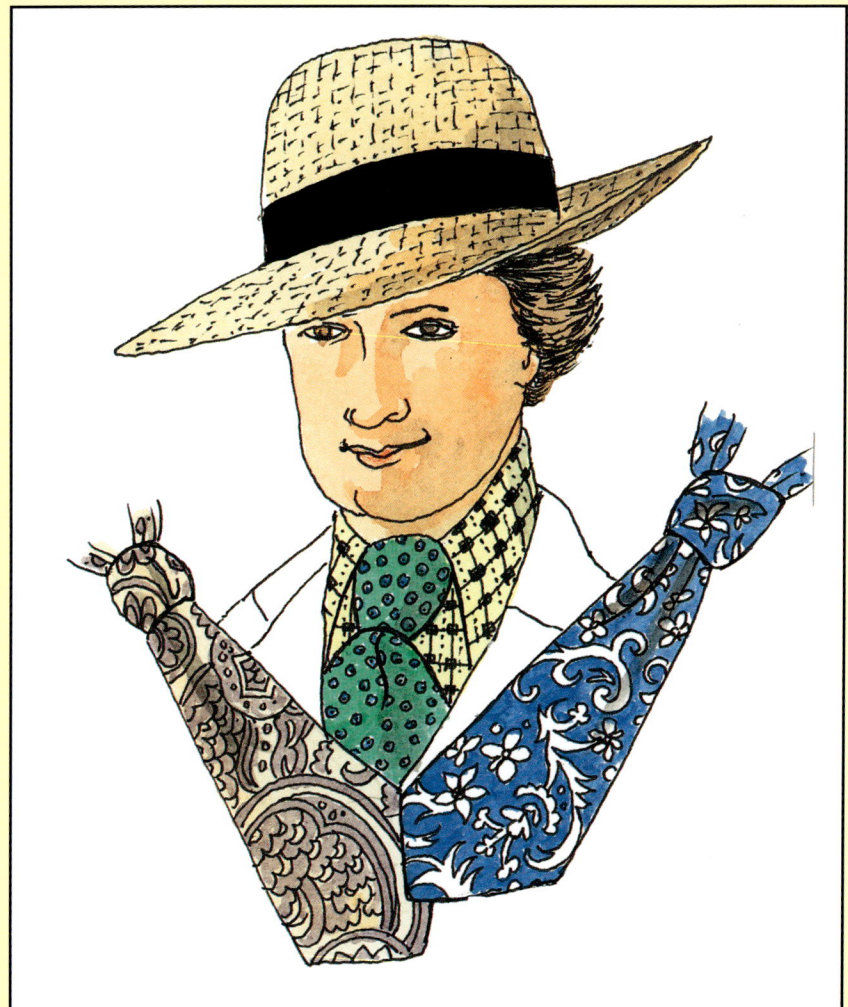

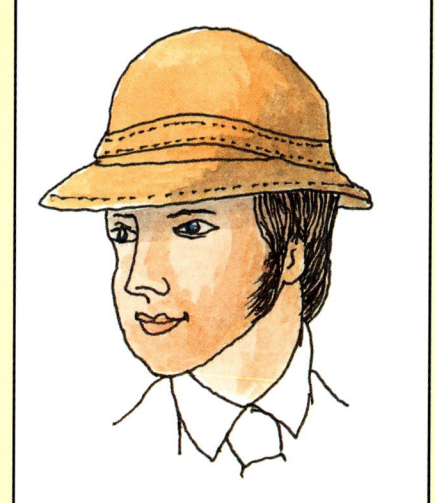

Stitched felt hat. Other hats included the fur "Cossack" and those in Tyrolean-style.

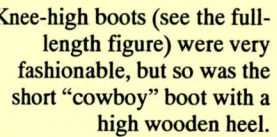 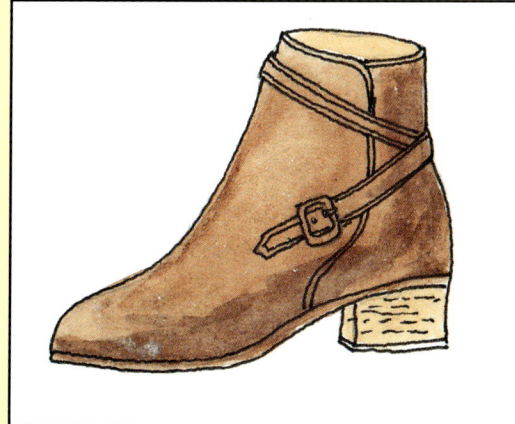

Knee-high boots (see the full-length figure) were very fashionable, but so was the short "cowboy" boot with a high wooden heel.

The 1970s saw the brightest-colored, most highly-patterned, high-collared shirts ever known, worn with similarly exotic neckties, which were very wide and tied in huge knots. Smart young men wore, hitherto thought to be elderly, Panama hats.

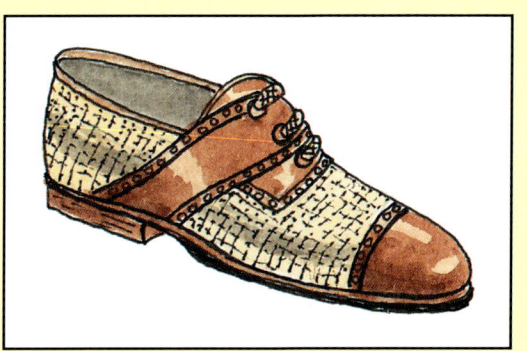

The 1920s and 1930s idea carried out in leather and tweed.

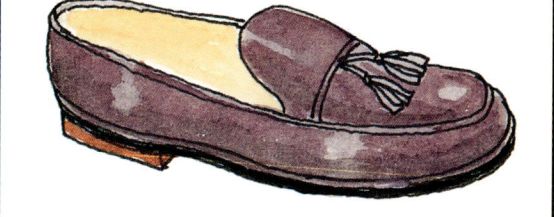

A shallow leather, low heeled slip-on which, in several colors, could be tasseled or plain.

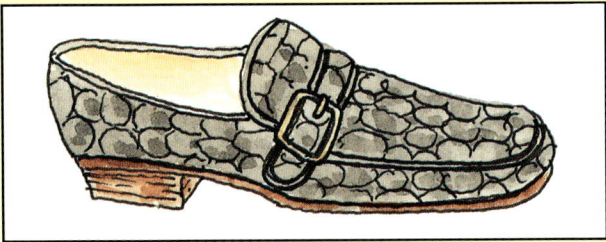

A buckled, real or fake crocodile slip-on, with a leather sole and heel.

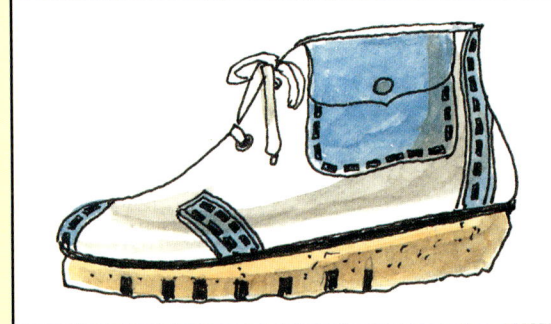

Anticipating its later, almost universal, popularity among the young: a leather or man-made material "trainer," with a thick crêpe sole.

With the loosening of sexual stereotypes, the prevalence of unisex clothes and the "Peacock revolution" still in evidence, it was no longer considered effeminate (except by conventional people, as with handbags) for men to wear a lot of jewelry. As well as identity and chain bracelets, adornment consisted of medallions and jewels worn on chains around the neck...the more the merrier. Here, a gold locket and a ball of turquoises is shown. Men also wore cameo and onyx rings, as well as cuff-links made out of antique, Art Nouveau, and Art Deco buttons.

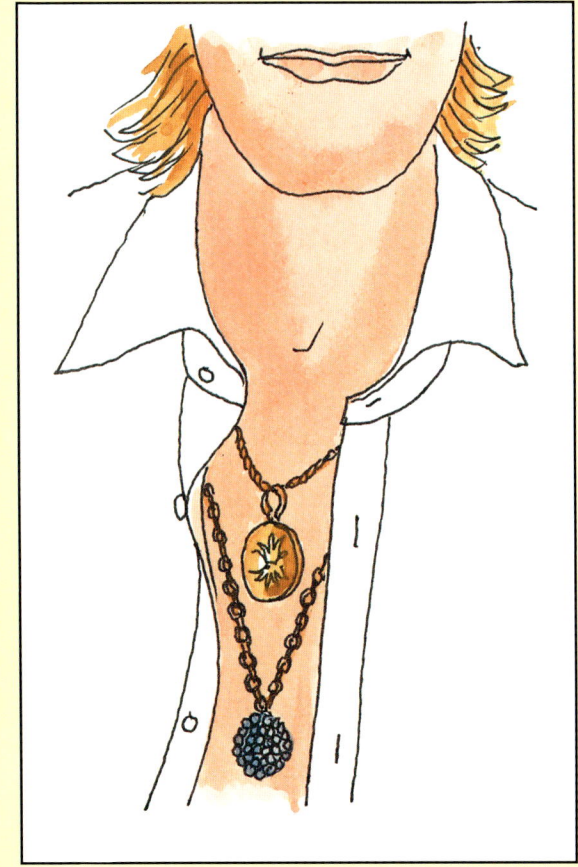

 Apart from a few men who, from approximately 1800 to 1850, had carried "miser" purses (even then, probably mostly in their pockets), for the first time in sartorial history, in the 1970s it was not thought of as effeminate for a man to be seen with a small leather handbag. Larger bags, as in the full-length figure, were also popular.

173

Select Bibliography

Amphlett, H. Hats: *A History of Fashion Headwear*. London. Richard Sadler, 1974.
Armstrong, Nancy. *Fans: A Collectors' Guide*. London. Souvenir Press. 1984.
Battersby, Martin. *Art Deco Fashion*. Academy Editions. New York. St Martin's Press, 1974.
Black, J. Anderson. *A History of Fashion*. London. Orbis Publishing, 1975.
Blum, Stella, edited by. *Paris Fashions of the 1890s*. New York. Dover Publications, 1984.
Boehn, Max Von. *Modes and Manners of the Nineteenth Century*. London. J.M. Dent. New York. E.P. Dutton & Co, 1927.
Buck, Anne. *Victorian Costume and Accessories*. London. Herbert Jenkins, 1961.
Byrde, Penelope. *The Male Image: Men's Fashions in Britain, 1300-1970* London. Batsford, 1977.
Caulfield, S.F.A. and Saward, Blanche C. *Encyclopedia of Victorian Needlework, Vol II*. New York. Dover Publications, 1972.
Chénounce, Farid. (Translated from the French by Deke Dusinberre). *A History of Men's Fashions*. Paris. Flammarion, 1993.
Clark, Fiona. *Hats*. London. Batsford, 1982.
Cumming, Valerie. *Gloves*. London. Batsford, 1982.
Cunnington, C. Willet & Philis. *Handbook of English Costume in the 19th Century*. London. Faber and Faber, 1959.
Cunnington, C. Willet. *English Women's Clothing in the 19th Century*. London, Faber and Faber, 1938.
_____. *English Women's Costume in the Present Century*. London. Faber and Faber, 1952.
Davenport, Millia. *The Book of Fashion*. New York. Crown, 1956.
Dorner, Jane. *Fashion in the Twenties & Thirties*. London. Ilsa Allen, 1973.
Ewing, Elizabeth. *History of Twentieth Century Fashion*. London. Batsford, 1986.
Farrell, Jeremy. *Umbrellas and Parasols*. London. Batsford, 1985.
Foster, Vanda. *Bags and Purses*. London, Batsford, 1985.
Fullée, Caroline. *20th Century Jewellery*. London. The Apple Press, 1990.
Gernsheim, Alison. *Fashion and Reality*. London. Faber and Faber, 1963.
Glynn, Predence and Ginsburg, Madeline. *In Fashion: Dress in the 20th Century*. London. Allen & Unwin, 1978.
Holland, Vyvian. *Hand Coloured Fashion Plates, 1770-1899*. London. Batsford, 1955.

Kennett, Frances. *The Collectors' Book of Twentieth Century Fashion*. London. Granads, 1983.
Klepper, Erhard. *Costume Through the Ages*. London, Thames & Hudson, 1963.
Kybalova, Ludmila. *The Pictorial Encyclopedia of Fashion*. London. Paul Hamlyn, 1968.
Laver, James. (Introduced by). *Costume Illustration. The Nineteenth Century*. London. Victoria and Albert Museum, 1947. (Introduced by.)
_____. *Costumes Through the Ages*. London. Thames & Hudson, 1963.
Marzy, Diana de. *The History of Haute Couture, 1850-1950*. London. Frederick Muller, 1984.
McDowell, Colin. *Directory of Twentieth Century Fashion*. London. Frederick Muller, 1984.
O'Day, Deirdre. *Victorian Jewellery*. London. Charles Letts, 1974.
Peter, Mary. *Collecting Victorian Jewellery*. London. Macgibbon and Kee. 1970.
Poynder, Michael. *The Pride Guide to Jewellery, 300 BC - 1050 AD*. Suffolk, England. Antique Collectors' Club, 1988.
Probert, Christina. *Shoes in Vogue*. London. Thames & Hudson, 1981.
Robinson, Julian. *The Golden Age of Style: Art Deco Fashion Illustration*. Orbis, 1974.
_____. *The Fine Art of Fashion. An Illustrated History*. Australia. Bay Books. No date - c. 1980s. *Fashion in the '40s*. London. Academy Editions. New York. St Martin's Press, 1976.
Ruby, Jennifer. *The 1960s and 1970s*. London. Batsford, 1989.
Squire, Geoffrey. *Dress, Art and Society, 1560-1970*. London. Studio Vista, 1974.
Swann, June. *Shoes*. London. Batsford, 1982.
Torrens. D. *Fashion Illustrated: A Review of Women's Dress, 1920-1950*. London. Studio Vista, 1974.
Waller, Jane, (Edited by.) *A Man's Book. Fashion in the Man's world in the 20s and 30s*. London. Duckworth, 1977.
Warren, Geoffrey. *Fashion Accessories Since 1500*. London. Unwin Hyman, 1987.
Magazines and Journals. These are very good reference sources, including the advertisements in many of them; along with fashion plates, there are so many that it is impossible to list them. However, among the most important are *Gazette du Bon Ton, Journal des Dames et Des Modes,* American, British and French *Vogue,* American *Harper's Bazaar,* and British *Harper's Bazaar.*

Price Guide

This price guide represents an estimate of items similar to those shown. Where prices are not given, it is because there was no basis upon which to set an estimate.

6	L	$675-725		BC	$175-225	43	TL	$200-225		TR	$165-185			$225-250 (dress, left lady)		$75-85 (hat, center lady)
7	L	$325-425		TR	$160-185		BL	$85-95		BR	$75-95			$125-185 (hat, right lady)		$110-135 (suit, center lady)
	C	$350-375		CR	$115-125		TC	$225-250	58	L	$50-150 (hatpins)			$225-300 (dress, right lady)		$75-85 (hat, right lady)
	TR	$350-375		BR	$115-125		BC	$85-95		TR	$85-125 (depending on catch)		R	$125-185		$85-95 (suit, right lady)
	BR	$185-225	29	L	$575-625		TR	$160-185		BR	$110-135	73	L	$110-125 (hat)		
8	L	$400-500	30	L	$175-225		BR	$225-250	59	L	$375-425			$85-95 (stole)	85	L	$95-110
	R	$150-165		C	$125-150	44	L	$425-475	60	BC	$45-65 (hair ribbon)			$85-95 (muff)		C	$95-110
9	L	$95-130	31		$200-225 (hat)	45	TL	$125-150			$65-75 (bow for neck)		BC	$110-125		R	$85-95
10	R	$575-625			$525-625 (dress)	46	L	$185-225 (hat)	61	L	$275-350		TR	$110-125	86	L	$95-110
11	TL	$275-325			$110-115 (parasol)			$375-425 (coat)		R	$200-250	74	TL	$95-120		TC	$110-125
	BC	$325-350	32	TL	$275-325		R	$225-250	62	TL	$175-225		BL	$95-115		BC	$85-95
	TR	$350-375		TC	$115-135	47	L	$185-225		BL	$125-150		TC	$95-115		R	$95-125
12	L	$225-250		BC	$225-250		TC	$110-125		C	$185-225		BC	$55-65	87	L	$125-150
	TC	$65-85		R	$200-225		BC	$185-225		TR	$150-185		TR	$95-135		TC	$45-60 (top)
	R	$120-165	33	TL	$65-75		TR	$115-135		BR	$115-175		BR	$65-75		TC	$45-60 (bottom)
13	R	$525-575		BL	$85-110		BR	$85-95	63	L	$115-150 (cape)	75	L	$175-225	88	L	$75-85 (hat, left lady)
14	TL	$65-95		TR	$75-85 (umbrella)	48	TL	$85-95		L	$300-375 (dress)		C	$95-120			$175-200 (dress, left lady)
	BC	$95-150			$85-95 (bag)		BC	$85-125 (bag)	64	L	$95-115		R	$85-95			$175-200 (dress, right lady)
	TR	$165-185		BR	$115-135		TC	$85-95 (umbrella)	65	L	$250-275	76	L	$95-110			
16	L	$675-725	34	L	$525-575		TR	$85-110	66		$115-125 (hat, left lady)	77	L	$65-75 (hat)	89	TL	$95-110
	R	$625-675	35	BC	$115-125		BR	$65-75			$95-115 (umbrella, left lady)			$175-225 (dress)		TR	$95-110
17	BL	$375-400	36		$225-250 (hat)	49		$45-55 (hat)			$225-300 (dress, left lady)		BC	$75-95		BR	$85-95
	TR	$250-275			$450-525 (dress)		L	$85-95 (jabot & cuffs)			$115-125 (hat, right lady)		TR	$95-110	90	L	$85-95
18	TL	$375-400			$50-75 (parasol)		R	$250-500 (sterling)			$225-300 (dress, right lady)	78	TL	$95-120		C	$65-75
	BL	$175-200	37	L	$275-325	50	L	$400-450	67	L	$85-110		BC	$65-75		R	$85-110
	BC	$175-200		C	$275-325	51	TL	$150-165		BC	$125-175		TR	$85-95	91	L	$95-110 (hat)
	TR	$95-125		R	$275-325		C	$95-110		R	$115-125	79	L	$95-110 (hat)			$150-175 (dress)
	BR	$95-125	38	TL	$110-125		TR	$85-95 (top)	68	L	$110-125			$45-55 (silk ruff)		BC	$95-110
19	L	$95-125		TC	$110-115			$45-85 (bottom)		TC	$115-135		C	$75-85		TR	$65-75
	TC	$95-125		BC	$150-165	52	L	$150-165 (umbrella)		BC	$95-115		R	$65-75	92	TL	$95-110
	BC	$165-200		TR	$110-115			$375-425 (suit)		R	$95-115	80	L	$150-175		BL	$85-95
20	L	$625-675		BR	$85-110		R	$175-225	69	TL	$95-135		TC	$165-185		TC	$95-110
21	TL	$95-115	39	TL	$75-85	53	L	$175-225		BL	$65-75		BC	$165-185		BC	$85-95
	BL	$160-185		C	$115-150		TC	$110-125		TC	$85-95 (left)	81	L	$85-110 (hat)		TR	$65-85
22	L	$425-475		BR	$75-85		BC	$130-150			$85-95 (right)			$225-250 (poiret, $1500-2500)		RC	$85-95
23	TL	$175-225	40	L	$375-425		TR	$75-85		R	$95-125		R	$95-115		BR	$75-85
	BC	$225-250	41	TL	$95-110		BR	$110-115	70	L	$95-110 (hat)	82	L	$65-75	93	L	$185-225
	TR	$225-250		BL	$185-225	54	L	$300-375			$175-225 (dress)		TC	$65-75		R	$65-75
	BR	$175-225	42	L	$225-250 (hat, left lady)	55	TC	$85-95		R	$95-110		BC	$85-95	94	TL	$85-95
24	L	$175-200			$375-475 (dress, left lady)		R	$50-75 (gloves)	72	L	$125-185 (hat, left lady)		BR	$95-110		TR	$95-110
	TC	$95-115			$225-250 (hat, right lady)			$85-95 (bag)				83	L	$65-85		BR	$65-85
	R	$125-150			$375-425 (dress, right lady)			$85-95 (fan)				84	L	$65-75 (hat, left lady)	95	L	$65-85 (hat)
25	L	$575-625				56	L	$95-110 (hat)						$85-95 (suit, left lady)			$150-225 (suit)
26	BL	$110-125						$300-375 (dress)									
27	L	$375-425				57	TL	$95-110									
28	L	$275-325		R	$275-325		BL	$95-110									
	TC	$225-250					C	$85-95									

Page	Pos	Price
	R	$65-85 (hat)
		$45-55 (scarf)
96	TL	$95-110
	BL	$110-125
	TR	$95-110
	BR	$95-110
97	TL	$95-110
	BL	$75-85
	TC	$55-65 (hat)
		$35-40 (fur; not fashionable)
	C	$55-75
	BC	$85-95
	TR	$65-75
	CR	$85-95
	BR	$35-45
98	TL	$65-75
	BL	$75-95
	C	$110-185
	R	$50-110
99	L	$125-150 (left lady)
		$125-150 (right lady)
	TR	$95-125
	BR	$85-110
100	TL	$110-125
	BL	$85-90
	C	$95-110 (cap)
		$85-95 (lappets)
101	L	$35-45 (hat, left lady)
		$75-85 (dress, left lady)
		$75-85 (hat, right lady)
		$110-125 (dress, right lady)
102	TL	$75-80
	BL	$35-45
	BC	$35-45
	TR	$55-60
	BR	$75-85
103	TL	$45-55
	BL	$35-45
	TC	$45-50
	C	$65-75
	TR	$30-35
	BR	$45-55
105	L	$95-125 (left lady)
		$95-125 (right lady)
	TR	$45-50
	BR	$95-110
107	L	$45-50 (hat)
		$45-55 (dress)
	BC	$65-70
	TR	$55-65
108	L	$75-80
	TC	$35-40 (hat)
		$35-40 (muff)
	TR	$65-75
	BR	$65-75
109	L	$55-65
	TC	$45-50
110	L	$45-50 (hat)
		$85-95 (dress)
	BC	$45-55
	TR	$65-75
111	TL	$25-30 (scarf-left lady)
		$35-40 (scarf-right lady)
	TC	$65-70
	BC	$45-55
	BR	$55-65 (scarf)
		$20-25 (gloves)
		$45-55 (bag)
112	TL	$65-75
	BL	$35-45
	C	$35-45
	TR	$25-35
	BR	$25-35
113	L	$40-45 (hat, left lady)
		$95-120 (coat, left lady)
		$85-110 (coat, right lady)
114	L	$35-45
	C	$35-45
	TR	$35-40
	BR	$35-40
115	L	$35-40 (hat)
		$85-110 (dress)
	C	$45-55
	R	$45-50
		$30-35 (fur)
116	L	$55-65
	TC	$45-55
	BC	$85-110
	TR	$35-45 (brassiere)
		35-45 (padding)
	BR	$25-35
117	L	$55-65 (hat)
		$85-110 (suit)
	BC	$35-45
	TR	$55-65
	BL	$?
118	BL	$?
	TC	$30-35
	BC	$75-85
	TR	$20-25 (gloves)
		$45-65 (bag)
119	L	$45-55 (hat)
		$20-25 (gloves)
		$85-110 (dress)
	C	$45-55
120	L	$20-25 (gloves)
	TR	$65-85
	BR	$65-75
121	L	$85-110 (suit-left lady)
		$65-85 (right lady)
122	TL	$35-40
	C	$55-65
	TR	$65-85
123	TL	$35-40
	BL	$45-50
	TC	$35-40
	BC	$15-20 (gloves)
		$35-45 (bag)
		$20-25 (scarf)
	R	$45-50
124	TL	$45-50
125	L	$85-95 (left lady)
		$65-85 (right lady)
	R	$25-30
126	C	$55-60
	TR	$45-50
	BR	$45-50
127	L	$325-600 (Dior)
		$375-600 (Chanel)
	C	$30-35
	TR	$30-35
	BR	$30-35
128	TL	$20-25
	BL	$30-35
	C	$35-45 (hat)
		$25-30 (muffler)
	TR	$65-70
	BR	$35-40
129	L	$50-60 (left lady)
		$75-85 (center lady)
		$55-75 (right lady)
	R	$30-35
130	TL	$25-30
	BL	$25-30
	TC	$65-75
	BC	$65-75
	TR	$45-50
	BR	$45-50
131	L	$55-65 (left lady)
		$45-55 (center lady)
		$55-65 (right lady)
132	TL	$35-40
	BL	$35-40
	TC	$35-40
	BC	$45-50
	TR	$25-30
133	TL	$25-30
	BL	$35-40
	TC	$35-40
	BC	$25-30
134	TL	$65-85
	BL	$75-85
	C	$115-125
	TR	$35-45
	BR	$35-45
135	L	$75-95 (left lady)
		$45-65 (right lady)
136	TL	$25-35
	BL	$15-20 (stockings)
		$35-45 (shoes)
	TC	$25-30
	TR	$25-30
	BR	$35-45
137	L	$85-110
	R	$15-20 (hat)
		$15-20 (gloves)
138	TL	$20-25
	TC	$50-65
	BC	$30-35 (hat)
		$15-20 (earrings)
	R	$65-85
139	L	$20-25 (hat)
		$85-110 (coat)
		$20-25 (bag)
	BC	$30-35 (hat)
		$15-25 (scarf)
	TR	$30-35
	R	$65-85
140	TL	$45-55
	BL	$30-35
	C	$30-40
	TR	$25-30
141	L	$75-85 (left lady)
		$65-75 (right lady)
	R	$35-45
142	TL	$55-65
	BL	$45-55
	C	$35-45 (top)
		$55-65 (bottom)
	TR	$35-45
	BR	$35-45
143	L	$25-30
144	L	$85-125 (hat)
		$150-185 (coat)
		$150-175 (vest)
	CT	$85-125
	BC	$95-110
	TR	$75-80
	BR	$75-80
145	L	$185-225 (left man)
		$55-75 (right man-hat)
		$150-175 (right man-suit)
	TC	$150-175
	BC	$55-75
	R	$85-125 (left)
		$85-110 (right)
146	L	$85-90 (hat)
		$185-250 (suit)
	BC	$75-95
	TR	$75-95
		$75-95
147	TL	$95-110
	BL	$40-45
	TC	$25-35
	BC	$150-175
148	L	$185-250 (suit-left)
		$185-250 (suit-right)
	BC	$95-125
	R	$75-95
149	TL	$165-185 (cane)
		$75-95 (hat)
	TC	$85-110
	BC	$50-60
	R	$50-60
150	L	$95-125 (hat)
		$185-250 (suit)
	R	$95-110
151	TL	$65-85
	TC	$75-85
	BC	$15-20
	R	$75-85
152	L	$65-75 (hat)
		$185-225 (suit)
	BC	$65-75
	R	$65-85
153	TL	$85-110
	BL	$75-85
	TR	$65-85
	CR	$65-85
	BR	$15-25
154	L	$185-225 (suit-left)
		$185-225 (suit-right)
	TR	$55-60
		$65-85
155	TL	$65-75
	BL	$25-35
	TC	$15-20 (collar)
		$30-35 (cravat)
	BC	$25-35 (socks)
		$65-85 (shoes)
	TR	$95-110
156	L	$150-175
	R	$65-75
157	TL	$45-55 (hat)
		$15-25 (collar)
	BL	$65-75
	TC	$65-80
	TR	$150-175
	BR	$85-150 (cane)
158	L	$150-175
	R	$85-110
159	L	$60-75
	BC	$85-95
	TR	$95-110
	BR	$65-75
160	L	$145-165 (suit-left)
		$135-155 (suit-right)
161	TL	$55-60
	BL	$65-75
	BC	$65-75
	TR	$55-60
	BR	$65-75
162	L	$145-155 (left man)
		$145-155 (right man)
	BR	$55-60
163	L	$25-30
	TC	$55-60
	BC	$65-70
	TR	$75-80
	BR	$65-70
164	L	$75-85 (left man)
		$75-85 (right man)
165	TL	$55-60
	TC	$65-75
	BC	$65-75
	R	$65-75
166	L	$35-40 (vest-left man)
		$75-85 (left man)
		$65-75 (center man)
		$45-65 (right man)
167	TL	$65-75
	CL	$65-75
	BL	$65-75
	R	$20-25
168	L	$85-95 (left man)
		$85-95 (right man)
	BR	$50-55
169	TL	$25-30
	BL	$85-95
	TR	$85-95
	BR	$125-150
170	TL	$35-40
	BR	$25-45
171	L	$95-125 (left man)
		$85-110 (right lady)
	BR	$35-40
172	TL	$45-55 (hat)
		$20-30 (tie)
	BL	$85-95
	TR	$35-40
	CR	$45-55
	BR	$40-45
173	TL	$15-20
	C	$45-55
	BL	$35-45
	R	$25-30 (top necklace)
		$25-35 (bottom necklace)